W9-AVR-599

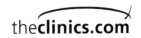

NEUROLOGIC CLINICS

Neck and Back Pain

GUEST EDITOR
Kerry H. Levin, MD

May 2007 • Volume 25 • Number 2

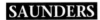

An Imprint of Elsevier, Inc.
PHILADELPHIA   LONDON   TORONTO   MONTREAL   SYDNEY   TOKYO

W.B. SAUNDERS COMPANY
A Division of Elsevier Inc.

1600 John F. Kennedy Blvd., Suite 1800, Philadelphia, PA 19103-2899

http://www.theclinics.com

NEUROLOGIC CLINICS
May 2007
Editor: Donald Mumford

Volume 25, Number 2
ISSN 0733-8619
ISBN 1-4160-4338-1
978-1-4160-4338-6

Copyright © 2007 by Elsevier Inc. All rights reserved. No part of this publication may be reproduced or transmitted in any form or by any means, electronic or mechanical, including photocopy, recording, or any information retrieval system, without written permission from the Publisher.

Single photocopies of single articles may be made for personal use as allowed by national copyright laws. Permission of the publisher and payment of a fee is required for all other photocopying, including multiple or systematic copying, copying for advertising or promotional purposes, resale, and all forms of document delivery. Special rates are available for educational institutions that wish to make photocopies for non-profit educational classroom use. Permissions may be sought directly from Elsevier's Rights Department in Philadelphia, PA, USA: phone: (+1) 215 239 3804, fax: (+1) 215 239 3805, e-mail: healthpermissions @elsevier.com. Requests may also be completed on-line via the Elsevier homepage (http://www.elsevier.com/locate/permissions). In the USA, users may clear permissions and make payments through the Copyright Clearance Center, Inc., 222 Rosewood Drive, Danvers, MA 01923, USA; phone: (978) 750-8400, fax: (978) 750-4744, and in the UK through the Copyright Licensing Agency Rapid Clearance Service (CLARCS), 90 Tottenham Court Road, London WIP 0LP, UK; phone: (+44) 171 436 5931; fax: (+44) 171 436 3986. Other countries may have a local reprographic rights agency for payments.

Reprints. For copies of 100 or more of articles in this publication, please contact the Commercial Reprints Department, Elsevier Inc., 360 Park Avenue South, New York, New York 10010-1710. Tel.: (212) 633-3813, Fax: (212) 462-1935, e-mail: reprints@elsevier.com.

The ideas and opinions expressed in *Neurologic Clinics* do not necessarily reflect those of the Publisher. The Publisher does not assume any responsibility for any injury and/or damage to persons or property arising out of or related to any use of the material contained in this periodical. The reader is advised to check the appropriate medical literature and the product information currently provided by the manufacturer of each drug to be administered to verify the dosage, the method and duration of administration, or contraindications. It is the responsibility of the treating physician or other health care professional, relying on independent experience and knowledge of the patient, to determine drug dosages and the best treatment for the patient. Mention of any product in this issue should not be construed as endorsement by the contributors, editors, or the Publisher of the product or manufacturers' claims.

Neurologic Clinics (ISSN 0733-8619) is published quarterly by Elsevier Inc., 360 Park Avenue South, New York, NY 10010–171. Months of issue are February, May, August, and November. Business and editorial offices: 1600 John F. Kennedy Blvd., Suite 1800, Philadelphia, PA 19103-2899. Customer Service Office: 6277 Sea Harbor Drive, Orlando, FL 32887–4800. Accounting and circulation offices: 6277 Sea Harbor Drive, Orlando, FL 32887-4800. Periodicals postage paid at New York, NY, and additional mailing offices. Subscription prices are $198.00 per year for US individuals, $313.00 per year for US institutions, $99.00 per year for US students, $248.00 per year for Canadian individuals, $367.00 per year for Canadian institutions, $259.00 per year for international individuals, $367.00 per year for international institutions and $132.00 for Canadian and foreign students/residents. To receive student/resident rate, orders must be accompanied by name of affiliated institution, date of term, and the *signature* of program/residency coordinator on institution letterhead. Orders will be billed at individual rate until proof of status is received. Foreign air speed delivery is included in all *Clinics* subscription prices. All prices are subject to change without notice. POSTMASTER: Send address changes to *Neurologic Clinics*, Elsevier Periodicals Customer Service, 6277 Sea Harbor Drive, Orlando, FL 32887-4800. **Customer Service: 1-800-654-2452 (US). From outside of the US, call 1-407-345-4000.**

Neurologic Clinics is also published in Spanish by Nueva Editorial Interamericana S.A., Mexico City, Mexico.

Neurologic Clinics is covered in *Current Contents/Clinical Medicine, Index Medicus, EMBASE/Excerpta Medica,* and *PsycINFO,* and *ISI/BIOMED.*

Printed in the United States of America.

GUEST EDITOR

KERRY H. LEVIN, MD, Director, Neuromuscular Center of the Neurological Institute, Cleveland Clinic, Cleveland; Acting Chairman, Department of Neurology, Cleveland Clinic, Cleveland; Professor of Medicine, Cleveland Clinic Lerner College of Medicine of Case Western Reserve University, Cleveland, Ohio

CONTRIBUTORS LIST

MANZOOR AHMED, MD, Staff Radiologist, Department of Radiology, Louis Stokes Veterans Administration Medical Center, Cleveland, Ohio

EDWARD C. BENZEL, MD, Staff Physician, Cleveland Clinic Foundation, Cleveland Clinic Spine Institute, Cleveland Clinic for Spine Health, Cleveland, Ohio

DAVID A. CHAD, MD, Professor of Neurology and Pathology, University of Massachusetts Medical School, Worcester, Massachusetts; Director MDA and MDA-ALS Clinics, University of Massachusetts Memorial Health Care; Attending Neurologist, University of Massachusetts Memorial Health Care, Worcester, Massachusetts

EDWARD COVINGTON, MD, Head, Section of Pain Medicine, Neurological Institute, Cleveland Clinic, Cleveland, Ohio

MICHAEL W. DEVEREAUX, MD, Professor of Neurology, Department of Neurology, University Hospitals of Cleveland/Case Western Reserve University, Cleveland, Ohio; and Chief Medical Officer, University Hospitals Health System, Richmond Heights Hospital, Richmond Heights, Ohio

AJIT A. KRISHNANEY, MD, Associate Staff, Cleveland Clinic Spine Institute, Department of Neurosurgery, Cleveland Clinic for Spine Health, Cleveland, Ohio

LISA S. KRIVICKAS, MD, Associate Professor of Physical Medicine and Rehabilitation, Harvard Medical School; and Associate Chief of Physical Medicine and Rehabilitation, Massachusetts General Hospital, Boston, Massachusetts

KERRY H. LEVIN, MD, Director, Neuromuscular Center of the Neurological Institute, Cleveland Clinic, Cleveland; Acting Chairman, Department of Neurology, Cleveland Clinic, Cleveland; Professor of Medicine, Cleveland Clinic Lerner College of Medicine of Case Western Reserve University, Cleveland, Ohio

ALEC L. MELEGER, MD, Director, Pain Medicine Fellowship, Spaulding Rehabilitation Hospital, Boston; and Clinical Instructor in Physical Medicine and Rehabilitation, Harvard Medical School, Boston, Massachusetts

MICHAEL T. MODIC, MD, Chairman, Division of Radiology, Cleveland Clinic Foundation, Cleveland, Ohio

JOHN PARK, MD, Resident, Cleveland Clinic Spine Institute, Department of Neurosurgery, Cleveland Clinic for Spine Health, Cleveland, Ohio

DAVID W. POLSTON, MD, Associate Staff, Department of Neurology, Cleveland Clinic, Cleveland, Ohio

ELIZABETH M. RAYNOR, MD, Associate Professor of Neurology, Harvard Medical School; and Director, EMG Laboratory, Department of Neurology, Beth Israel Deaconess Medical Center, Boston, Massachusetts

DEVON I. RUBIN, MD, Assistant Professor, Mayo Clinic College of Medicine, Rochester, Minnesota; Consultant, Department of Neurology; and Director, EMG Laboratory, Department of Neurology, Mayo Clinic, Jacksonville, Florida

ANDREW W. TARULLI, MD, Instructor in Neurology, Harvard Medical School; and Research Fellow, Division of Neuromuscular Diseases, Department of Neurology, Beth Israel Deaconess Medical Center, Boston, Massachusetts

BRYAN TSAO, MD, Department of Neurology, Loma Linda University, Loma Linda, California

DEBORAH A. VENESY, MD, Vice Chairman, Department of Physical Medicine and Rehabilitation, Cleveland Clinic, Cleveland, Ohio

CONTENTS

important to minimize unnecessary tests and identify patients who require more urgent intervention. Patient education, pain control, and physical therapy are the first line of therapy. Patients who have protracted pain or significant functional deficits may require a more thorough evaluation, including imaging, electrodiagnostic testing, and, possibly, surgical referral. This article outlines the basic clinical, diagnostic, and therapy considerations in the evaluation of cervical radiculopathy.

Lumbosacral radiculopathy is one of the most common disorders evaluated by neurologists and is a leading referral diagnosis for the performance of electromyography. Although precise epidemiologic data are difficult to establish, the prevalence of lumbosacral radiculopathy is approximately 3% to 5%, distributed equally in men and women. Degenerative spondyloarthropathies are the principal underlying cause of these clinical syndromes and are increasingly commonplace with age. Men are most likely to develop symptoms in their 40s, whereas women are affected most commonly between ages 50 and 60. The clinical presentation and initial management of lumbosacral radiculopathies of various etiologies are discussed.

Lumbar spinal stenosis may be congenital or acquired. A classic clinical presentation is described as neurogenic claudication. Physical signs of sensory loss, weakness, and attenuation of reflexes often are mild and limited in distribution. Neuroimaging of the lumbosacral spine with MRI and electrodiagnostic (electromyographic [EMG]) tests are the most informative diagnostic modalities. Conservative management often is successful, but surgical decompression may be indicated in refractory cases.

In this article, non-neurologic causes of neck and back pain are reviewed. Musculoskeletal pain generators include muscle, tendon, ligament, intervertebral disc, articular cartilage, and bone. Disorders that can produce neck and back pain include muscle strain, ligament sprain, myofascial pain, fibromyalgia, facet joint pain, internal disc disruption, somatic dysfunction, spinal fracture, vertebral osteomyelitis, and polymyalgia rheumatica. Atlantoaxial instability and atlanto-occipital joint pain are additional causes of neck pain. Back pain resulting from vertebral compression fracture, Scheuermann's disease, spondylolysis and spondylolisthesis, pregnancy, Baastrup's disease, sacroiliac joint dysfunction, and sacral stress fracture is discussed.

are used widely, seldom have they been subjected to the scrutiny of careful randomized and controlled clinical trials. The costs of complementary treatments, such as spinal manipulation, massage therapy, and acupuncture, now are reimbursed by many medical insurance providers, but these modalities lack much scientific support. Physical medicine and complementary treatment modalities and some of the scientific studies aimed at assessing their effectiveness are reviewed.

Chronic nonmalignant pain is less a symptom of a disease than a disease in itself. Accordingly, successful treatments rely less on identifying underlying pathology than on treating neural causes of pain amplification, psychologic causes of disability, and the sequelae of deconditioning and psychiatric illness. The outcome, when such treatment is provided, is remarkably favorable.

FORTHCOMING ISSUES

RECENT ISSUES

THE CLINICS ARE NOW AVAILABLE ONLINE!

Access your subscription at
www.theclinics.com

ELSEVIER
SAUNDERS

Neurol Clin 25 (2007) xi–xii

NEUROLOGIC
CLINICS

Preface

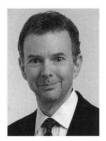

Kerry H. Levin, MD
Guest Editor

Neck and back disorders are pervasive medical problems in our society. These disorders are seen in every neurologist's practice and occur in every neurologist's family. It was estimated in 1997 that $25 billion per year was spent in the United States on medical care for back pain and an additional $50 billion was spent for disability and lost productivity. It has been stated that low back pain is the second leading cause for medical visits. Patients go to chiropractors, family practitioners, internists, rheumatologists, physiatrists, orthopedists, neurosurgeons, and neurologists for their spine disorders.

Over the last 10 to 20 years, clinical, neuroradiologic, and surgical and nonsurgical interventional approaches to the diagnosis and treatment of spine conditions have proliferated, and thousands of articles have been published on these subjects. The number of careful scientific studies on these topics remains relatively small, however. For the practitioner, it is difficult to find the "best" strategy for a given patient, because so many experts recommend so many different approaches. In addition to the traditional medical treatments, alternative approaches have entered the mainstream. Complementary treatments, such as spinal manipulation, massage therapy, and acupuncture, are reimbursed by several medical insurance providers. However, the little scientific scrutiny that has been applied to assessing their effectiveness has not been widely publicized to the professions or lay public.

The purpose of this issue is to review the current understanding and practice of the neurologic care of spinal disorders. Wherever possible, systematic reviews and controlled studies have been highlighted to aid in the analysis of

0733-8619/07/$ - see front matter © 2007 Elsevier Inc. All rights reserved.
doi:10.1016/j.ncl.2007.02.005

neurologic.theclinics.com

the effectiveness of current diagnostic and therapeutic approaches. Covered topics include basic anatomic concepts, elements of an appropriate history and examination, diagnostic modalities, such as imaging and electromyography, specific treatment approaches, and chronic pain assessment and management.

I wish to extend my gratitude to all the experts who contributed to this issue. I would like to acknowledge the editorial assistance provided by Donald Mumford, *Clinics* development editor for WB Saunders/Elsevier, and his editorial staff.

Kerry H. Levin, MD
Neuromuscular Center of the Neurological Institute
Department of Neurology
Cleveland Clinic, 9500 Euclid Avenue
Cleveland, OH 44195, USA

E-mail address: levink@ccf.org

ELSEVIER
SAUNDERS

Neurol Clin 25 (2007) 331–351

NEUROLOGIC
CLINICS

Anatomy and Examination of the Spine

Michael W. Devereaux, MD[a,b]

[a]Department of Neurology, University Hospitals of Cleveland/Case Western Reserve
University, 11100 Euclid Avenue, Cleveland, OH 44106, USA
[b]University Hospitals Health System, Richmond Heights Hospital 27100 Chardon Road,
Richmond Heights, OH 44143-1116, USA

A review of the anatomy of the spine in a few pages must, by necessity, be abridged. This article concentrates on clinically relevant anatomy. For a more expansive discussion, the reader is referred to the most recent edition of Gray's anatomy [1].

Vertebral column

The structures that form the spinal column must be rigid enough to support the trunk and the extremities, strong enough to protect the spinal cord and cauda equina and anchor the erector spinae and other muscles, and yet sufficiently flexible to allow for movement of the head and trunk in multiple directions. The anatomic organization of the spinal column and related structures allows for all of this, but at a price, because the combined properties of rigidity and mobility can lead to many problems, particularly at the level of the cervical and lumbar spine.

The spinal column is composed of 7 cervical, 12 thoracic, 5 lumbar, and 5 fused sacral vertebra, along with 5 coccygeal bones. The cervical, thoracic, and lumbar vertebrae are similar in structure except for the first (atlas) and second (axis) cervical vertebrae. Each "standard" vertebra is composed of a body, two pedicles, two lamina, four articular facets, and a spinous process. The atlas is composed of a ring of bone without a body, whereas the axis has an odontoid process around which the atlas rotates. Between each pair of vertebrae are two openings, the foramina, through which pass a spinal nerve, radicular blood vessels, and the sinuvertebral nerves (recurrent meningeal nerves) (Fig. 1). Each foramen is bordered superiorly and inferiorly by pedicles, anteriorly by the intervertebral disc and adjacent vertebral body surfaces, and posteriorly by the facet joint.

E-mail address: Michael.Devereaux@UHhospitals.org

0733-8619/07/$ - see front matter © 2007 Elsevier Inc. All rights reserved.
doi:10.1016/j.ncl.2007.02.003   *neurologic.theclinics.com*

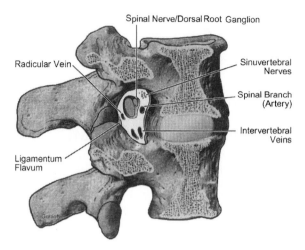

Spinal Nerve/Dorsal Root Ganglion

Radicular Vein

Sinuvertebral
Nerves

Spinal Branch
(Artery)

Intervertebral
Veins

Ligamentum
Flavum

Fig. 1. The foremen. (*From* Levin KH, Covington EC, Devereaux MW, et al. Neck and low back pain. Continuum (NY) 2001;7:9; with permission.)

The spinal canal itself is formed posterolaterally by the laminae and ligamentum flavum, anterolaterally by the pedicles, and anteriorly by the posterior surface of the vertebral bodies and intervertebral discs. The midsagittal (anterior-posterior) diameter of the cervical canal from C1 to C3 is usually approximately 21 mm (range 16–30 mm), and from C4 to C7 the diameter is approximately 18 mm (range 14–23 mm). The midsagittal diameter of the cervical spinal cord is 11 mm at C1, 10 mm from C2 to C6, and 7 to 9 mm below C6. The midsagittal diameter of the cervical cord normally occupies approximately 40% of the midsagittal diameter of the cervical canal in healthy individuals. This cervical canal midsagittal diameter is decreased by 2 to 3 mm with extension of the neck, which is of clinical importance in the context of hyperextension injuries in an individual with a congenitally narrow spinal canal, especially in the presence of additional narrowing caused by cervical spondylosis. Under such circumstances an acute cervical myelopathy may result. With regard to the lumbar canal, the midsagittal diameter is approximately 18 mm. Narrowing as a result of spondylosis coupled with extension can compromise the cauda equina and the accompanying vasculature, producing the symptoms of neurogenic claudication.

The facet (zygapophyseal) joint, unlike the intervertebral disc, is a true synovial joint. Although it contributes—to a limited extent—to the support of the spinal column, this joint's main function is to maintain stability of the spinal column by guiding the direction of vertebral movement, a function that depends on the plane of the facet joint surface, which varies throughout the spinal column. The joint is subject to degenerative change that results in enlargement, which, in association with thickening of the ligamentum flavum, can contribute to canal stenosis as a component of spondylosis. It is innervated by branches from the posterior ramus of the spinal nerve. The exact role of the facet joint in the production of back pain, particularly low back pain, remains somewhat controversial [2].

The intervertebral disc

The intervertebral disc is a cartilaginous and articulating structure between the vertebral bodies. Intervertebral discs have the dual role of providing the primary support for the column of vertebral bones while possessing enough elasticity to permit the required mobility of the spine (flexion, extension, and rotation). The aggregate of discs together accounts for 25% to 30% of the overall length (height) of the spine. Each disc is comprised of a ring of elastic collagen, the annulus fibrosus, which surrounds the gelatinous nucleus pulposus (Fig. 2). The collagen fibers of the annulus are arranged obliquely in alternating directions, in layers (lamellae), which allows for flexibility while maintaining strength. Fifteen to 25 lamellae comprise the annulus [3]. Collagen fibers continue from the annulus into the adjacent tissues, which ties this structure to each vertebral body at its rim, to the anterior and posterior longitudinal ligaments, and to the hyaline cartilage endplates superiorly and inferiorly. The cartilage endplates in turn lock into the osseus vertebral endplates via the calcified cartilage [4].

The nucleus pulposus is a self-contained, pliable gelatinous structure that is 88% water in a healthy young disc. It is essentially a hydraulic system that provides support and separates the vertebrae, absorbs shock, permits transient compression, and allows for movement. As a result of the aging process and injury to the disc, increasing amounts of fibrous tissue replace the highly elastic collagen fibers of the young, normal, uninjured disc. The older disc is less elastic, and its hydraulic recoil mechanism is weakened [4].

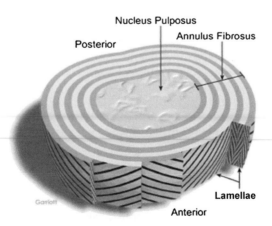

Fig. 2. The intervertebral disk. (*From* Levin KH, Covington EC, Devereaux MW, et al. Neck and low back pain. Continuum (NY) 2001;7:11; with permission.)

By the fifth decade of life, the annulus becomes fissured, with transformation into fibrous bodies separated by softer substances. Ultimately the disc deteriorates into a desiccated, fragmented, and frayed annulus fibrosus surrounding a fibrotic nucleus pulposus [4,5].

The intervertebral disc is avascular by the third decade of life, and nutrition is delivered to the disc by diffusion. The nucleus pulposus in the normal adult disc has no nerve supply. The outer lamellae of the annulus fibrosus contains nerve endings derived from the sinuvertebral nerves (recurrent meningeal nerves), however [4,6–9].

There is debate in the literature regarding nociceptive nerve supply to the intervertebral disc and what role the disc plays as a generator of back pain. Korkala and colleagues [8] showed that the nerve endings entering the annulus fibrosus do not contain substance P and are not nociceptors. The authors noted that nociceptive nerve endings are located in the posterior ligament adjacent to the disc. Palmgren and colleagues [9], in a study of normal human lumbar intervertebral disc tissue, demonstrated that nerve endings could be found at a depth of a few millimeters, whereas neuropeptide markers (eg, substance P) revealed nociceptive nerves only in the outermost layers of the annulus fibrosus. This study lends support to the concept that the normal intervertebral disc is almost without innervation.

This finding leads to the question of the mechanism of primary discogenic pain, particularly in the lumbar spine. Damage to the intervertebral disc can produce pain, but no consensus exists on the responsible mechanisms. Radial tears and fissures in the annulus fibrosus occur as the disc ages. This change has been linked to the ingrowth of blood vessels and nerve fibers, leading to the concept that the ingrowth of these nerve endings may be the pathoanatomic basis for discogenic pain [6,10]. First, if the ingrowth of nociceptive nerve fibers into the intervertebral disc may be the neuroanatomic substrate for discogenic pain, then why are most degenerative discs not a source of pain? For example, discography of degenerative discs does not uniformly induce pain [10]. Because disc degeneration per se is not the basis for discogenic pain, contributing factors must be at play. Possibly a combination of focal damage to the annulus fibrosus, inflammation, neoinnervation, and nociceptor sensitization is necessary to induce discogenic pain [11].

Ligaments of the vertebral column

Several ligaments lash the vertebrae together and, along with the intrinsic paraspinous muscles, control and limit spinal column motion. From a clinical perspective, some of the ligaments are more important than others.

The posterior longitudinal ligament stretches from the axis (named the membrane of tectoria in the "high" cervical spine) to the sacrum and forms the anterior wall of the spinal canal. It is broad throughout the cervical and thoracic portions of the spine. At the L1 vertebral level it begins to narrow, however, and at L5 it is one-half its original width. It is attached firmly to each intervertebral disc by hyalin cartilage endplates, but only in the midline by a septum to the periosteum of each vertebra. The open space between the posterior longitudinal ligament and the vertebral body is the anterior epidural space, which is important in disc herniation. The narrowing of the ligament in the lumbar spine inadequately reinforces the lumbar disc, which creates an inherent structural weakness. This narrowing, coupled with the great static and kinetic stress placed on the lumbar discs, contributes to their susceptibility to injury and herniation.

The ligamenta flava is composed of a series of strong paired elastic ligaments that span the space between the laminae, attached to the anterior inferior surface of the laminae above and the posterior superior margin of the laminae below. Each component stretches laterally, joining the facet joint capsule. The ligament stretches under tension, which permits flexion of the spine. It contains few, if any, nociceptive nerve fibers. It can be clinically important because with age it can thicken and, along with other spondylotic degenerative changes, can contribute to canal stenosis, which produces myelopathy in the cervical spine and cauda equina compression in the lumbar spine.

Other ligaments that contribute to the stabilization of the spine include the anterior longitudinal ligament, the ligamentum nuchae from the occiput to the cervical vertebra, the infraspinous ligaments, and the supraspinous ligaments. The occipitovertebral ligaments are dense, broad, and strong and connect the occiput to the atlas. These ligaments permit up to 30° of flexion and extension around the atlanto-occipital joint. The stability of the atlantoaxial joints depends almost entirely on ligaments. The transverse ligament of the atlas helps to contain the odontoid process in place. It is actually stronger than the odontoid process, which means that the odontoid process fractures before the ligament is torn. The paired alar ligaments attach on either side of the apex and extend to the medial side of the occipital condyles. The main function of these ligaments is limitation of rotation, keeping in mind that in the atlas axis there is approximately 90° of the 160° of total head rotation capacity.

The paraspinous muscles

With the exception of the atlas and axis, the range and type of movement in each segment of the spine is determined by the facet joints, but spine stability and the control of spinal movement depend on muscles and ligaments. The movement itself, of course, depends on muscle.

The spinal muscles are arranged in layers. The deeper layers comprise the intrinsic, true back muscles, as defined by their position and innervation by the posterior rami of the spinal nerves. This is in contrast to the more superficial extrinsic muscles, which insert on the bones of the upper limbs and are innervated by anterior rami of the spinal nerves.

The intrinsic muscles are also divided into superficial and deep groups. The superficial layer is comprised of the paraspinous erector spinae group, which spans the entire length of the spine from the occiput to the sacrum, and the splenius muscles of the upper back and neck. This superficial group functions collectively primarily to maintain erect posture. Deep to the erector spinae is the transversospinalis muscle group, which is composed of muscles made up of several smaller muscles that run obliquely and longitudinally. In essence, they form a system of guy ropes that provide lateral stability to the spine, contribute to maintenance of an erect posture, and rotate the spine. Deepest of all are the interspinal and intertransverse muscles, which are composed of numerous small muscles involved in the maintenance of posture.

The multiple subdivisions of muscle mass, numerous connective tissue planes, and multiple attachments of tendons over small areas of vertebral periosteum help to explain the prevalence of neck and back pain while simultaneously explain the difficulty in precisely localizing the source of that pain. Taking into account this difficulty in identifying muscle and tendon injury as the source of pain and the fact that there are other generators of low back pain besides muscles (eg, fascia, ligaments, facet joint, intervertebral disc), it is no wonder that according to Deyo and colleagues [12], the source of acute low back pain cannot be identified in 85% of patients. It also should be noted that when muscle is the source of pain, the pathophysiologic pain-generating process is unclear. In the clinic, muscle spasm is often the diagnosis made. Muscle spasm is generally defined as a contraction of muscle that cannot be voluntarily released and is associated with electromyographic activity. Johnson and others [13,14] have taken issue with increased muscle activity as a source of paraspinous pain, noting a lack of electromyographic evidence indicative of muscle spasm.

Vascular supply to the spinal column and contents

The vertebral column and its contents receive blood supply from segmental medullary arteries. These arteries originate from the vertebral arteries in the cervical spine and from the posterior intracostal and lumbar arteries in the thoracic and lumbar portions of the spine, which ultimately originate from the aorta. Branches enter into the spinal column through the foramina. Some of the anterior branches are large, such as the great anterior segmental medullary artery of Adamkiewicz, and anastomose with longitudinal spinal cord vessels to form a pial plexus on the surface of the cord. The segmental spinal arteries send anterior and posterior radicular branches to the spinal cord along the ventral and dorsal roots. The importance of the segmental arterial blood supply to the spinal cord is amply demonstrated in patients with a dissection of the aorta, with resultant occlusion of paired branches feeding segmental branches to the spinal column and cord and resultant ischemic injury to the cord.

In addition to the segmental arties, the longitudinal paired posterior spinal arteries and the single anterior spinal artery originate from the distal vertebral arteries. Although they run the length of the surface of the spinal cord, they alone cannot supply the spinal cord and anastomose with segmental vessels along their entire length.

The importance of the anterior spinal artery in the cervical cord is well known to clinicians. Hyperextension injuries to the neck in association with cervical spondylosis and canal stenosis can result in occlusion of the anterior spinal artery and ischemia to the anterior two thirds of the cord. Therapeutic cervical manipulation has been associated with mechanical injury to the spinal cord and distal vertebral artery dissection, which results in posterior cerebral circulation distribution strokes [15].

The nerve supply to the spinal column and related structures

One of the most frustrating aspects of neck and back pain for the physician and patient is the difficulty in arriving at a precise cause. As in the case of acute low back pain, a definite diagnosis cannot be established in 85% of patients because of weak associations between symptoms, pathologic changes, and imaging results [12]. It is widely assumed that much nonradiating neck and low back pain is secondary to musculoligamentous injury and degenerative changes.

Localized cervical and lumbosacral pain is mediated primarily through the posterior primary ramus and the sinuvertebral (recurrent meningeal) nerves. The sinuvertebral nerves supply structures within the spinal canal. They arise from the rami communicantes and enter the spinal canal by way of the intervertebral foramina [16]. Branches ascend and descend one or more levels, interconnecting with the sinuvertebral nerves from other levels and innervating the anterior and posterior longitudinal ligaments, the anterior and posterior portion of the dura mater, and blood vessels, among other structures (Fig. 3). This system also may supply nociceptive branches to degenerated intervertebral discs.

Branches of the posterior ramus provide sensory fibers to fascia, ligaments, periosteum, and facet joints (Box 1). The source of deep somatic neck and low back pain can be the vertebral column itself, the surrounding muscle, tendons, ligaments, and fascia, or a combination thereof.

Radicular pain, unlike spondylogenic pain, is not mediated by sinuvertebral nerves or the posterior rami, but rather by proximal spinal nerves. Two major factors are involved in the generation of radicular pain: compression and inflammation. Compression of the nerve root produces local ischemia with possible alteration in axoplasmic transport and edema. Ischemia may have a particular impact on large mechanoreceptor fibers. Because of their large diameter, these fibers have greater metabolic activity and are more sensitive to reduced blood flow. This reduction can result in the loss of inhibitory pain impulses and lead to preferential nociceptive input into the spinal cord.

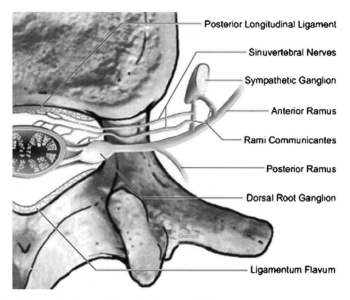

Fig. 3. The sinuvertebral nerve. (*From* Levin KH, Covington EC, Devereaux MW, et al. Neck and low back pain. Continuum (NY) 2001;7:13; with permission.)

Compression alone can produce paresthesia and some radicular pain; however, compression and traction in the presence of chronic inflammation produces more prominent radicular pain. The origin of the inflammatory response itself may be neurogenic or immunologic. In the case of disc

---

Box 1. Pain-sensitive tissues in the spine

Skin, subcutaneous tissue, and adipose tissue
Capsules of facet and sacroiliac joints
Ligaments: longitudinal spinal, interspinous (mainly posterior), flaval (minimal innervation – probably not clinically significant), and sacroiliac
Periosteum: vertebral bodies and arches
Dura mater and epidural fibroadipose tissue
Arterioles that supply spinal and sacroiliac joints and vertebral cancellous bone
Veins: epidural and paravertebral
Paravertebral muscles: perivascular unmyelinated nerve endings in the adventitial sheaths of intramuscular blood vessels

---

Data from Levin KH, Covington EC, Devereaux MW, et al. Neck and low back pain. Continuum (NY) 2001;7:13.

herniation with nerve root compression, the normally avascular nucleus pulposus comes into contact for the first time with the immune defense mechanism, which results in autoimmune-induced inflammatory response in the region of the spinal nerve.

Radicular, radiating pain secondary to disc herniation is the product of spinal nerve compression and local inflammation. The normal disc itself may not contain nociceptive nerve fibers and is insensitive to pain. When the nucleus pulposus ruptures through the annulus fibrosus, there is little or no localized pain until nociceptive fibers of the sinuvertebral nerves in the lateral posterior ligament and the dura of the nerve root sleeves are stimulated. This stimulation generates localized back and neck pain. Understanding the role of (1) the sinuvertebral system and the posterior rami in the generation of localized spine pain and (2) the spinal nerve and the generation of radiating pain helps to explain why patients with disc herniation develop sciatica only approximately one third of the time. The following clinical situations also can be more easily understood on this basis:

- Disc herniation visualized on a neuroimaging procedure in the absence of a history of radicular pain [17,18].
- Weakness in a radicular distribution without significant radicular pain secondary to disc herniation, with compression of the ventral root only
- Nonradiating low back pain secondary to disc herniation (with radicular pain perhaps developing months or years later)

One last generator of spine pain, viscerogenic referred pain (pain that arises from organs that share segmental innervation with structures in the lumbosacral spine), sometimes eludes clinical neurologists. The quality of pain is often, but not always, different (eg, cramping in quality). Organs that can refer pain to the low back and sometimes mid-spine include the aorta, pancreas, duodenum, ascending and descending colon, rectum, kidney, ureter, bladder, and pelvic organs. The abdominal examination is important in the evaluation of the patient who is experiencing low and mid-back pain.

Neurologic history

History

The history is of critical importance in assessing patients with symptoms believed to be secondary to cervical and lumbar spine disorders, especially in persons with a nonfocal neurologic examination. The differential diagnosis is frequently based solely on the history in these patients.

Pain profile

Onset

In most instances, patients who present with a history of acute onset of neck and low back pain have a history of preceding pain, often for weeks or months or longer. This is also the case in patients with the acute onset of radicular pain. The acute onset of cervical or lumbosacral radicular pain in the absence of any prior history of neck and low back pain is the exception rather than the rule.

Quality

Variable, nonradiating musculoskeletal back pain is often described as being deep and aching, whereas radicular pain is usually described as sharp, jabbing, or lancinating in quality.

Location

Musculoskeletal pain is usually localized to the paraspinous regions. In the neck, it is generally maximally felt in the paracervical regions, at times spreading into the shoulders and scapular regions. Lumbosacral pain tends to be maximal in the paraspinal regions, spreading at times to the flanks and into the buttocks. When cervical roots are involved, the pain generally radiates into the upper extremity. Occasionally the distribution of the pain alone may be enough to allow localization to a specific cervical root (Table 1). In the case of lumbosacral radiculopathy, the pain usually radiates into one or

Table 1
Symptoms and signs associated with cervical radiculopathy

Root	Pain distribution	Dermatomal sensory distribution	Weakness	Affected reflex
C4	Upper neck	"Cape" distribution shoulder/arm	None	None
C5	Neck, scapula, shoulder, anterior arm	Lateral aspect of arm	Shoulder abduction	Biceps Brachioradialis
			Forearm flexion	
C6	Neck, scapula, shoulder, lateral arm, and forearm into first and second digits	Lateral aspect forearm and hand and first and second digits	Shoulder abduction	Biceps Brachioradialis
			Forearm flexion	
C7	Neck, shoulder, lateral arm, medial scapula, extensor surface forearm	Third digit	Elbow extension Finger extension	Triceps
C8	Neck, medial scapula, medial aspect arm and forearm into fourth and fifth digits	Distal medial forearm to hand and fourth and fifth digits	Finger: abduction adduction flexors	Finger flexors

Data from Levin KH, Covington EC, Devereaux MW, et al. Neck and low back pain. Continuum (NY) 2001;7:7–43.

both lower extremities. The distribution of the pain also can occasionally point to the specific root involved (Table 2). For example, "high" lumbar (L2, L3) radiculopathic pain does not radiate distal to the knee, whereas the pain of an L4 radiculopathy can radiate to the medial leg distal to the knee. L5 and S1 radiculopathies tend to produce pain that radiates into the posterolateral thigh and posterolateral leg and often involves the foot. Pain may be maximum in the medial (L5 radiculopathy) or lateral aspect of the foot (S1 radiculopathy).

Duration

Mechanical low back pain generally has a duration of days to weeks. Radicular pain often resolves more gradually over 6 to 8 weeks. An extensive neurodiagnostic evaluation is generally not necessary in this setting. A patient who presents with a history of chronic low back pain, however, requires a careful history to rule out a new problem superimposed over chronic symptoms that, in the proper setting, may require an immediate neurodiagnostic evaluation.

Severity

As all clinicians recognize, the severity of pain is often difficult to interpret because it can be colored by several factors, including a patient's

Table 2
Symptoms and signs associated with lumbar radiculopathy

Root	Pain distribution	Dermatomal sensory distribution	Weakness	Affected reflex
L1	Inguinal region	Inguinal region	Hip flexion	Cremasteric
L2	Inguinal region and anterior thigh	Anterior thigh	Hip flexion Hip adduction	Cremasteric Thigh adductor
L3	Anterior thigh and knee	Distal anteromedial Thigh, including knee	Knee extension Hip flexion Hip adduction	Patellar Thigh adductor
L4	Anterior thigh, medial aspect leg	Medial leg	Knee extension Hip flexion Hip adduction	Patellar
L5	Posterolateral thigh Lateral leg Medial foot	Lateral leg, dorsal foot, and great toe	Dorsiflexion foot/toes Knee flexion Hip extension	
S1	Posterior thigh and leg and lateral foot	Posterolateral leg and lateral aspect of foot	Plantar flexion foot/toes Knee flexion Hip extension	Achilles

Data from Levin KH, Covington EC, Devereaux MW, et al. Neck and low back pain. Continuum (NY) 2001;7:7–43.

personality. Severe low back and neck pain that is not relieved when the patient is recumbent suggests metastatic cancer, pathologic vertebral fracture, or infection of a vertebra, disc, or the epidural space.

Time of day

Cervical and lumbar radiculopathy frequently present upon awakening in the morning. Nonradiating pain that tends to be dull during the day is often the result of mechanical disorders (eg, muscle strain, degenerative disc disease/spondylosis). Tumors of the spine and spinal cord often produce pain that persists and occasionally increases in the supine position; patients with lumbar and cervical tumors may have increased pain in bed at night.

Associated symptoms

Several cervical spine disorders that cause localized and radiating pain into an upper extremity also may produce symptoms secondary to an associated cervical myelopathy (eg, weakness and paresthesia in the lower extremities) and sphincter dysfunction. In the case of low back pain, the patient should be questioned about abdominal pain and intestinal or genitourinary symptoms.

Triggers

Valsalva maneuvers (eg, coughing, sneezing, and bearing down at stool) often transiently aggravate lumbosacral and cervical radicular pain. In the case of cervical radicular pain, lateral head movements to the side of the radiating pain—and sometimes to the opposite side—may aggravate the pain. Low back radicular pain is generally made worse by sitting and standing and often is relieved by lying supine. If pain persists or increases in the supine position, the possibility of spinal metastatic cancer or infection must be considered. In the case of lumbar canal stenosis, neurogenic claudication can be brought on by standing erect and walking.

Motor symptoms

In the face of pain, distinguishing between weakness and guarding by the history alone can be difficult. In the case of low back and lower extremity pain, however, weakness is suggested by a history of a foot slap when walking or of falls secondary to a lower extremity "giving way." With neck pain radiating into an upper extremity, a history of difficulty writing with the symptomatic extremity and difficulty elevating the limb may be useful clues as to the presence of true accompanying weakness. Although weakness is usually best appreciated on a neurologic examination, the history is a useful adjunct in helping to separate weakness from guarding secondary to pain.

Sensory disturbances

Patients with radiculopathy often report numbness, tingling, and even coolness in the involved extremity. At times, symptoms suggest dysesthesia and allodynia. The distribution of a sensory disturbance by history, particularly of numbness and tingling, may be even more useful in determining the presence and localization of a radiculopathy than the sensory examination itself.

Bladder and bowel disturbances

Symptoms of a hypertonic bladder (ie, urgency, frequency, nocturia, and incontinence of bladder [or occasionally of bowels]) are often found in association with cervical myelopathy. Sphincter disturbances also may appear with cauda equina compression and, when acute, always must serve as a warning of the need for urgent surgical intervention.

Risk factors

Although various risk factors have been associated with an increased incidence of neck and low back pain, knowledge of these risk factors is not necessarily helpful in evaluating individual patients. Risk factors are better established for low back pain than neck pain, but many risk factors are common to both, including the following:

- Increasing age
- Heavy physical work, particularly long static work postures, heavy lifting, twisting, and vibration
- Psychosocial factors, including work dissatisfaction and monotonous work
- Depression
- Obesity
- Smoking
- Severe scoliosis ($>80\%$)
- Drug abuse
- History of headache

Several other factors are commonly thought to increase the risk of low back and neck pain but probably do not, including

- Anthropometric status (height, body build)
- Posture, including kyphosis, lordosis, and scoliosis $<80\%$
- Leg length differences
- Gender
- State of physical fitness (although not a predictor of acute low back pain, fit individuals have a lower incidence of chronic low back pain and tend to recover more quickly from episodes of acute low back pain than unfit individuals).

The pain patient at risk

Although most patients who present with neck and back pain do not need immediate diagnostic evaluation and initially should be treated conservatively, certain historical features should lead to the consideration of an immediate and thorough study of the patient with new onset neck/back pain with or without radiating pain into extremity. These historical features include the following factors:

- Age > 50
- Body temperatures > 38°C
- Neuromuscular weakness
- Significant trauma before the onset of pain
- History of malignancy
- Pain at rest in the recumbent position
- Unexplained weight loss
- Drug and alcohol abuse (increased risk of infection and possibly unremembered trauma)

Evaluation in the emergency room

Neurologists generally do not see patients early in the course of low back pain. Occasionally, however, a neurologist may be called to the emergency room. It is clear that patients who present to the emergency room with the acute onset of focal neurologic deficits, such as weakness in the lower extremities or bladder and bowel disturbances, require an immediate and detailed evaluation, usually including a neuroimaging procedure. Patients who present with severe low back pain and abdominal symptoms also should be evaluated for a leaking aortic aneurysm or other acute abdominal disorders.

Physical examination

The experienced neurologist knows that the neurologic examination of the patient with neck and low back pain can be altered by the pain itself. For example, when testing strength, guarding must be taken into account. Tendon reflexes may be suppressed as a result of poor relaxation of a limb as a consequence of pain. Preparing the patient by explaining each step of the examination in advance may reduce anxiety and encourage relaxation, thereby reducing guarding and enhancing the reliability of the examination itself.

General examination

The necessity for a general physical assessment in the patient who complains of back pain cannot be underestimated. The presence of a low-grade fever, for example, may signal infection that involves the vertebral column, the epidural space, or the surrounding muscle (eg, psoas abscess). Inspection of the skin for lesions may yield diagnostic information (Box 2). Changes in the rectal examination, including sphincter tone, anal "wink," and the bulbocavernosus reflex, may reflect changes in the spinal cord or cauda equina, whereas an abnormal prostate may lead to a diagnosis of prostate cancer with spinal metastases.

Box 2. Skin lesions and spine pain

Psoriasis—psoriatic arthritis
Erythema nodosum—inflammatory disease, cancer
Café-au-lait spots—neurofibromatosis
Hydradenitis suppurativa—epidural abscess
Vesicles—herpes zoster
Needle marks (intravenous drug abuse)—vertebral column
  infections
Subcutaneous masses—neurofibroma, lymphadenopathy

Data from Levin KH, Covington EC, Devereaux MW, et al. Neck and low back
pain. Continuum (NY) 2001;7:18.

The abdominal examination may be particularly important. The presence of abdominal tenderness, organomegaly, or a pulsatile abdominal mass with a bruit in a patient with low back pain should immediately direct an urgent diagnostic evaluation, which may lead to a potentially lifesaving diagnosis, such as a leaking abdominal aortic aneurysm. In patients with low back pain and claudication, evaluation of the peripheral pulses in both lower extremities is essential to help distinguish neurogenic claudication from vascular claudication.

Neurologic examination

Low back pain

Inspection of the low back can be of value. The presence of a tuft of hair over the lumbar spine suggests diastematomyelia/spina bifida occulta. Percussion may produce pain over an infected area or at the site of a malignancy. Palpation of the paraspinous muscles may demonstrate spasm as a cause, or accompaniment, of acute low back (and neck) pain. The concept of spasm itself as a cause of back pain has been challenged.

Posture while standing may be altered by a herniated lumbar disc. Splinting with list away from the painful lower extremity is seen with lateral lumbar disc herniation, whereas list toward the painful side can be seen with medial herniation. Tilting the trunk to the side opposite the list can cause additional nerve root compression, with resultant accentuation of radicular distribution pain. Patients with neurogenic claudication secondary to compression of the cauda equina may tend to stand and walk with the trunk flexed forward, which reduces compression by widening the anteriorposterior dimension of the lumbar canal. Walking with the trunk extended may accentuate the symptomatology. Lumbar spine mobility is usually reduced in patients with low back pain, but because there is such wide variability as a result of conditioning and age, a measurement of degrees of mobility is usually not useful. Evaluation of the gait is of fundamental importance to seeking, for example, evidence of

- An antalgic gait that favors the side of a lumbar radiculopathy
- "Foot slap" (ie, foot drop) secondary to weakness of dorsiflexors of the foot, found with an L5 radiculopathy
- Trendelenburg gait ("drop" of ipsilateral side of pelvis as foot is lifted), which signals proximal (unilateral or bilateral) lower extremity weakness.

Neuromechanical tests are an important adjunct to the traditional neurologic examination in patients with low back pain and sciatica.

- **Straight leg raising test:** With the patient in the supine position, the symptomatic lower extremity is slowly elevated off the examining table. The spinal nerve and its dural sleeve, tethered by a herniated disc, are stretched when the lower extremity is elevated between 30° and 70°. This movement accentuates the radiating pain ("sciatica"). Increased pain at less than 30° and more than 70° is nonspecific (Fig. 4).
- **Lasegue test:** A variation of the straight leg raising test. With the patient in the supine position, the symptomatic lower extremity is flexed to 90° at the hip and knee. The knee is then slowly extended, which produces radiating pain with L5 and S1 nerve root compression.

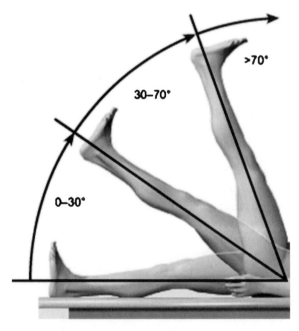

Fig. 4. The straight leg raising test. (*From* Levin KH, Covington EC, Devereaux MW, et al. Neck and low back pain. Continuum (NY) 2001;7:20; with permission.)

- **Bragard's sign (test):** After a positive straight leg raising test, the elevated extremity is lowered to the point of pain resolution. The foot is then dorsiflexed by the examiner. If this movement recreates the pain, the test is positive (Fig. 5).
- **Contralateral ("well") straight leg raising test:** Performed on the asymptomatic lower extremity, this test has specificity but low sensitivity for disc herniation.
- **Prone straight leg raising test:** With the patient in the prone position, the symptomatic lower extremity is slowly extended at the hip by the examiner. Accentuation of pain in the anterior thigh suggests a "high" lumbar (L2, L3) radiculopathy (Fig. 6).
- **Valsalva test:** This maneuver increases intrathecal pressure, which accentuates radicular pain in the presence of spinal nerve compression and inflammation.
- **Brudzinski test:** With the patient supine, the head is flexed by the examiner, which aggravates radicular pain in the presence of spinal nerve compression.
- **Patrick's (Faber) test:** The lateral malleolus of the symptomatic lower extremity is placed on the patella of the opposite extremity, and the symptomatic extremity is slowly externally rotated. Accentuation of pain favors a lesion of the hip or sacroiliac joint as the cause for the pain (Fig. 7).
- **Gaenslen test:** With the patient supine and the symptomatic extremity and buttock slightly over the edge of the examination table, the asymptomatic lower extremity is flexed at the hip and knee and brought to the chest. The symptomatic lower extremity is extended at the hip to the floor. Increased nonradiating low back and buttock pain indicates sacroiliac joint disease (Fig. 8).
- **Waddell test:** Excessive sensitivity to light pinching of the skin in the region of the low back pain suggests a functional component.

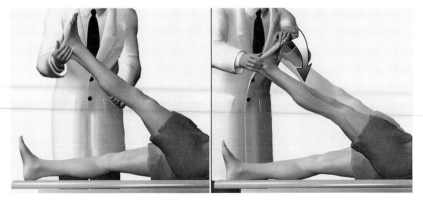

Fig. 5. Bragard's sign. (*From* Levin KH, Covington EC, Devereaux MW, et al. Neck and low back pain. Continuum (NY) 2001;7:20; with permission.)

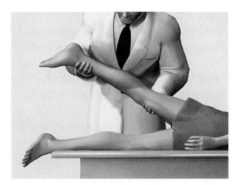

Fig. 6. Prone straight leg raising test. (*From* Levin KH, Covington EC, Devereaux MW, et al. Neck and low back pain. Continuum (NY) 2001;7:21; with permission.)

Lumbosacral root testing is the essence of the neurologic examination in patients with back pain and a suspected lumbosacral radiculopathy. Each myotome and dermatome must be carefully evaluated (Table 2). There are several pitfalls to be avoided in this portion of the examination. Guarding secondary to pain may simulate weakness, but this is usually diffuse and not specific to a given myotome. Reflexes may be suppressed secondary to poor relaxation. The sensory examination is usually less useful than the history of the distribution of paresthesia, particularly early in the course of a radiculopathy.

Neck pain

Inspection of the head and neck, noting reduced spontaneous head movement, head tilt, and neck deformity all raise the possibility of an underlying vertebral disorder or deformity. Palpation and percussion of the neck, as

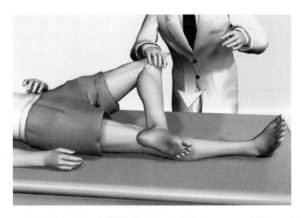

Fig. 7. Faber maneuver. (*From* Levin KH, Covington EC, Devereaux MW, et al. Neck and low back pain. Continuum (NY) 2001;7:22; with permission.)

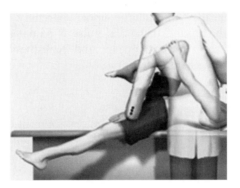

Fig. 8. Gaenslen test. (*From* Levin KH, Covington EC, Devereaux MW, et al. Neck and low back pain. Continuum (NY) 2001;7:22; with permission.)

with the low back, have a low yield with regard to identifying a specific process, but paracervical tenderness or other changes such as palpation of a mass offer support of the diagnosis of a vertebral column disorder.

Gait assessment is also important in patients with neck pain, because evidence of myelopathy may appear. Unilateral or bilateral spastic, ataxic, spastic-ataxic, or Trendelenberg gait all signal a possible cervical myelopathy.

Neuromechanical tests, as with low back and lower extremity pain, are useful in the assessment of patients with neck and upper extremity pain.

- **Spurling test:** The head is inclined toward the side of the painful upper extremity and then compressed downward by the examiner. Pain and paresthesia that radiate into the symptomatic extremity strongly suggest nerve root compression, usually secondary to disc herniation. (It should be noted that lateral head movement away from the symptomatic extremity sometimes can accentuate pain and paresthesia in the symptomatic upper extremity, secondary to stretching a compressed nerve root.)
- **Traction ("distraction") test:** Lifting (traction) on the head may relieve cervical spinal nerve compression and reduce upper extremity pain and paresthesia.
- **Valsalva test:** As with low back pain, the Valsalva maneuver with resultant increased intrathecal pressure can accentuate neck and upper extremity symptoms.
- **Lhermitte's test:** In patients with myelopathy that affects the posterior columns, neck flexion can produce paresthesia, usually in the back but sometimes into the extremities. As is familiar to neurologists, Lhermitte's sign is most commonly associated with an inflammatory process, such as multiple sclerosis but it is sometimes noted with spinal cord compression.
- **Adson's and hyperabduction tests:** Long used in the evaluation of suspected thoracic outlet syndrome, these tests are nonspecific and unreliable. With the patient sitting erect and the upper extremities at the

side (Adson) or the symptomatic upper extremity abducted and extended (hyperabduction), the radial pulse is palpated. The test results are positive if the pulse disappears and paresthesia develops in the hand of the symptomatic extremity.

Cervical root and spinal cord tests

As with the evaluation of low back pain, cervical root testing is central to the neurologic evaluation of a patient with neck and upper extremity pain. In addition to cervical root involvement, the possibility of associated spinal cord compression makes the examination of the lower extremities essential.

Motor examination

In additional to evaluating the strength of each cervical myotome for evidence of a cervical radiculopathy as such, assessment of strength and tone of the lower extremities is required to rule out a cervical myelopathy.

Reflexes

Cervical radiculopathy and myopathy in combination may result in loss of a tendon reflex at the level of the lesion with heightened reflexes below the level of the lesion. All reflexes may be lost with an acute myelopathy during periods of diaschisis ("spinal shock").

Sensation

In addition to testing for a dermatomal pattern of sensory loss, a segmented checking for "cord" level also should be sought. Spinal cord compression may be associated with paresthesia and sensory disturbance confined to the upper extremities as a result of a so-called *central cord syndrome* with involvement primarily of decussating anterior sensory fibers [19].

Sympathetic function

Lesions in the superior thoracic spine may affect the T2 spinal nerve and produce pain in the upper back, shoulder, and proximal upper extremity along with an ipsilateral Horner's syndrome.

Summary

A careful history and physical examination are of primary importance in the evaluation of a patient with spine pain and related symptoms. It can be the difference between sending a patient home with a conservative treatment plan and admitting the patient for an immediate evaluation and possible surgery. In this same vein, the history and physical examination can determine if an expensive evaluation is necessary immediately or whether conservative treatment is appropriate first.

References

[1] Williams A, Newell RLM. Back and macroscopic anatomy of the spinal cord. In: Standing S, editor. Gray's anatomy. 39th edition. New York: Elsevier Churchill Livingstone; 2005. p. 727–87.

[2] Jackson R. The facet syndrome: myth or reality? Orthop Clin North Am 1992;279:110–21.

[3] Boos N, Weissbach S, Rohrbach H, et al. Classification of age-related changes in lumbar intervertebral discs. Spine 2002;27:2631–44.

[4] Roberts S, Evans H, Trivedi J, et al. History and pathology of the human intervertebral disc. J Bone Joint Surg Am 2006;88(Suppl 2):10–4.

[5] Battie MC, Videman T. Lumbar disc degeneration: epidemiology and genetics. J Bone Joint Surg Am 2006;88(Suppl 2):3–9.

[6] Brisby H. Pathology and possible mechanisms of nervous system response to disc degeneration. J Bone Joint Surg Am 2006;88(Suppl 2):68–71.

[7] Levin KH, Covington EC, Devereaux MW, et al. Neck and low back pain. Continuum (N Y) 2001;7:1–205.

[8] Korkala O, Gronblad M, Liese P, et al. Immunohistochemical demonstration of nociceptors in the ligamentous structures of the lumbar spine. Spine 1985;10:156–7.

[9] Palmgren T, Gronblad M, Virri J, et al. An immunohistochemical study of nerve structures in the annulus fibrosus of human normal lumbar intervertebral discs. Spine 1999;24:2075–9.

[10] Coppes M, Marani E, Thomeer R, et al. Innervation of "painful" lumbar discs. Spine 1997; 22:2342–9.

[11] Lotz JC, Ulrich JA. Innervation inflammation and hypermobility may characterize pathologic disc degeneration: review of animal model data. J Bone Joint Surg Am 2006;88(Suppl 2):76–82.

[12] Deyo RA, Cherkin D, Conrad D, et al. Cost controversy crises: low back pain and the health of the public. Annu Rev Public Health 1992;12:141–55.

[13] Johnson EW. The myth of skeletal muscle spasm [editorial]. Am J Phys Med 1989;68:1.

[14] Mense S, Simons D. Muscle pain understanding is nature, diagnosis and treatment. Baltimore (MD): Lippincott, Williams & Wilkins; 2001. p. 117–8.

[15] Devereaux MW. The neuro-ophthalmologic complications of cervical manipulation. J Neuroophthalmol 2000;20:236–9.

[16] Groen GJ, Baljet B, Drukker J. Nevers and nerve plexuses of the human vertebral column. Am J Anat 1990;188:282–96.

[17] Boden SD, Davis DO, Dina TS, et al. Abnormal magnetic resonance scans of the lumbar spine in asymptomatic subjects: a prospective investigation. J Bone Joint Surg Am 1990; 72:403–8.

[18] Jensen M, Brant-Zawadzki M, Obuchowski N, et al. Magnetic resonance imaging of the lumbar spine in people without back pain. N Engl J Med 1994;331:69–73.

[19] Voskuhl R, Hinton R. Sensory impairment in the hands secondary to spondylotic compression of the cervical spinal cord. Arch Neurol 1990;47:309–11.

ELSEVIER
SAUNDERS

NEUROLOGIC
CLINICS

Neurol Clin 25 (2007) 353–371

Epidemiology and Risk Factors for Spine Pain

Devon I. Rubin, MD[a,b,*]

[a]Mayo Clinic College of Medicine, 200 First Street, SW, Rochester, MN 55905, USA
[b]Department of Neurology, Mayo Clinic, 4500 San Pablo Road, Jacksonville, FL 32224, USA

Pain in the low back and neck is one of the most common medical problems in the adult population. It is estimated that between 70% and 80% of adults experience an episode of low back pain at least once during their lifetime [1,2]. This high prevalence and widespread nature of the problem affect physicians throughout the medical specialties and it is estimated that between 2% and 5% of the population seeks medical attention annually because of back pain. Patients seek medical consultation not only from their primary care physicians but also from various physician and nonphysician subspecialists, including neurologists, neurosurgeons, orthopedic surgeons, physiatrists, rheumatologists, physical therapists, and chiropractors. In many instances, patients who have back and neck pain make up the largest proportion of patients for many of these specialists. Furthermore, it is estimated that back pain is the most common reason for limitation of activity in the younger population and is the most frequent cause of absences from work [1,3–5].

Although the evaluation and treatment of back pain is one of the most common reasons for patients to seek medical attention, accurate assessment of the true incidence and prevalence is difficult. The literature is full of studies performed during the past several decades focusing on the epidemiology of back and neck pain. The wide methodologic variability of the studies, however, poses several challenges in interpreting the results. For example, the cohorts from which the epidemiology of back and neck pain have been studied vary widely and have consisted of patients in the general population or in subpopulations (such as those seen in general medical practices or in specific work environments), in largely or sparsely populated cities, in the United States or in other countries, in young or old individuals, and in

* Department of Neurology, Mayo Clinic, 4500 San Pablo Road, Jacksonville, FL 32224.
E-mail address: rubin.devon@mayo.edu

0733-8619/07/$ - see front matter © 2007 Elsevier Inc. All rights reserved.
doi:10.1016/j.ncl.2007.01.004
neurologic.theclinics.com

individuals involved in a variety of occupations. Another interpretive challenge lies in the inconsistency and lack of standardization of the case definition used to define back pain in different studies, the criteria used to define the severity of the symptoms, and the variability in the duration of low back pain used in the studies. Attempts to standardize the definition of back pain have led to improvements in the quality of the studies, but even with standardized definitions, comparisons are difficult. Furthermore, most studies rely on self-reporting the experience of back or neck pain, which is subjective and prone to inaccuracies because of reliance on patient recollection. As a result of these many variables, extrapolating the results of the studies in the literature to determine the most "accurate" prevalence and incidence rates is difficult and generalizing the findings may be impossible.

Regardless of the exact prevalence of back and neck pain, spine problems undoubtedly pose a major medical problem to society. There are many different causes of back pain; however, a specific cause rarely is identified in the majority of patients. Nonetheless, the identification of factors that may lead to increased risk for development of back or neck pain is important to ultimately guide individuals who may be more predisposed to experiencing pain in the use of potential preventative measures. This articlea article reviews the epidemiology and risk factors for neck and back pain. Because neck pain is less common and disables a smaller proportion of the population than low back pain, the epidemiology and risk factors for neck pain are studied much less extensively than for low back pain. As a result, the focus of the article predominantly is on low back pain.

Epidemiology

The burden of low back and neck pain to society can be estimated in epidemiologic studies evaluating the prevalence and incidence of the conditions. The prevalence refers to the number of patients in a population who experience pain at a certain point in time. Prevalence can be defined as the number of people who have pain at a defined point or period of time divided by the total defined population during that time. Prevalence is measured at a single point in time (point prevalence) or over a specific period of time (period prevalence), such as during 1 month, 1 year, or throughout an entire lifetime (cumulative lifetime prevalence). The incidence refers to the number of patients who experience a new episode of pain over a specific period of time, such as over a 1-year period. Although both parameters assess the burden of the problem, estimation of the incidence focuses on new-onset or first-time development of acute back or neck pain.

Incidence of developing back pain

Most studies that focus on the epidemiology of back pain have concentrated on identifying the prevalence, but the incidence for developing a new episode of pain also has been studied. The annual incidence of developing an episode of low back pain is reported as low as 4% and as high as 93% [6–8]. In an epidemiologic survey of adults, ages 20 to 69, in Saskatchewan, Canada, 19% of 318 individuals who did not have a history of back pain over a period of 6 months before the study developed an episode of low back pain over a 1-year period, and most episodes were reported as mild in severity [8]. In another population-based study of adults from a single small town in Israel, a similar 1-year incidence of 18% was found for developing low back pain that interfered with regular daily activities and lasted at least 24 hours [9]. When assessed over a 3-year period, the incidence of developing low back pain of any degree or duration in 148 randomly selected Veterans Affairs (VA) outpatients was 67%, whereas 44% self-reported experiencing an episode of "moderately severe" pain [10].

Contrary to the high rates reported in some studies, a longitudinal study of adults in a Canadian population demonstrates the risk for developing new onset of back pain over 2 years to be only 8% for males and 9% for females, with an overall incidence of approximately 45 per 1000 person years [11]. Similarly, a large study of more than 2000 adults who were free of low back pain during the month before the study found a 12-month cumulative incidence of only 3% to 5% for a new episode of low back pain for which patients consulted a physician. The 12-month cumulative incidence was approximately 30% for an episode of back pain, however, for which patients did not consult a physician [6]. These studies suggest that the incidence of developing any type of back pain over a 1- to 2-year period may be high, whereas that of developing pain that is more severe and limits daily activities or requires medical attention is lower.

Prevalence of low back pain

One of the challenges in comparing different studies on prevalence of back pain is the variation in study populations and in the many factors that may affect the development of back pain. For example, differences in the ages of the populations studied, activity level, psychosocial function, physical features, and other health status all potentially may contribute to differences in the prevalence of back pain in the population. Controlling for all of these variables to compare different epidemiologic studies is unrealistic. Despite the varying prevalence rates, many studies show that low back pain is a common and frequent problem in the general adult population.

The prevalence rates reported for low back pain in the population vary widely. It is estimated that 15% to 20% of adults experience back pain during a single year and 50% to 80% experience at least one episode of back pain during an individual lifetime [1,12,13]. A systematic review of studies in the literature evaluating the prevalence of low back pain between 1966 and 1998 notes that the methods of data collection, sample sizes, response

rates, and prevalence time frames varied widely, even when strict methodologic criteria were used to include only high-quality studies [14]. In this evidence-based review, the ranges for prevalence rates reported were 12% to
30% for point prevalence studies, 22% to 65% for 1-year prevalence studies,
and 11% to 84% for lifetime prevalence studies [14]. In a similar methodologic literature review during a shorter but similar time period, Loney and
Stratford [15] reported the point prevalence rates for any duration of low
back pain at the time of the surveys to be 4% to 33%, whereas the point
prevalence rates for low back pain lasting greater than 2 weeks were lower.

Prevalence of neck pain

There are fewer population-based epidemiologic studies on neck pain. It
is estimated that one fifth of the adult population experiences neck pain over
a 1-year period and two thirds experience neck pain at least once during
their lifetime [16,17]. Other community-based studies report 6-month prevalence rates for neck pain of approximately 40% in the working population
[18,19]. Approximately 18% of the general population visits a health care
professional annually for neck pain and approximately 5% of patients
who have neck pain report significant disability from the pain [16,20]. Disability from neck pain seems less common than for back pain but still can be
a significant burden in the population. The prevalence of neck pain increases
with age and is more common in women than men [21].

Prevalence in different age groups

Children and adolescents

Most epidemiologic studies of spine pain have focused on adults and
working populations, and back pain in the childhood or adolescent period
has been investigated in less detail. Although generally it is believed that
back pain is uncommon in children and adolescents, several studies have attempted to estimate the prevalence in this population and to determine if the
presence of pain at a young age predicts the presence in adulthood [22]. The
prevalence of low back pain in younger individuals is variable. In a study of
adolescents between ages 11 and 15, 11% to 50% self-reported experiencing
pain in their back [23]. The age of onset of back pain in children is approximately 13 to 14 years, after which the prevalence rates may increase and become similar to the adult prevalence rates in the older adolescent population
[22–24]. Although the evidence is conflicting, genetic predisposition, socioeconomic status, athletic activities, the presence of scoliosis, and increased
height are factors suggested to increase the risk for back pain in children
[22,25].

Neck pain also is a problem in the adolescent age group, with 15% to
30% experiencing neck pain [26,27]. Symptoms in adolescence are shown
to predict morbidity from neck pain in adulthood [26].

Elderly

Despite the growing elderly population, few epidemiologic studies have focused on the presence of back pain in the older population. In a survey of adults age 65 years or older, however, back pain was considered to be one of the most important factors to affect individual state of health [28]. Back and neck pain is a common problem in the older population, and the prevalence of low back pain in the older population (>65 years) may be higher than in younger adults. Several studies show that approximately one fifth of visits to physicians for back problems occur in patients more than 65 years old [29,30].

Bressler and colleagues [31] systematically reviewed the literature between 1966 and 1999 for studies assessing low back pain in patients older than 65 years and found the prevalence in the general community to be 13% to 49%. In older patients evaluated in a medical practice setting, the prevalence was slightly higher, at 23% to 51%. In a study of individuals ages 70 to102, the 1-month prevalence rate of back pain was 25% [32]. Other studies report similar findings, with "frequent" back pain over a 1-year period occurring in approximately one third of the older population [33]. Back pain consistently is shown to be more frequent in older women than men [32,33]. The prevalence of back pain decreases significantly in women over age 85 and men over age 90 [33,34]. The reason for this decline in the oldest patients may be related to recall bias, the acceptance of some pain as "natural," less reporting of their pain, or a lesser degree of physical activity. Despite a high prevalence of back pain in the elderly, most patients experience only intermittent or episodic pain rather than constant or progressive pain [35]. In one survey of patients between ages 68 and 100, however, 22% of responders indicated that they experienced back pain "on most days" [34]. Nonetheless, functional limitation was reported in approximately only 7% of older patients who had back pain, and most patients were not impaired significantly by the pain [33].

The frequency of neck pain decreases after age 50 [19]. The prevalence of neck pain in older patients (>70 years) is slightly less than low back pain in one population-based study, with a reported 1-month prevalence of 11% for neck pain compared with 15% for low back pain [35]. The likelihood of experiencing neck and low back pain together, however, is high in older individuals [35]. Although the prevalence of low back pain is shown to be higher in older women than men, no gender differences are found with respect to the prevalence of neck pain [31,35].

The studies that evaluate the frequency of back and neck pain in the elderly may underestimate the true prevalence rates for several reasons. Factors that may lead to underreporting in this age group include the presence of cognitive impairment, depression, and decreased pain perception. In addition, elderly patients may have an attitude of not wishing to burden their caregivers and, therefore, may not complain of pain [31].

Course of low back and neck pain

The course of back and neck back pain refers to the progression, stabilization, or resolution of pain after the initial onset and diagnosis. Similar to the difficulty in determining the prevalence, defining the typical clinical course of pain in the population is challenging. Differences in the terminology used to define the course of pain, etiologies, treatments, and outcome parameters confound comparison of prognostic studies. For example, in some studies, a good outcome may be considered when patients no longer seek medical attention or return to work, even though the pain may persist, whereas others define a good outcome based on complete resolution of pain.

It generally is believed that most episodes of low back pain are self-limiting. It is estimated that approximately 50% of patients who have acute low back pain no longer are disabled after 2 weeks and 70% recover by 1 month. Furthermore, nearly 90% of patients recover from an acute episode of pain by 3 months, leaving only 10% of patients who continue to seek medical care after 3 months [1,36]. With respect to the prevalence of episodes of pain lasting various durations, the 1-year prevalence of pain lasting longer than 2 weeks is 15% and pain lasting 3 to 6 months occurs in only 5% to 10% of patients who have back pain [12].

Several studies have attempted to determine the course of back pain, with similar reported rates of recovery and progression to chronic pain. In one study of 530 patients who had low back pain of varying degrees of severity, resolution of the pain was reported in 27% during a 1-year period [8]. Another review of the prevalence studies in the literature that assessed the course of back pain found that between 42% and 75% of subjects continued to experience pain 1 year after onset and between 44% and 78% of subjects experienced relapses of pain [13]. Another study followed adults who experienced an episode of back pain lasting less than 2 weeks for 12 months, measuring predominantly days absent from work and the degree of complete recovery of pain, and found that 45% of patients continued to complain of low back pain at the 1-year follow-up, although 50% returned to work within 8 days after evaluation [37]. Although these finding may be interpreted as indicating that back pain resolves completely within 3 months in most patients, alternatively they may indicate only that patients continue to experience pain but simply do not require further medical attention.

The findings in the literature support the concept that recurrent episodes of back pain are common and having experienced a prior episode of low back pain consistently is a strong predictor of future episodes [3,6,7]. In many instances, new or first-time episodes often develop into longer and possibly more disabling episodes over time and eventually into chronic back pain. The definition of chronic back pain is variable but typically refers to pain persisting beyond 3 months. Much research has been undertaken to determine the prevalence of chronic back pain and variable rates are reported. One study finds that 79% of patients who have a new episode of back pain experience chronic pain, with many experiencing pain lasting more than 1 year in duration [36]. In a longitudinal study of patients in the United Kingdom, 20% of patients who did not experience chronic pain when surveyed in 1996 experienced chronic back pain when surveyed 4 years later [38]. In the initial survey, however, nearly 60% of patients experienced pain somewhere other than in their back, suggesting that previous chronic pain or poorer general health is predictive of the development of chronic back pain [38]. Other studies also find that the point prevalence rates of low back pain is higher in patients who have experienced previous episodes of low back pain compared with those who do not have a history of low back pain.

Several other predictors for the transition from acute to chronic back pain are proposed, including the initial duration of the first episode of back pain and the severity of pain. The risk for developing chronic disability from back pain becomes higher when the duration of the initial episode of back pain exceeds 14 days [39]. The longer the initial episode of back pain lasts, the less likely that patients return to work; fewer than 50% of patients return to work after experiencing back pain lasting longer than 6 months [40]. Patients who have a prior history of absenteeism from work because of an episode of back pain, older age, or a prior history of low back pain likely have a poorer outcome after a single episode of pain and more likely have persistent or chronic low back pain after an initial episode [37,41]. Patients who have more severe baseline pain are less likely to experience resolution compared with those who have mild baseline pain (10% versus 36% with resolution) [39]. Other studies suggest that women are more likely to experience "persistent" chronic back pain than men, but age had no effect on the development of chronic pain [38].

The course of neck pain has been evaluated less frequently than that of low back pain. A 1-year prevalence rate of 11% is reported for neck pain last more than 1 month. Persistent pain at 6 to 12 months after an episode of neck pain has been reported in 10% to 37% of individuals, and in one survey approximately half of the patients who experienced pain at one point in time continued to experience pain at a 1-year follow-up [42–45]. Recurrent episodes of neck pain are common and occur in approximately one quarter of individuals [44]. These findings indicate that the course of neck pain often is one of periods of remission and exacerbation rather than one of complete resolution.

Risk factors for back pain

Despite the variability in the prevalence rates reported for back and neck pain in the general population, it is evident that spine pain is a common and significant medical condition with a tremendous social and economic impact on society. Back pain is a leading cause of absenteeism from work, temporary disability, and workers' compensation; therefore, the financial costs to society are enormous. Identifying factors that may increase the risk for or predispose individuals to the development of back pain is critical in attempting to reduce the prevalence and ultimately the social impact of this problem.

Many studies have attempted to identify and evaluate the contribution of multiple different demographic, physical, socioeconomic, psychologic, and occupational factors to the development of spine pain. There is a significant limitation in interpreting the literature on risk factors, because many of the studies rely on self-reported parameters and on statistical correlations of association among large cohorts of the population. Many factors are implicated in the predisposition to the development of pain. One review notes that more than 55 different individual factors and 24 work-related factors have been studied in relation to back pain [46]. Most of these factors, however, are assessed only in single or small studies, with weak and nonreproducible evidence to support a definite association. Several risk factors are evaluated more thoroughly and the results of these risk factors are discussed in more detail (Box 1) [5,11]. Although not studied in as much detail as back pain, similar risk factors for neck pain are identified [21].

Box 1. Risk factors for back pain

Demographic factors
Age
Gender
Socioeconomic status and education level

Health factors
Body mass index (BMI)
Tobacco use
Perceived general health status

Occupational factors
Physical activity, such as bending, lifting, or twisting
Monotonous tasks
Job dissatisfaction

Psychologic factors
Depression

Spinal anatomy factors
Anatomic variations
Imaging abnormalities

Demographic factors

Age

The prevalence of back pain in different age groups is discussed earlier in this article. The highest rates of back pain consistently are found in the adult population from the third to the sixth decades, with those experiencing new onset of back pain more likely to be in the third decade [5,7,11,47]. A systematic review of the literature comparing the prevalence of low back pain in different age groups finds lower prevalence rates in younger adult patients (ages 20–35) with rates increasing with age until ages 60 to 65, after which there is a decline in the frequency of pain [12,15]. Older patients more likely experience persistent or intermittent neck and low back rather than new onset of pain than younger individuals [7,45]. As noted previously, the presence of low back pain in adolescence seems to be a risk factor for the development of low back pain in adulthood [48].

The causal relationship between age and the development of back pain is not entirely clear. The high prevalence of back pain in younger adults may be related to the fact that the younger population is more physically active in general than older population and the activity may predispose them to developing pain (discussed later) or the effect of back pain on their daily lifestyle may be more pronounced and, therefore, cause them to seek medical attention more often. With increasing age, more stress and anatomic changes in the spinal structures also could result in a predisposition for experiencing more chronic and persistent pain.

Gender

Back and neck pain poses a significant problem for men and women. Although several studies suggest that women are more predisposed to experiencing back pain than men, the literature does not consistently identify significant differences in the incidences between genders [11,49]. In the older age population, women have a higher prevalence of low back pain than men, possibly related to a higher risk for osteoporosis involving the spine [31]. Several reports indicate that women are more likely than men to use health care for back pain, take more sick days from work, have a poor outcome after a single episode of low back pain, and develop persistent, chronic pain lasting more than 3 months [38,41,49].

Neck pain is reported more frequently in women than in men, and women are more likely to seek medical attention from a health care professional [19]. Chronic or persistent neck pain over a 1-year period is reported with similar frequency in men and women [45].

Socioeconomic status and level of education

Low socioeconomic status and a lower level of education are associated with disability retirement from back pain [50–52]. In a systematic review of the literature, Dionne and colleagues [51] found a consistent association of increased prevalence of back pain with low educational status. There seemed to be a stronger effect, however, of education on the duration and recurrence of back pain than on the onset of pain. Furthermore, the course of back pain was less favorable in those who had low educational status, with a poorer outcome in those patients. The incidence of disability retirement from back pain was seven- to tenfold higher in unskilled workers compared with skilled workers in a higher social class [50]. Similarly, the incidence of disability increased by 22- to 25-fold in patients who had less than or equal to 7 years of education compared with those who had college degrees. In addition, patients who had a low level of education demonstrated more misconceptions about low back pain and endorsed pain beliefs associated with poorer ability to adjust to chronic pain [52].

There are several proposed mechanisms that may account for the relationship between low educational status and back pain. There is a direct relationship between education and socioeconomic status, because the amount of formal education contributes to the types of jobs individuals may secure and, subsequently, the types of jobs influence their socioeconomic status. The association between socioeconomic status and the development of back pain disability is not understood completely, although a correlation between socioeconomic status and other environmental factors, such as cigarette smoking, obesity, chronic stressful events, dietary habits, and physical occupations may play a role.

Health factors

Obesity

Obesity or high BMI (>30 BMI) is an independent predictor of the development of low back pain and disability from pain [1,53,54]. The association of BMI on the development of back pain may be stronger in women than men [55]. Vogt and colleagues [53] reviewed the prevalence and risk factors in postmenopausal women who had back pain and found that postmenopausal women who had low back pain had a higher BMI and weighed approximately 2 to 3 kg more than those who did not have back pain.

Smoking

Smoking is suggested as a risk factor for the development of back pain, although the supportive evidence for this association is modest at best. Smoking has an impact on the musculoskeletal system by several mechanisms, including increasing the risk for osteoporosis and fractures, decreasing bone density, and increasing degenerative changes in the spine. Several studies identify a higher prevalence of back pain in smokers compared with nonsmokers [56–60]. For example, one study finds that individuals who began smoking at age 16 and continued to smoke moderately or heavily for 17 years had a 90% higher relative risk for back pain at age 33 than nonsmokers [60]. In another study, smoking for more than 15 years is associated with a higher risk for sciatic pain, but volume of smoking is not a contributing factor, whereas another study finds that smoking volume and duration were associated with chronic back pain [61,62]. Because most studies do not control for other possible associated variables, the evidence for a clear causal link between back pain and smoking is not strong. An indirect stressor effect related to chronic coughing in smokers also is proposed to account for the possible association with back pain [55]. In contrast, other studies show that smoking is not associated with a significantly increased risk for back pain [9,11,55]. It remains unclear whether or not smoking is a definite risk factor for developing pain.

Health status

Self-rated health status is an important predictor of the development of back pain in men and women [3,11,35,55,63]. Patients who have a perception of poorer health are more prone to back pain [11,41,55,63]. In one prospective, longitudinal study of back pain in Canadian adults, the strongest risk factor for the development of back pain was a self-rated poor overall health status [11]. Croft and colleagues [55] studied a large population that had low back pain in the United Kingdom and also found that poor general health at baseline was the strongest predictor of a new episode of back pain.

Patients who have back pain experience many co-occurring health problems and comorbidities, including bone and joint diseases, migraine headaches, pulmonary diseases, cardiac diseases, and gastrointestinal diseases [32]. The relationship between these comorbidities and back pain is unclear, but this association may account for the self-reported poor health status found in individuals experiencing back pain. Therefore, in the studies that demonstrate a relationship between the perception of poor health and back pain, it is likely that the presence of back pain is one of many factors that lead to the perception of poor health status rather than a direct causal relationship.

Occupational factors

Occupational and leisurely physical activity

Repetitive physical activities may produce cumulative stress on the spine and lead to the development of back pain. Athletic activities or repetitive physical maneuvers that occur with manual labor occupations are suggested to predispose individuals to back pain [1,64]. It is estimated that 37% of low back pain worldwide is attributable to occupational risk factors [65]. A systematic review of the literature to assess the evidence related to the type of physical activity on the development of back pain concludes that there is moderate evidence to support a relationship between heavy physical work and manual handling techniques and pain but no evidence for an association with prolonged standing or sitting [64]. The type, degree, and duration of physical activity that individuals perform on a regular basis may affect the development of back pain; however, studies assessing the level of physical activity as a predictor of back pain report conflicting results.

The types of physical activity performed, from occupational and recreational standpoints, potentially may play a role in the development of neck and low back pain. Occupations that consist of manual material handling, such as heavy lifting, moving, carrying, bending, or twisting; those that include long-term static positions, such as sitting; and those that have high exposure to low-frequency whole-body vibration are perceived to apply more stress on the structures in the spine and are a risk factor for back pain [1,64]. Similarly, work-related risk factors for the development of neck pain include neck flexion, arm posture, sitting for more than 95% of the working time, twisting or bending of the trunk, and hand-arm vibration [66,67]. Professions, such as those in sales, clerical work, repair, service, and transportation, more likely are associated with back pain than other professional occupations [5]. Several types of occupations are stratified according to level of risk for stress on the back; those that are at a low risk include managers, professionals, and clerical or sales workers, whereas higher-risk professions include operators, service workers, and farmers [65]. The degree of acute physical load applied to the back and the cumulative or long-term load to the back may play a role in the development of pain [64]. Adults whose job requires standing or walking for more than 2 hours per shift and women who lift or move more than 25 pounds are more than twice as likely to consult a general practitioner for back pain than those whose jobs are more sedentary and do not require lifting [68].

Another risk factor identified as predicting the progression from acute to chronic occupational back pain is the need to lift for at least 75% of the work day [69]. In workers returning to their occupation after experiencing an episode of back pain, those who were unable to return with light duties on return to work and those who were required to lift for most of the day were at a higher risk for developing chronic pain [69].

In some cases, the perception of the degree of physical demand, rather than the actual degree of activity, may be associated with pain. In one survey of 715 patients who were granted back pain disability, the strongest predictor for developing back pain disability was the patients' perception that their work was "physically demanding" [63]. Subjects who reported physically demanding work frequently were at higher risk for disability than those who reported infrequent physically demanding work.

Several studies have surveyed athletes in various types of sporting activities to assess the prevalence of back pain, with conflicting results [64]. When assessed according to specific sports, no increased risk for back pain was seen in golf, cycling, or athletic training [64]. In a study of cross-country skiers and rowers, the 1-year prevalence of self-reported low back pain was higher than in nonathletic controls [70]. Back pain appeared more often during periods of training and competition.

In contrast to the evidence suggesting that physical stress may lead to the development of back pain, other studies report that a lower level of physical activity is associated with an increased risk for back pain [32]. In one study, a lower baseline level of sporting activities is associated with a higher likelihood of experiencing back pain episodes [9]. In a another study, however, of a cohort of adults in the general population evaluating the association of low back pain and self-reported level of physical activity compared with their peers, the perceived level of leisurely physical activity in the subjects who had back pain was not significantly different than those who did not have pain [55]. The causative nature of a lower physical activity level and back pain is unclear, and the presence of back pain may be the cause of limitation of physical function rather that a result.

Job satisfaction

Studies also have attempted to assess the role of work satisfaction with the development of back pain. Although some studies suggest that workplace dissatisfaction is a predictor of back pain, others show that level of work satisfaction is not associated with an increased risk for back pain [9,69,71]. In a study of a large population of aircraft employees, the degree of work satisfaction was associated significantly with back pain, with subjects who had low work satisfaction 2.5 times more likely to report a back injury than those who had high job satisfaction [72].

The psychologic work environment also is associated with the experience of neck and shoulder pain [67]. Secretaries who reported a "poor" psychologic work environment with poor social support at work were found to have a higher relative risk for experiencing frequent neck pain compared with those who reported a "good" work environment [73].

Psychologic factors: depression

There is a strong association between back and neck pain and depression [10,74–78]. The experience of pain involves a complex interaction of physical, emotional, cognitive, and behavioral components. The ability to cope with pain relies on emotional and psychologic capabilities, and underlying depression may affect the mechanism of coping adversely, thereby leading to an increased perception or experience of pain. Patients who experience pain, particularly when the precise cause cannot be determined, often feel hopeless and helpless. The inability to obtain timely or effective relief for the pain may result further in depression and anxiety. In the acute phase of back pain, a natural emotional reaction, such as anxiety or worry about the cause of the pain, may occur. As the pain persists, increasing behavioral or psychologic reactions may develop, including anger, depression, and somatization. Psychologic changes and depression become more prominent as back pain becomes more chronic. In individuals who have chronic pain, a complex interaction between the physical, psychologic, and social environments may develop and patients may adopt a "sick role," where interaction with their environment, social obligations, and normal responsibilities become more difficult [79]. Patients who have chronic back pain are approximately 6 times more likely to be depressed than pain-free individuals [78]. A genetic predisposition to symptoms of back pain and to depression or anxiety also is suggested as playing a role [80].

In 2000, Linton [77] systematically reviewed the literature related to the interaction between psychologic factors and the development of back or neck pain and came to several conclusions. First, a significant relationship between stress, distress, anxiety, mood, and depression and neck and back pain was identified consistently. Second, this relationship existed independently of other variables. Third, psychosocial variables have more impact than biomedical factors on back pain disability and are linked to the transition from acute to chronic pain disability. In addition, cognitive factors, such as attitude, passive coping, and fear-avoidance beliefs, also were related to the development of pain and disability.

Depression, as identified by patient report, also is a predictor of developing low back pain rather than a response to the experience of pain. Several studies demonstrate that depression is an independent risk factor for the development of back or neck pain and those individuals who have self-reported depression are twice as likely to develop back pain [10,81]. The degree of pain may correlate with the development of depression, and individuals who have more severe pain have a higher likelihood of depression [78].

Spinal anatomy factors

Several anatomic factors can affect the spine, including congenital abnormalities, degenerative changes, scoliosis, osteoporosis, and disk herniations. Congenital vertebral abnormalities, such as a transitional vertebra or spina bifida occulta, may be contributors to back pain. The presence of a transitional lumbosacral vertebra refers to a total or partial fusion of the transverse process of the lowest lumbar vertebra to the sacrum. A review of approximately 800 radiographs from male patients who had a 4-week or more history of low back pain found congenital vertebral abnormalities in 10%, with approximately half being transitional vertebrae and half spina bifida occulta [82]. Transitional vertebrae are found in approximately 8% to 30% of young and middle-aged men. The evidence regarding the association between a transitional vertebrae and the development of low back pain is conflicting [83–86]. In several studies, a transitional vertebra is shown to be the cause of back pain [83–85]. Increased prevalence of disk protrusion or extrusion above the transitional vertebra or altered biomechanics associated with asymmetric transitional vertebrae may account for the pain. Other studies find no association between the presence of a transitional vertebra and any type of low back pain [86].

The association between disk abnormalities on imaging studies and back pain is the subject of controversy. Disk disruption is found in approximately 40% of a population with low back pain [87]. Several studies conclude, however, that the presence of lumbar disk abnormalities often is seen in asymptomatic subjects and does not predict the development of low back pain [88–90]. In an assessment of 148 asymptomatic VA outpatients followed over a 3-year period, the incidence of low back pain was 67%, and no significant association was found between the development of low back pain and MRI findings, including endplate changes, disk degeneration, annular tears, or facet degeneration [10]. Another study finds disk degeneration on MRI in 39% of working males, between ages 20 and 58, with a higher frequency of disk degeneration in the older patients, but failed to find an association between lumbar disk degeneration on MRI and the presence of low back pain [91]. The findings of disk extrusion (but not protrusion) or central spinal stenosis more likely are associated with the development of pain [10].

In a study evaluating the association between radiographic cervical spine degenerative changes and neck pain or disability, no significant differences were found in the degree of pain between patients who did or did not have radiographic cervical spine degeneration [92].

Summary

Low back and neck pain remains a common problem and one of enormous social, psychologic, and economic burden. Low back pain afflicts individuals of all ages, from adolescent to elderly populations, and is a major cause of disability in the adult working population. The risk factors for the development of spine pain are multidimensional, with physical attributes, socioeconomic status, general medical health and psychologic state, and occupational environmental factors all playing a role in contributing to the risk for experiencing pain.

References

[1] Andersson GB. Epidemiology of low back pain. Acta Orthop Scand Suppl 1998;281:28–31.
[2] Frymoyer JW. Back pain and sciatica. N Engl J Med 1988;318:291–300.
[3] Biering-Sorensen F, Thomsen C. Medical, social and occupational history as risk indicators for low back trouble in a general population. Spine 1986;11:720–5.
[4] Frank JW, Kerr MS, Brooker AS, et al. Disability resulting from occupational low back pain: I. What do we know about primary prevention? A review of the scientific evidence on prevention before disability begins. Spine 1996;21:141–56.
[5] Hurwitz EL, Morgenstern H. Correlates of back problems and back related disability in the United States. J Clin Epidemiol 1997;50:669–81.
[6] Papageorgiou AC, Croft PR, Thomas E, et al. Influence of previous pain experience on the episode incident of low back pain: results from the South Manchester Back Pain Study. Pain 1996;66:181–5.

[7] Waxman R, Tennant A, Helliwill P. A prospective followup study of low back pain in the community. Spine 2000;25:2085–90.

[8] Cassidy JD, Cote P, Carroll LJ, et al. Incidence and course of low back pain episodes in the general population. Spine 2005;30:2817–23.

[9] Jacob T. Low back pain incident episodes: a community based study. Spine J 2006;6:306–10.

[10] Jarvik JG, Hollingworth W, Heagerty PJ, et al. Three-year incidence of low back pain in an initially asymptomatic cohort: clinical and imagıng risk factors. Spine 2005;30:1541–8.

[11] Kopec JA, Sayre EC, Esdaile JM. Predictors of back pain in a general population cohort. Spine 2004;29:70–7.

[12] Lawrence RC, Helmick CG, Arnett FC, et al. Estimates of the prevalence of arthritis and selected musculoskeletal disorders in the United States. Arthritis Rheum 1998;41:778–99.

[13] Hestbaek L, Leboef-Yde C, Manniche C. Low back pain: what is the long term course? A review of studies of general patient populations. Eur Spine J 2003;12:149–65.

[14] Walker BF. The prevalence of low back pain: a systematic review of the literaturefrom 1965 to 1998. J Spinal Disord 2000;13:205–17.

[15] Loney PL, Stratford PW. The prevalence of low back pain in adults: a methodological review of the literature. Phys Ther 1999;79:384–96.

[16] Cote P, Cassidy JD, Carroll L. The Saskatchewan Health and Back Pain Survey: the prevalence of neck pain and related disability in Saskatchewan adults. Spine 1998;23:1689–98.

[17] Croft PR, Lewis M, Papageorgiou AC, et al. Risk factors for neck pain: a longitudinal study in the general population. Pain 2001;93:317–25.

[18] Eckberg K, Karlsson M, Axelson O, et al. Cross-sectional study of risk factors for symptoms in the neck and shoulder area. Ergonomics 1995;38:971–80.

[19] Leclerc A, Niedhammer I, Landre M, et al. One-year predictive factors for various aspects of neck disorders. Spine 1999;24:1455–62.

[20] Linton SJ. Risk factors for neck and back pain in a working population in Sweden. Work Stress 1990;4:41–9.

[21] Cote P, Cassidy JD, Carroll L. The factors associated with neck pain and its related disability in the Saskatchewan population. Spine 2000;25:1109–17.

[22] Salminem JJ, Erkintalo M, Laine M, et al. Low back pain in the young. A prospective three-year follow-up study of subjects with and without low back pain. Spine 1995;20:2101–7.

[23] Burton KA, Clarke RD, McClune TD, et al. The natural history of low back pain in adolescents. Spine 1996;21:2323–8.

[24] Fairbank JCT, Pynsent PB, van Poortvliet JA, et al. Influence of anthropometric factors and joint laxity in the adolescent back pain. Spine 1984;9:461–4.

[25] Kovacs FM, Abraira V, Zamora J, et al. The transition from acute to subacute and chronic low back pain. Spine 2005;30:1786–92.

[26] Hertzberg A. Prediction of cervical and low back pain based on routine school health examinations. Scand J Prim Health Care 1985;3:247–53.

[27] Vikat A, Rimpela M, Salminem JJ, et al. Neck or shoulder pain and low back pain in Finnish adolescents. Scand J Public Health 2000;28:164–73.

[28] Cooper JK, Kohlmann T. Factors associated with health status of older Americans. Age Ageing 2001;30:495–501.

[29] Cypress BK. Characteristics of physician visits for back symptoms: a national perspective. Am J Public Health 1983;73:389–95.

[30] Hart LG, Deyo RA, Charkin DC. Physician office visits for low back pain: frequency, clinical evaluation, and treatment patterns from a U.S. national survey. Spine 1995;20:11–9.

[31] Bressler HB, Keyes WJ, Rochon PA, et al. The prevalence of low back pain in the elderly: a systematic review of the literature. Spine 1999;24:1813–9.

[32] Hartvigsen J, Christensen K, Frederiksen H. Back pain remains a common symptom in old age. A population-based study of 4486 Danish twins aged 70-102. Eur Spine J 2003;12:528–34.

[33] Cecchi F, Debolini P, Lova RM, et al. Epidemiology of back pain in a representative cohort of Italian persons 65 years of age and older. Spine 2006;31:1149–55.

[34] Edmond SL, Felson DT. Prevalence of back symptoms in elders. J Rheumatol 2000;27: 220–5.

[35] Hartvigsen J, Christensen K, Frederiksen H. Back and neck pain exhibit many common features in old age: a population-based study of 4,486 Danish twins 70-102 years of age. Spine 2004;29:576–80.

[36] Croft PR, Macfarlane GJ, Papageorgiou AC, et al. Outcome of low back pain in general practice: a prospective study. BMJ 1998;316:1356–9.

[37] Schiottz-Christensen B, Nielsen GL, Hansen VK, et al. Long-term prognosis of acute low back pain in patients seen in general practice: a 1-year prospective follow-up study. Fam Pract 1999;16:223–32.

[38] Smith BH, Elliott AM, Hannaford PC, et al. Factors related to the onset and persistence of chronic back pain in the community. Results from a general population follow-up study. Spine 2004;29:1032–40.

[39] Kovacs FM, Gestoso M, Del Real MTG, et al. Risk factors for non-specific low back pain in schoolchildren and their parents: a population based study. Pain 2003;103:259–68.

[40] Waddell G. A new clinical model for the treatment of low back pain. Spine 1987;12:523–7.

[41] Thomas E, Silman AJ, Croft PR, et al. Predicting who develops chronic low back pain in primary care: a prospective study. BMJ 1999;318:1662–7.

[42] Pietri-Taleb F, Riihimaki H, Viikari-Juntura E, et al. Longitudinal study on the role of personality characteristics and psychological distress in neck trouble among working men. Pain 1994;58:261–7.

[43] Makela M, Heliovaara M, Sievers K, et al. Prevalence, determinants and consequences of chronic neck pain in Finland. Am J Epidemiol 1991;134:1356–67.

[44] Cote P, Cassidy JD, Carroll LJ, et al. The annual incidence and course of neck pain in the general population: a population-based cohort study. Pain 2004;112:267–73.

[45] Hill J, Lewis M, Papageorgiou AC, et al. Predicting persistent neck pain: a 1-year follow-up of a population cohort. Spine 2004;29:1648–54.

[46] Hildebrandt VH. A review of epidemiological research on risk factors of low back pain. In: Buckle PE, editor. Musculo-skeletal disorders at work. London: Taylor & Francis; 1987. p. 9–16.

[47] Reigo T, Timpka T, Tropp H. The epidemiology of back pain in vocational age groups. Scand J Prim Health Care 1999;17:17–21.

[48] Hestbaek L, Leboeuf-Yde C, Kyvik KO, et al. The course of low back pain from adolescence to adulthood. Spine 2006;31:468–72.

[49] Linton SJ, Hellsing AL, Hallden K. A population-based study of spinal pain among 35–45-year-old individuals. Spine 1998;23:1457–63.

[50] Hagen KB, Holte HH, Tambs K, et al. Socioeconomic factors and disability retirement from back pain. A 1983–1993 population-based prospective study in Norway. Spine 2000;25: 2480–7.

[51] Dionne CE, Von Korff M, Deyo RA, et al. Formal education and back pain: a review. J Epidemiol Community Health 2001;55:455–68.

[52] Goubert L, Crombez G, Bourdeaudhuij ID. Low back pain, disability and back pain myths in a community sample: prevalence and interrelationships. Eur J Pain 2004;8:385–94.

[53] Vogt MT, Lauerman WC, Chirumbole M, et al. A community based study of postmenopausal white women with back and leg pain: health status and limitations in physical activity. Journal of Gerontology Series A–Biological Sciences & Medical Sciences 2002;57:M544–50.

[54] Webb R, Brammah T, Lunt M, et al. Prevalence and predictors of intense, chronic, and disabling neck and back pain in the UK general population. Spine 2003;28:1195–202.

[55] Croft PR, Papageorgiou AC, Thomas E, et al. Short term physical risk factors for new episodes of low back pain: prospective evidence from the South Manchester Back Pain Study. Spine 1999;24:1556–61.

[56] Deyo RA, Bass JE. Lifestyle and low back pain. The influence of smoking and obesity. Spine 1989;14:501–6.

[57] Ernst E. Smoking: a cause of back trouble? Br J Rheumatol 1993;32:239–42.

[58] Liira JP, Shannon HS, Chambers LW, et al. Long-term back problems and physical work exposures in the 1990 Ontario Health Survey. Am J Public Health 1996;86:382–7.

[59] Kostova V, Kileva M. Back disorders (low back pain, cervicobrachial and lumbosacral radicular syndromes) and some related risk factors. J Neurol Sci 2001;192:17–25.

[60] Power C, Frank J, Hertzman C, et al. Predictors of low back pain onset in a prospective British study. Am J Public Health 2001;91:1671–8.

[61] Leboeuf-Yde C, Kyvik K, Bruun N. Low back pain and lifestyle: part I. Smoking: information from a population-based sample of 29,424 twins. Spine 1998;23:2207–13.

[62] Miranda H, Viikari-Juntura E, Martikainen R, et al. Individual factors, occupational loading, and physical exercise as predictors of sciatic pain. Spine 2002;27:1102–9.

[63] Hagen KB, Tambs K, Bjerkedal T. A prospective cohort study of risk factors for disability retirement because of back pain in the general working population. Spine 2002;27:1790–6.

[64] Hoogendoorn WE, van Poppel MN, Bongers PM, et al. Physical load during work and leisure time as risk factors for back pain. Scand J Work Environ Health 1999;25:387–403.

[65] Punnett L, Pruss-Ustun A, Nelson DI, et al. Estimating the global burden of low back pain attributable to combined occupational exposures. Am J Ind Med 2005;48:459–69.

[66] Ariens GA, van Mechelen W, Bongers PM, et al. Physical risk factors for neck pain. Scand J Work Environ Health 2000;26:7–19.

[67] Ariens GAM, Bongers PM, Douwes M, et al. Are neck flexion, neck rotation, and sitting at work risk factors for neck pain? Results of a prospective cohort study. Occup Environ Med 2001;58:200–7.

[68] Macfarlane GJ, Thomas E, Papageorgiou AC, et al. Employment and physical work activities as predictors of future low back pain. Spine 1997;22:1143–9.

[69] Fransen M, Woodward M, Norton R, et al. Risk factors associated with the transition from acute to chronic occupational back pain. Spine 2002;27:92–8.

[70] Bahr R, Andersen SO, Loken S, et al. Low back pain among endurance athletes with and without specific back loading—a cross-sectional survey of cross country skiers, rowers, orienteerers, and nonathletic controls. Spine 2004;29:449–54.

[71] Davis KG, Heaney CA. The relationship between psychosocial work characteristics and low back pain: underlying methodological issues. Clin Biomech 2000;15:389–406.

[72] Bigos SJ, Battie MC, Spengler DM, et al. A prospective study of work perceptions and psychosocial factors affecting the report of back injury. Spine 1991;16:1–6.

[73] Linton SJ, Kamwendo K. Risk factors in the psychosocial work environment for neck and shoulder pain in secretaries. J Occup Med 1989;31:609–13.

[74] Leino P, Magni G. Depressive and distress symptoms as predictors of low back pain, neck-shoulder pain, and other musculoskeletal morbidity: a 10-year follow-up of metal industry employees. Pain 1993;53:89–94.

[75] Von Korff M, Simon G. The relationship between pain and depression. Br J Psychiatry Suppl 1996;(30):101–8.

[76] Adams MA, Mannion AF, Dolan P. Personal risk factors for first-time low back pain. Spine 1999;24:2497–505.

[77] Linton SJ. A review of psychological risk factors in back and neck pain. Spine 2000;25: 1148–56.

[78] Currie SR, Wang JL. Chronic back pain and major depression in the general Canadian population. Pain 2004;107:54–60.

[79] Gatchel JR. Psychological disorders and chronic pain: cause-and-effect relationships. In: Gatchel RJ, Turk DC, editors. Psychological approaches to pain management: a practitioner's handbook. New York: Guilford; 1996. p. 3–52.

[80] Reichborn-Kjennerud T, Stoltenberg C, Tams K, et al. Rack-neck pain and symptoms of anxiety and depression: a population-based twin study. Psychol Med 2002;32:1009–20.

[81] Carroll LJ, Cassidy JD, Cote P. Depression as a risk factor for onset of an episode of troublesome neck and low back pain. Pain 2004;107:134–9.
[82] Taskaynatan MA, Izci Y, Ozgul A, et al. Clinical significance of congenital lumbosacral malformations in young male population with prolonged low back pain. Spine 2005;30:E210–3.
[83] Avimadje M, Goupille P, Jeannou J, et al. Can an anomalous lumbo-sacral or lumbo-iliac articulation cause low back pain? A retrospective study of 12 cases. Rev Rhum Engl Ed 1999;66:35–9.
[84] Jonsson B, Stromqvist B, Egund N. Anomalous lumbosacral articulations and low-back pain: evaluation and treatment. Spine 1989;14:831–4.
[85] Brault J, Smith J, Currier B. Partial lumbosacral transitional vertebra resection for contralateral facetogenic pain. Spine 2001;26:226–9.
[86] Luoma K, Vehmas T, Rajninko R, et al. Lumbosacral transitional vertebra. Relation to disc degeneration and low back pain. Spine 2004;29:200–5.
[87] Schwartzer AC, Aprill CN, Derby R, et al. The prevalence and clinical features of internal disc disruption in patients with chronic low back pain. Spine 1995;20:1878–83.
[88] Boden SD, Davis DO, Dina TS, et al. Abnormal magnetic-resonance scans of the lumbar spine in asymptomatic subjects: a prospective investigation. J Bone Joint Surg Am 1990;72:403–8.
[89] Jensen MC, Brant-Zawadzki MN, Obuchowski N, et al. Magnetic resonance imaging of the lumbar spine in people without back pain. N Engl J Med 1994;331:69–73.
[90] Van Tulder MW, Assendelft WJ, Koes BW, et al. Spinal radiographic findings and nonspecific low back pain. A systemic review of observational studies. Spine 1997;22:427–34.
[91] Savage RA, Whitehouse GH, Roberts N. The relationship between the magnetic resonance imaging appearance of the lumbar spine and low back pain, age, and occupation in males. Eur Spine J 1997;6:106–14.
[92] Peterson C, Bolton J, Wood AR, et al. A cross-sectional study correlating degeneration of the cervical spine with disability and pain in United Kingdom patients. Spine 2003;28:129–33.

ELSEVIER
SAUNDERS

NEUROLOGIC
CLINICS

Neurol Clin 25 (2007) 373–385

Cervical Radiculopathy

David W. Polston, MD

Department of Neurology, Cleveland Clinic, 9500 Euclid Avenue,
Cleveland, OH 44195, USA

Neck pain commonly is derived from a variety of nonspecific musculo-skeletal causes, including direct trauma, progressive structural changes with or without associated systemic disease (eg, rheumatoid arthritis), chronic stress or strain injury, and degenerative conditions [1,2]. Cervical radiculopathy is a distinct consideration in the evaluation of any patients who have neck pain and may be defined simply as an abnormality of a nerve root, which originates in the cervical spine. James Parkinson (1755–1824) is credited with the first clinical description of this disorder, in 1817, but he attributed it to "a rheumatic affectation of the deltoid muscle" and the clinical scenario subsequently has been well described in large patient series for more than 50 years [3].

Incidence rates for cervical radiculopathy from a population-based study in Rochester, Minnesota, indicate an overall rate of 83.2 per 100,000, with a higher incidence in men than women (107.3 per 100,00 versus 63.4 per 100,000, respectively) and peak incidence in the sixth decade of life in both genders [3]. Compared with the reported annual incidence of neck pain (14.6%) in a Canadian-based cohort, cervical radiculopathy is less common, but a systematic approach to its evaluation when encountered is no less important [4]. This article addresses those considerations that are somewhat unique to cervical radiculopathy in the assessment of patients who have neck pain.

Brief anatomic review

Eight pairs of cervical nerve roots are formed directly from multiple tiny rootlets that originate directly from the spinal cord. These tiny rootlets coalesce immediately within the intraspinal canal and form the dorsal (sensory) and the ventral (motor) roots. These join together just before passing through the intervertebral foramen and form the spinal nerve

E-mail address: polstod@ccf.org

0733-8619/07/$ - see front matter © 2007 Elsevier Inc. All rights reserved.
doi:10.1016/j.ncl.2007.01.012

neurologic.theclinics.com

root. On exiting the foramen, the nerve root splits into the small posterior ramus and the larger anterior ramus (Fig. 1). In contrast to the roots, there are only seven cervical vertebrae, so cervical roots 1–7 exit via the foramen above the corresponding vertebra whereas the eighth root exits below the seventh cervical vertebra and above the first thoracic vertebra. An abnormality at the C6-7 neuroforamen, therefore, causes a lesion of the C7 root.

In general, it is as the cervical nerve roots enter the neuroforamina that they are most susceptible to injury. The neuroforamen are bordered anteromedially by the uncovertebral joint, posterolaterally by the facet joint, superiorly by the pedicle of the vertebral body immediately above, and inferiorly by the pedicle of vertebral body immediately below. The medial section of the foramen is derived from the intervertebral disks and the vertebral endplates. The roots originate in close proximity to the level at which they exit the intraspinal canal. Consequently, the cervical roots generally pass through the canal in a somewhat more horizontal fashion than the lumbar roots. This arrangement causes the neuroforamen to originate more medially and the cervical root and the cervical spinal cord to be in close proximity, thereby susceptible to abnormalities of these medial structures (eg, osteophytes or disk herniations) [5,6].

Clinical evaluation

The hallmark clinical manifestations of cervical radiculopathies are pain, sensory loss, and motor weakness in the distribution of the affected nerve

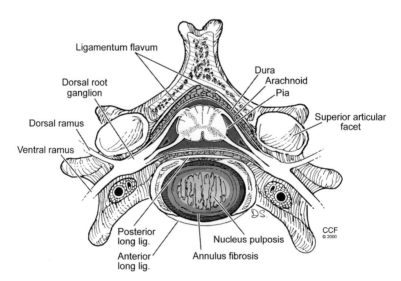

Fig. 1. Section of the cervical spine. (*From* Levin KH. Electrodiagnostic approach to the patient with suspected radiculopathy. Neurol Clin 2002;20:398. *Courtesy of* Cleveland Clinic Foundation, Cleveland, OH.)

root [7]. Antecedent events and putative risk factors, such as physical exertion or heavy lifting, previous cervical or lumbar radiculopathy, smoking, and trauma, are reported. Patients also frequently develop radiculopathy, however, with no apparent causative or predisposing factors identified [3,8,9]. Classically, patients present with some degree of discomfort or pain that may have developed in an acute to subacute manner. The timing of onset may vary according to the cause and clinically may be helpful in predicting the underlying pathology. Disk herniations may develop suddenly, whereas root lesions related to spondylosis may develop more slowly. The description of the pain itself varies considerably and may be multifaceted, with aching, lancinating, or burning qualities.

The distribution of the discomfort and physical findings may vary depending on the nerve root involved (Table 1). Historical studies correlating radiographic, clinical, and surgical data indicate that C7 root lesions are the most common. A 1957 analysis of 100 cervical radiculopathies found the C7 nerve root involved in 69% of cases. The C6 (19%), C8 (10%), and C5 (2%) were involved much less frequently [10]. A population-based analysis of cervical radiculopathies in Olmsted County, Minnesota, suggested comparable results (Table 2). Lesions of the upper cervical roots (C2, C3, and C4) are uncommon and generally give rise to no motor deficit.

In addition to the routine neurologic assessment of strength, tone, muscle bulk, and reflexes, several provocative tests are described. These tests

Table 1
Symptoms and signs associated with cervical radiculopathy

Root	Pain distribution	Dermatomal sensory distribution	Motor deficit	Reflex abnormality
C4	Upper neck	"Cape distribution" Shoulder/upper arm	Usually none	None
C5	Neck, scapula, shoulder and anterior arm	Lateral aspect of arm	Shoulder abduction Forearm flexion	Biceps Brachioradialis
C6	Neck scapula, shoulder, lateral arm and forearm into thumb and 2nd digit	Lateral aspect of the forearm, hand, thumb and 2nd digit	Shoulder Abduction Forearm flexion Forearm pronation	Biceps Brachioradialis
C7	Neck, shoulder, lateral arm, medial scapula and extensor surface of the forearm	Dorsal lateral forearm and hand and 3rd digit	Elbow extension Wrist extension	Triceps
C8	Neck, medial scapula, medial aspect of the arm, forearm and into the 4th and 5th digits	Medial forearm, hand and to the 4th and 5th digits	Finger abduction Finger adduction Finger flexion	Finger flexors

Adapted from Levin KH, Covington, ED, Deveraux MW, et al. Neck and back pain. Continuum 2001;7:15; with permission.

Table 2
Frequency comparison for surgically confirmed cervical radiculopathy

	Yoss et al	Radhakrishnan et al
	n = 100	n = 561
C5	2%	6.6%
C6	19%	17.6%
C7	69%	46.3%
C8	10%	6.2%
C5, C6	N/A	10.3%
C6, C7	N/A	8.4%

Abbreviation: N/A, lesions not localized in this manner.

Data from Yoss RE, Corbin KB, Maccarty CS, et al. Significance of symptoms and signs in localization of involved root in cervical disk protrusion. Neurology 1957;7:673–83; and Radhakrishnan K, Litchy WJ, O'Fallon WM, et al. Epidemiology of cervical radiculopathy. A population-based study from Rochester, Minnesota, 1976 through 1990. Brain 1994;117: 325–35.

are designed to mechanically induce or alleviate patient symptoms that are the result of anatomic changes in the spine. Spurling's maneuver may be the one known most widely [11]. It is performed by an examiner slightly rotating and laterally bending the head and then applying approximately 7 kg of force to the head. This test is considered positive if it provokes symptoms. Other maneuvers also are used, such as Valsalva's maneuver and neck distraction. The usefulness of all of these tests, however, remains unproved [12].

Radiculopathy may coexist with cervical myelopathy, particularly in the setting of cervical spondylosis, and should be considered in the evolution of any patients who have neck pain. Direct questioning, therefore, for symptoms suggestive of myelopathy and close inspection for physical signs of myelopathy should be done routinely (Box 1). Additionally, ominous or potentially life-threatening conditions (eg, abcess or cancer metastases) may cause cervical radiculopathy, so red flags (such as fever, chills, history of cancer, intravenous drug abuse, and so forth) should suggest to an examiner that more urgent attention may be necessary.

Etiologic considerations

Compressive radiculopathies are the most common type of cervical root lesion encountered. Given their proximity to the mobile structural components of the spine, cervical nerve roots are susceptible to a variety of injuries and mechanical distortions. Causes of compressive cervical radiculopathy vary according to the age of the population. Radiculopathies seen in the younger population most often are related to disk herniation resulting in direct pressure on an exiting nerve, whereas those in older patients most

---

Box 1. Clinical features suggestive of myelopathy

Symptoms
Clumsiness of the upper or lower limbs
Generalized sensory disturbances
Stiffness of the upper or lower limbs
Urinary urgency
Bladder or bowel incontinence
Lhermitte's sign
Frequent falls

Examination findings
Hyperreflexia
Hoffmann's sign
Increased tone or spasticity
Extensor plantar responses (Babinski's signs)
Gait abnormalities

---

often are related to foraminal narrowing resulting from the formation of osteophytes (spondylosis) [6]. Overall, spondylosis accounts for approximately 70% and disk herniation accounts for approximately 20% of all cervical radiculopathies [3]. Focal masses, such as tumors or infectious processes, also may cause compressive lesions but less frequently.

Disk herniations

The herniation of an intervertebral disk most often is related to the degenerative processes of aging but may occur after trauma. Degeneration of the disk is a process associated with progressive loss of the proteoglycan matrix within the disk. This leads to loss of the elasticity and hydration of the nucleus pulposus (the center portion of the disk). Additionally, the anulus fibrosis (the outer portion of the disk) undergoes degeneration, resulting in cracks or fissures in its lamellated structure. These processes and the mechanical loading forces applied over time may predispose adults to disk herniation [13].

Disk herniations may be classified according to the anatomic locations relative to the vertebra: central, paracentral, lateral, and far lateral. Central herniations may give rise to compression of the cervical cord, whereas paracentral herniations may give rise to hemicord compression (Brown-Séquard syndrome). Far lateral and lateral disk herniations may result in compression of the exiting nerve root (and in some cases the dorsal root ganglion), giving rise to weakness in the myotomal distribution of the affected nerves [14,15].

Cervical spondylosis

The naturally occurring degenerative changes within the spine often are asymptomatic. The alteration of the biochemical composition of the intervertebral disk may lead to redistribution of the axial load supported by the cervical spine and loss of the separation of the vertebral bodies [13]. These factors plus the development of osteophytes may culminate in compression of the neural structures, leading to pain and functional loss. The non-neural structures likely also are pain generators and give rise to mechanical or nonradicular neck pain that results from innervation of some of these structures by the sinuvertebral (recurrent meningeal) nerves, which are derived from rami communicantes of the ventral rami [7].

Because nerve root compression and severe degenerative spine disease may be asymptomatic, all of the factors that contribute to the generation of pain are not yet understood. Recent studies suggest, however, that local biochemical changes related to inflammatory mediators, such as nitric oxide, interleukins, and prostaglandins, play a role [12,16–18].

Extraspinal compressive radiculopathies

Lesions external to the cervical spinal canal giving rise to injury of the anterior primary rami are uncommon and may be difficult to diagnose. Two disorders (neurogenic thoracic outlet syndrome and postmedian sternotomy brachial plexopathy) historically have been classified as lesions of the brachial plexus but likely are related to injury of the cervical anterior primary ramus after emerging from the foramen [19,20].

Neurogenic thoracic outlet syndrome clinically results in wasting of the hand, with varying degrees of sensory disturbance and pain. It is caused by a congenital anomaly that generally consists of a tight tissue band extending from the first thoracic rib to an elongated C7 transverse process or, alternatively, a rudimentary cervical rib. This band results in stretching of fibers originating from the T1 and to a much lesser extent the C8 anterior primary rami (Fig. 2A, B). Because this is a postganglionic lesion, clinically and electrophysiologically, the sensory fibers that originate from these rami are involved [21].

Postmedian sternotomy lesions may occur after cardiac surgery. The clinical appearance is that of a C8 radiculopathy. Although the causal mechanism is not well understood, it likely is related to an occult fracture of the first thoracic rib, which lies immediately inferior to the C8 ventral ramus (see Fig. 2C) [22]. These lesions generally manifest postoperatively as weakness and sensory disturbances in the distribution of the C8 nerve root. As a result of several factors, these lesions may not come to clinical attention until long after the procedure and because of the distribution of the symptoms, postmedian sternotomy lesions may be mistaken for an ulnar neuropathy (at the elbow). Consequently, clinicians should keep these lesions in mind when evaluating cardiac patients in the postoperative period [22].

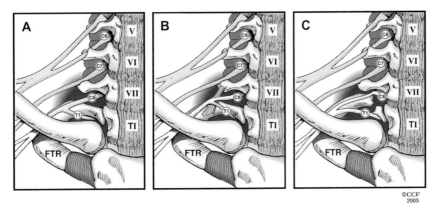

©CCF
2003

Fig. 2. Pathogenesis of neurogenic thoracic outlet syndrome and postmedian sternotomy lesions. (*A*) Normal anatomy. (*B*) The C8 and T1 nerve roots in relation to the congenital ligamentous band in neurogenic thoracic outlet syndrome. (*C*) The injured C8 nerve root in relation to the fractured first thoracic rib in postmedian sternotomy lesions. Roman numerals, level of vertebral body. Circled numbers, cervical root. FTR, first thoracic rib. (*From* Wilbourn AJ. Brachial plexus lesions. In: Dyck PJ, Thomas PK, editors. Peripheral Neuropathy. 4th ed. Philadelphia: Elsevier Saunders; 2005. p. 1360. *Courtesy of* Cleveland Clinic Foundation, Cleveland, OH.)

Noncompressive radiculopathies

Cervical root lesions not related to compression are important to consider, particularly in patients who have predisposing or chronic illnesses. Potential causes of noncompressive radiculopathies are outlined (Box 2). These lesions may be related to inflammatory changes within the nerve,

---

Box 2. Potential causes of non-compressive radiculopathies

Infection
Herpes zoster
HIV
Cytomegalovirus
Borrelia burgdorferi (Lyme disease)

Inflammatory
Vasculitis
Sarcoidosis
Diabetic radiculoplexus neuropathy (diabetic radiculopathy/
    Bruns-Garland syndrome)
Neuralgic amyotrophy (Parsonage-Turner syndrome)

Neoplastic
Carcinomatous meningitis
Lymphoma

the associated connective tissue, and supporting blood vessels or to direct infiltration by the offending agent.

With these lesions, a medical history or physical examination suggestive of predisposing conditions (eg, a history of diabetes mellitus or skin lesions suggestive of herpes zoster) usually, but not always, is noted. Additionally, these conditions often affect the nervous system in a more generalized manner or cause systemic abnormalities. Therefore, signs of a more generalized neurologic or systemic disease raise the possibility of these conditions. Occasionally, these possibilities may not be considered until alternative diagnoses (eg, spondylosis) are excluded by imaging. Nevertheless, awareness of these possibilities is important, as disease specific treatment is available for many of these disorders.

Diagnostic considerations

In general, laboratory testing has little or no value. If a systemic or infectious disorder is considered, limited testing to evaluate the specific possibilities in question is appropriate.

Imaging

It is suggested that given the prevalence of cervical spondylosis (>90% by the seventh decade), imaging studies are used too frequently in patients who have isolated neck pain [23,24]. In cases of neurologic deficits or abnormalities suggestive of radiculopathy, however, imaging potentially can be helpful in determining the cause. In some cases, a definite cause cannot be determined, but assessing the level of abnormality may assist with surgical planning, if indicated.

Conventional radiographs often are the first diagnostic tests requested in the evaluation of neck pain. These may be helpful in assessing for bony abnormalities, such as fractures or instability, particularly in cases associated with trauma. They are less useful in the evaluation of radiculopathy, however, because of their low sensitivity and specificity in determining the presence or absence of root lesions [25,26].

MRI is the modality of choice in the assessment of cervical radiculopathy [27]. The inherent contrast between tissues and the various sequencing protocols available allows for differentiation between various types of soft tissue abnormalities and determination of the cervical level involved. CT myelography may have some advantages in distinguishing soft tissue from bony pathology but is more invasive [28].

Electrodiagnostic studies

Electrodiagnostic studies (nerve conduction studies and needle electromyography) commonly are used in the evaluation of neck pain, particularly if cervical radiculopathy is considered likely. The usefulness of these studies in the assessment of radiculopathy may vary considerably, depending on the age of the lesion in question, segmental level of the lesion, and diagnostic approach. In recent years, MRI has supplanted electrodiagnostic studies as the preferred initial diagnostic test. In the presence of clinical evidence of weakness, however, electrodiagnostic studies may provide valuable information regarding the presence of axon loss and the chronicity, activity, and severity of the denervation [29,30]. Electrodiagnostic studies also differentiate radiculopathy from mimics, such as rotator cuff disease and entrapment neuropathies.

Treatment

The initial approach to the management of cervical radiculopathy is nearly identical to that of patients who have nonspecific neck or back pain. There currently are no randomized, placebo-controlled trials available comparing the standard nonsurgical treatments [31]. Consequently, care plans are developed primarily based on cumulative experience, the services available locally, and the specific preferences of patients. Treatment plans should be designed to alleviate pain, improve function, and prevent recurrences [32]. They must be tailored to patients, considering their specific symptoms or functional limitations.

Activity modification

Patients should be educated regarding the cause of their pain and basic activity modifications that may improve it. Simple activity modifications to keep the head and neck in a midline and unflexed position may minimize stress on the cervical spine and thereby relieve pain and reduce root compression. The effectiveness of these measures, however, is unproved [9]. Cervical orthoses (or collars) sometimes are recommended for this same purpose but should be used for less than 1 to 2 weeks, given the counterproductive effects of prolonged immobilization [12,33].

In the past, complete bed rest had been advocated in the treatment of lumbar radiculopathy, but more recently, care providers encourage a rapid return to activity [34]. A similar approach in the acute period of cervical radiculopathy may be advisable but in the most severe cases, a reduced activity level may be necessary [32].

Medications

Nonsteroidal anti-inflammatory drugs (NSAIDs) and acetaminophen generally are the medications recommended most frequently early in the course of radiculopathy. These agents are believed to reduce the inflammatory response that may underlie the pain in these conditions [18]. NSAIDs have the potential for renal and gastric toxicity. This is important to remember in high-risk patients (eg, the elderly or those treated with anticoagulants); coadministration of gastric protective agents, such as proton pump inhibitors, may be needed.

Although not proved effective, steroids often are used in the acute period of radiculopathy as a pulse treatment. Many regimens are described but generally an initial oral dose (approximately 1 mg/kg of ideal body weight daily) is followed by a tapered reduction over 2 to 3 weeks. Steroids are associated with side effects, such as impaired glycemic control, worsening hypertension, and gastritis, but short-term use generally results in few long-term complications [9].

Epidural injections

Few randomized clinical trials are available and those available generally do not provide assessment with validated outcome measures [12]. Multiple studies suggest that these injections may be beneficial, with decreased pain reported in up to 60% of patients [35]. These procedures may have significant complications, although the current use of fluoroscopic guidance may minimize the risk [36,37]. This treatment modality is covered in detail in the article by Levin, elsewhere in this issue.

Traction

Traction has been described for centuries in the treatment of a variety of spine disorders. It generally involves the use of a system of pulleys or pneumatic devices to provide the force to allow separation of the cervical vertebra and relieve pressure [38–40]. In 1995, a systematic review of the literature regarding cervical traction identified only three randomized studies. Based on available data, no valid judgment regarding this treatment modality could be drawn [41]. Many devices are available, however, and many care providers consider this modality a standard of care [32].

Surgery

Several procedures are available for the treatment of cervical radiculopathy. The approach used varies according to the location of the lesion, patient age, the overall anatomic structure of the spine (appropriate lordosis versus kyphosis), and other factors, including surgeon preference [42]. Surgery may be considered for patients who have medically refractory pain or signs of myelopathy. Progressive neurologic deficit resulting from a root lesion is documented to improve with conservative management, so this alone may not be an adequate indication for surgery [43].

There are limited data from randomized controlled trials available to address the benefits of surgery versus conservative management. A recently updated report from the *Cochrane Database of Systemic Reviews* in 2001 found only two acceptable studies that address this issue. This review suggests that in one study of 81 patients, neurologic outcome in regard to pain, weakness, and sensory deficits improved in the short term (3 months), but at 1 year no differences between the surgical and nonsurgical groups could be seen. Consequently, it is unclear if the surgical risk is outweighed by any long-term benefit [44].

Recommendations

In general, the prognosis of radiculopathy is considered favorable, with most patients improving substantially over time [6,12,32]. Epidemiologic data suggest that up to 90% of patients improve with conservative treatment alone [3,45]. The natural history of this disorder remains somewhat unclear, however, given the lack of standardized criteria for the diagnosis of radiculopathy and limited long-term follow-up in many studies. Furthermore, the lack of comparative randomized, controlled trials assessing conservative and operative management complicates decision making and hinders the development of standardized evidence-based treatment guidelines. Despite these limitations, a systematic approach to the evaluation and treatment of cervical radiculopathy is necessary.

Initial evaluation always must include a careful history and thorough examination, for it is based on these that all further clinical decisions are made. In general, conservative treatment, combining the use of NSAIDs and physical therapy, is acceptable for the first 4 to 6 weeks in the absence of red flags or myelopathy [31]. If pain remains persistent at this point, then cervical MRI is appropriate. Even in the setting of severe disk herniations, regression generally occurs, and in cases of cervical spondylosis, the pain may remit spontaneously, so structural abnormalities alone are not an indication for surgical treatment [46]. Progressive neurologic deficits and intractable pain are indications for surgical consultation [47]. In the absence of these factors, however, conservative management likely yields long-term results similar to those of surgical patients.

Summary

Cervical radiculopathy is a condition encountered commonly, which, despite the use of ancillary imaging and electrodiagnostic tests, remains a clinical diagnosis for which there are no widely accepted or standardized criteria. Consequently, clinicians must be familiar with its clinical features and consider it in the differential diagnosis of any person who has the complaint of neck pain. Clinical improvement is the rule but diligence in assessment is necessary so that appropriate measures may be taken to alleviate pain and prevent potential long-term morbidity.

References

[1] Narayan P, Haid RW. Treatment of degenerative cervical disc disease. Neurol Clin 2001;19: 217–29.

[2] Jackson R. Cervical trauma: not just another pain in the neck. Geriatrics 1982;37:123–6.

[3] Radhakrishnan K, Litchy WJ, O'Fallon WM, et al. Epidemiology of cervical radiculopathy. A population-based study from Rochester, Minnesota, 1976 through 1990. Brain 1994;117: 325–35.

[4] Cote P, Cassidy JD, Carroll LJ, et al. The annual incidence and course of neck pain in the general population: a population-based cohort study. Pain 2004;112:267–73.

[5] Ahlgren BD, Garfin SR. Cervical radiculopathy. Orthop Clin North Am 1996;27:253–63.

[6] Malanga GA. The diagnosis and treatment of cervical radiculopathy. Med Sci Sports Exerc 1997;29:S236–45.

[7] Bogduk N. The anatomy and pathophysiology of neck pain. Phys Med Rehabil Clin N Am 2003;14:455–72.

[8] Kelsey JL, Githens PB, O'Conner T, et al. Acute prolapsed lumbar intervertebral disc. An epidemiologic study with special reference to driving automobiles and cigarette smoking. Spine 1984;9:608–13.

[9] Ellenberg MR, Honet JC, Treanor WJ. Cervical radiculopathy [comment]. Arch Phys Med Rehabil 1994;75:342–52.

[10] Yoss RE, Corbin KB, Maccarty CS, et al. Significance of symptoms and signs in localization of involved root in cervical disk protrusion. Neurology 1957;7:673–83.

[11] Spurling RG, Scoville WB. Lateral rupture of the cervical intervertebral discs: a common cause of shoulder and arm pain. Surg Gynecol Obstet 1944;78:350–8.

[12] Wainner RS, Gill H. Diagnosis and nonoperative management of cervical radiculopathy. J Orthop Sports Phys Ther 2000;30:728–44.

[13] Roh JS, Teng AL, Yoo JU, et al. Degenerative disorders of the lumbar and cervical spine. Orthop Clin North Am 2005;36:255–62.

[14] Levin KH, Covington ED, Devereaux MW, et al. Neck and back pain. Continuum, Philadelphia: Lippincott Williams and Wilkins; 2001;7(1):1–205.

[15] Epstein NE. Foraminal and far lateral lumbar disc herniations: surgical alternatives and outcome measures. Spinal Cord 2002;40:491–500.

[16] Kang JD, Georgescu HI, McIntyre-Larkin L, et al. Herniated lumbar intervertebral discs spontaneously produce matrix metalloproteinases, nitric oxide, interleukin-6, and prostaglandin E2. Spine 1996;21:271–7.

[17] Kang JD, Stefanovic-Racic M, McIntyre LA, et al. Toward a biochemical understanding of human intervertebral disc degeneration and herniation contributions of nitric oxide, interleukins, prostaglandin E2, and matrix metalloproteinases. Spine 1997;22: 1065–73.

[18] Rao R. Neck pain, cervical radiculopathy, and cervical myelopathy: pathophysiology, natural history, and clinical evaluation. Instr Course Lect 2003;52:479–88.

[19] Levin KH, Wilbourn AJ, Maggiano HJ. Cervical rib and median sternotomy-related brachial plexopathies: a reassessment. Neurology 1998;50:1407–13.

[20] Levin KH. Electrodiagnostic approach to the patient with suspected radiculopathy. Neurol Clin 2002;20:397–421.

[21] Wilbourn AJ. Thoracic outlet syndromes. Neurol Clin 1999;17:477–97.

[22] Wilbourn AJ. Brachial plexus lesions. In: Dyck PJ, Thomas PK, editors. Peripheral Neuropathy. 4th edition. Philadelphia: Elsevier Saunders; 2005. p. 1339–73.

[23] Ruggieri PM. Cervical radiculopathy. Neuroimaging Clin N Am 1995;5:349–66.

[24] Irvine DH, Foster JB, Newell DJ, et al. Prevalence of cervical spondylosis. Lancet 1965;14: 1089–92.

[25] Mink JH, Gordon RE, Deutsch AL. The cervical spine: radiologist's perspective. Phys Med Rehabil Clin N Am 2003;14:493–548.

[26] Friedenberg ZB, Edeiken J, Spencer HN, et al. Degenerative changes in the cervical spine. J Bone Joint Surg Am 1959;41:61–70.

[27] Nakstad PH, Hald JK, Bakke SJ, et al. MRI in cervical disk herniation. Neuroradiology 1989;31:382–5.

[28] Modic MT, Masaryk TJ, Mulopulos GP, et al. Cervical radiculopathy: prospective evaluation with surface coil MR imaging, CT with metrizamide, and metrizamide myelography. Radiology 1986;161:753–9.

[29] Wilbourn AJ, Aminoff MJ. AAEM minimonograph 32: the electrodiagnostic examination in patients with radiculopathies. american association of electrodiagnostic medicine. Muscle Nerve 1998;21:1612–31.

[30] Fisher MA. Electrophysiology of radiculopathies. Clin Neurophysiol 2002;113:317–35.

[31] Carette S, Fehlings MG. Clinical practice. Cervical radiculopathy. N Engl J Med 2005;353: 392–9.

[32] Wolff MW, Levine LA. Cervical radiculopathies: conservative approaches to management. Phys Med Rehabil Clin N Am 2002;13:589–608.

[33] Akeson WH. An experimental study of joint stiffness. J Bone Joint Surg Am 1961;43: 1022–34.

[34] Deyo RA, Weinstein JN. Low back pain [comment]. N Engl J Med 2001;344:363–70.

[35] Slipman CW, Lipetz JS, Jackson HB, et al. Therapeutic selective nerve root block in the non-surgical treatment of atraumatic cervical spondylotic radicular pain: a retrospective analysis with independent clinical review. Arch Phys Med Rehabil 2000;81:741–6.

[36] Waldman SD. Complications of cervical epidural nerve blocks with steroids: a prospective study of 790 consecutive blocks. Reg Anesth 1989;14:149–51.

[37] Cicala RS, Thoni K, Angel JJ. Long-term results of cervical epidural steroid injections. Clin J Pain 1989;5:143–5.

[38] Colachis SC Jr, Strohm BR. A study of tractive forces and angle of pull on vertebral inter-spaces in the cervical spine. Arch Phys Med Rehabil 1965;46:820–30.

[39] Colachis SC Jr, Strohm BR. Effect of duration of intermittent cervical traction on vertebral separation. Arch Phys Med Rehabil 1966;47:353–9.

[40] Colachis SC Jr, Strohm BR. Cervical traction: relationship of traction time to varied tractive force with constant angle of pull. Arch Phys Med Rehabil 1965;46:815–9.

[41] van der Heijden GJ, Beurskens AJ, Koes BW, et al. The efficacy of traction for back and neck pain: a systematic, blinded review of randomized clinical trial methods. Phys Ther 1995;75: 93–104.

[42] Epstein N. Posterior approaches in the management of cervical spondylosis and ossification of the posterior longitudinal ligament. Surg Neurol 2002;58:194–207.

[43] Ellenberg MR, Ross ML, Honet JC, et al. Prospective evaluation of the course of disc her-niations in patients with proven radiculopathy. Arch Phys Med Rehabil 1993;74:3–8.

[44] Fouyas IP, Statham PF, Sandercock PA, et al. Surgery for cervical radiculomyelopathy. Cochrane Database Syst Rev 2001;CD001466.

[45] Sampath P, Bendebba M, Davis JD, et al. Outcome in patients with cervical radiculopathy. prospective, multicenter study with independent clinical review. Spine 1999;24:591–7.

[46] Bush K, Chaudhuri R, Hillier S, et al. The pathomorphologic changes that accompany the resolution of cervical radiculopathy. A prospective study with repeat magnetic resonance im-aging [comment]. Spine 1997;22:183–6.

[47] Bartleson JD. Spine disorder case studies. Neurol Clin 2006;24:309–30.

ELSEVIER
SAUNDERS

Neurol Clin 25 (2007) 387–405

NEUROLOGIC
CLINICS

Lumbosacral Radiculopathy

Andrew W. Tarulli, MD[a,b],
Elizabeth M. Raynor, MD[a,b],*

[a]Harvard Medical School, 25 Shattuck Street, Boston, MA 02115, USA
[b]Department of Neurology, Beth Israel Deaconess Medical Center,
330 Brookline Avenue, TCC 810, Boston, MA 02215, USA

Lumbosacral radiculopathy is one of the most common disorders evaluated by neurologists and is a leading referral diagnosis for the performance of electromyography. Degenerative spondyloarthropathies are the principal underlying cause of these syndromes and are increasingly common with age. The clinical presentation and initial management of lumbosacral radiculopathies of various etiologies are discussed.

Epidemiology

Although precise epidemiologic data are difficult to establish, the prevalence of lumbosacral radiculopathy is approximately 3% to 5%, distributed equally in men and women [1,2]. Men are most likely to develop symptoms in their 40s, whereas women are affected most commonly between ages 50 and 60 [1].

Anatomy

Detailed spinal anatomy is discussed elsewhere in this issue by Devereaux; however, clinically relevant points are reviewed. There are five moveable lumbar vertebrae, five fused sacral vertebrae, and four fused coccygeal vertebrae [3] with intervertebral disks sandwiched between each of the lumbar vertebrae and between the fifth lumbar vertebra and sacrum. The moveable vertebrae are connected by paired facet joints between the articular processes of the pedicles and by the anterior and posterior longitudinal ligaments. The intervertebral foramina are formed by notches in the articular processes

---

* Corresponding author. Department of Neurology, Beth Israel Deaconess Medical Center, 330 Brookline Avenue, TCC 810, Boston, MA 02215.
E-mail address: eraynor@bidmc.harvard.edu (E.M. Raynor).

0733-8619/07/$ - see front matter © 2007 Elsevier Inc. All rights reserved.
doi:10.1016/j.ncl.2007.01.008

of adjacent pedicles of two vertebrae; the disk is anterior and medial to the foramen.

In adults, the spinal cord terminates at the L1-2 intervertebral level as the conus medullaris. The nerve roots descend from this point through the spinal canal as the cauda equina and exit eventually through the neural foramina at their respective intervertebral levels. Eleven pairs (five lumbar, five sacral, and one coccygeal) of spinal nerves emerge from the spinal cord in the lumbosacral region. Ventral roots, containing primarily motor fibers, arise from rootlets, which extend from the ventral gray matter of the spinal cord. Dorsal rootlets, carrying sensory information, extend centrally from the dorsal root ganglia that lie outside the spinal cord, within the neural foramen. Just distal to the intervertebral foramen, the dorsal and ventral roots unite to form a mixed spinal nerve, which divides into dorsal and ventral primary rami. The dorsal rami supply the paraspinal muscles and skin overlying the paraspinal region, whereas the ventral rami give rise to the lumbosacral plexus and, eventually, the individual nerves supplying the lower limbs and sacral region. The muscles supplied by a single spinal segment constitute a myotome; the skin region supplied by a single spinal segment is a dermatome.

History and physical examination

Performance of a careful history and physical examination is the initial and integral step in the diagnosis and management of lumbosacral radiculopathy. Lesion localization depends on demonstration of a segmental myotomal or dermatomal distribution of abnormalities; a working knowledge of the relevant anatomy is essential. Sciatica, the classic presenting symptom of lumbosacral radiculopathy, is characterized by pain in the back radiating into the leg. Patients variably describe this pain as sharp, dull, aching, burning, or throbbing. Pain related to disk herniation is exacerbated by bending forward, sitting, coughing, or straining and relieved by lying down or sometimes walking [4]. Conversely, pain related to lumbar spinal stenosis characteristically is worsened by walking and improved by forward bending. Pain that is exacerbated by or fails to respond to the recumbent position is a distinctive feature of radiculopathy produced by inflammatory or neoplastic lesions and other nonmechanical causes of back pain. The distribution of pain radiation along a dermatome may be helpful in localizing the level of involvement; when present, the dermatomal distribution of paresthesias is more specific [4].

In the majority of cases, lumbosacral radiculopathy is caused by compression of nerve roots from pathology in the intervertebral disk or associated structures. The differential diagnosis of lesions producing lumbosacral radiculopathy, however, is broad and includes neoplastic, infectious, and inflammatory disorders (Box 1). Important risk factors for serious underlying disease that should be sought in the history include age greater than 50,

Box 1. Causes of lumbosacral radiculopathy

Degenerative
  Intervertebral disk herniation
  Degenerative lumbar spondylosis

Neoplastic
  Primary tumors
  Ependymoma
  Schwannoma
  Neurofibroma
  Lymphoma
  Lipoma
  Dermoid
  Epidermoid
  Hemangioblastoma
  Paraganglioma
  Ganglioneuroma
  Osteoma
  Plasmacytoma
Metastatic tumors
Leptomeningeal metastasis

Infectious
  Herpes zoster (HZ)
  Spinal epidural abscess (SEA)
  HIV/AIDS-related polyradiculopathy
  Lyme disease

Inflammatory/metabolic
  Diabetic amyotrophy
  Ankylosing spondylitis
  Paget's disease
  Arachnoiditis
  Sarcoidosis

Developmental
  Tethered cord syndrome
  Dural ectasia

Other
  Lumbar spinal cysts
  Hemorrhage

previous history of cancer, unexplained weight loss, and failure to improve after 1 month of conservative therapy [5].

Aside from assessment of potential serious disease, the history is geared toward establishing the involvement of nerve roots and their anatomic level. Similarly, the aim of the physical examination is to elucidate motor, sensory, or reflex abnormalities in a radicular distribution relevant to the suspected clinical level. Sciatic nerve tension signs may provide supporting evidence of L5-S1 radiculopathy; however, they may be present with lesions of the lumbosacral plexus, sciatic nerve, or hip joint and in mechanical lower back pain [6–8]. With the patient supine and one hand on the iliac crest of the affected side, an examiner passively elevates the heel slowly while keeping the knee straight; the angle at which pain or paresthesias are produced and the distribution are noted. Dorsiflexion of the foot may increase symptoms. The straight leg raise test is positive if symptoms are produced between 30° and 70° [6]. In a similar fashion, the femoral nerve stretch test produces tension on the L3, L4 nerve roots. With a patient lying on the asymptomatic side and the lower limb flexed at the hip and knee, the symptomatic knee is extended passively at the hip [9]. Pain radiating into the anterior thigh with this maneuver suggests L3 or L4 radiculopathy.

Clinical presentation of monoradiculopathies

L1 radiculopathy

Disk herniation at this level is rare; consequently, L1 radiculopathy is extremely uncommon. The typical presentation is one of pain, paresthesias, and sensory loss in the inguinal region, without significant weakness. Infrequently, subtle involvement of hip flexion is noted. Muscle stretch reflexes (MSRs) are normal. Differential diagnostic considerations include ilioinguinal and genitofemoral neuropathies. Physical examination may help distinguish between these conditions, but imaging of the lumbosacral spine or pelvis often is required (Table 1).

L2 radiculopathy

Also rarely caused by disk herniation, L2 radiculopathy produces pain, paresthesias, and sensory loss in the anterolateral thigh. Weakness of hip flexion may occur; MSRs are normal. Lateral femoral cutaneous neuropathy (meralgia paresthetica) may mimic L2 radiculopathy; the presence of hip flexor weakness suggests radiculopathy rather than meralgia. Femoral neuropathy and upper lumbar plexopathy may present similarly.

L3 radiculopathy

Although more common than with higher lumbar roots, disk herniation is an uncommon cause of L3 radiculopathy. Pain and paresthesias involve

Table 1
Neurologic examination findings in monoradiculopathies

Root level	Pain	Sensory loss (paresthesias)	Motor abnormalities or weakness	Muscle stretch reflex abnormalities
L1	Inguinal region	Inguinal region	None	None
L2	Groin, anterior thigh	Anterolateral thigh	Iliopsoas	None
L3	Anterior thigh to knee, anterior leg	Medial thigh and knee	Quadriceps, iliopsoas, hip adductors	Knee jerk
L4	Medial foreleg	Medial lower leg	Tibialis anterior, quadriceps, hip adductors	Knee jerk
L5	Lateral thigh and lower leg, dorsum foot	Lateral lower leg, dorsum foot, great toe	Toe extensors and flexors, ankle dorsiflexor, everter and inverter, hip abductors	Internal hamstrings
S1	Posterior thigh, calf, heel	Sole, lateral foot and ankle, lateral two toes	Gastrocnemius, hamstrings, gluteus maximus, toe flexors	Ankle jerk
S2-4	Medial buttocks	Medial buttocks, perineal, perianal region	None unless S1-2 involved	Bulbocavernosus, anal wink. Ankle jerk if S1 involved

the medial thigh and knee, with weakness of hip flexors, hip adductors, and knee extensors; the knee jerk may be depressed or absent. L3 radiculopathy may be confused with femoral neuropathy, obturator neuropathy, diabetic amyotrophy, or upper lumbar plexopathy. Combined weakness of hip adduction and hip flexion differentiates L3 radiculopathy from femoral and obturator mononeuropathies.

L4 radiculopathy

Unlike the higher lumbar levels, L4 radiculopathy is produced most commonly by disk herniation. Spinal stenosis frequently involves this nerve root in conjunction with roots at adjacent spinal levels. Sensory symptoms involve the medial lower leg in the distribution of the saphenous nerve. As with L3 radiculopathy, knee extension and hip adduction may be weak; additionally, foot dorsiflexion weakness uncommonly may be observed. When present, ankle dorsiflexion weakness generally is less prominent than in L5 radiculopathy. The knee jerk may be depressed or absent. Lumbosacral plexopathy is the main differential diagnostic consideration; saphenous neuropathy also is a possibility in pure sensory syndromes.

L5 radiculopathy

The most common cause of L5 radiculopathy is intervertebral disk herniation. Foot drop is the salient clinical feature, with associated sensory symptoms involving the anterolateral leg and dorsum of the foot. In addition to weakness of ankle dorsiflexion, L5 radiculopathy commonly produces weakness of toe extension and flexion, foot inversion and eversion, and hip abduction. Common peroneal neuropathy closely mimics and must be distinguished from L5 radiculopathy. Physical examination is helpful in localization as weakness of foot eversion (mediated by the L5/peroneal-innervated peroneus muscles) in conjunction with inversion (mediated by the L5/tibial-innervated tibialis posterior) places the lesion proximal to the peroneal nerve. Lumbosacral plexopathy and sciatic neuropathy are important differential diagnostic considerations. The involvement of hip abductors (gluteus medius and minimus) indicates a lesion proximal to the sciatic nerve but does not differentiate L5 radiculopathy from lumbosacral plexopathy. Although there is no classic MSR abnormality associated with L5 radiculopathy, an asymmetric internal hamstring reflex can support its presence.

S1 radiculopathy

S1 radiculopathy also is caused commonly by intervertebral disk herniation, with associated weakness of foot plantar flexion, knee flexion, and hip extension. Subtle weakness of foot plantar flexion may be demonstrated by having patients stand or walk on their toes. Sensory symptoms typically involve the lateral foot and sole. The ankle jerk is depressed or absent. Sciatic neuropathy and lower lumbosacral plexopathy may mimic S1 radiculopathy. Both of these conditions, however, also are expected to affect L5-innervated muscles.

Lumbosacral polyradiculopathy and cauda equina syndromes

Multiple, contiguous nerve roots may be involved by compressive lesions affecting several individual nerve roots, either in the vertebral canal or the neural foramina; less frequently, infiltrating or inflammatory processes spreading along the meninges produce similar clinical syndromes. Lesions involving the cauda equina should be considered when nerve roots at more than two neighboring levels are involved, developing acutely or gradually. Acute cauda equina syndrome most often is the result of compression of the lower lumbar and sacral nerve roots by a large, central disk herniation, usually at L4-5. Sacral nerve roots, which lie medially in the cauda equina, often are affected disproportionately, leading to sacral polyradiculopathy with prominent bowel and bladder dysfunction and characteristic saddle anesthesia. Lumbar nerve roots also may be involved, resulting in leg weakness that can progress to paraplegia, depending on the extent of nerve root compromise. A true neurologic emergency, prompt recognition of cauda equina syndrome is necessary to preserve sphincter function and ambulation.

A more insidious manifestation of cauda equina dysfunction results from central spinal stenosis, creating a clinical syndrome of intermittent neurogenic claudication (discussed in Chad's article, elsewhere in this issue). The neurologic and electrodiagnostic examinations in these cases may demonstrate patchy lumbosacral polyradiculopathy but often are normal.

Differential diagnosis

The majority of lesions causing lumbosacral radiculopathy are compressive in nature and result from disk herniation or spondylosis with entrapment of nerve roots. It is important, however, to recognize a variety of other lesions that may produce lumbosacral radiculopathy, including several neoplastic, infectious, and inflammatory disorders (see Box 1).

Degenerative spine disorders

Acute disk herniation

Intervertebral disk herniation is the most common cause of lumbosacral radiculopathy in patients under age 50 [7]. At birth, the boundary between the gelatinous nucleus pulposus and the tough, surrounding annulus pulposus is distinct; with increasing age, the concentration of collagen in the disk increases and water content decreases [7]. As a result, clefts and fissures form in the disk and disruption of annular fibers occurs, predisposing to herniation of the nucleus pulposus [7]. Acute disk herniation produces symptoms by direct compression of the nerve roots and by inflammatory and ischemic mechanisms involving the roots and dorsal root ganglia [8]. The intervertebral disks affected most frequently are L4-5 and L5-S1, leading to L5 or S1 radiculopathies. Pain characteristically is of abrupt onset and intense, often precipitated by bending over or lifting. Patients may report of sciatica without back pain. Aggravation of pain with movement, particularly forward or lateral bending, or with Valsalva's maneuver is typical; usually, pain is relieved with recumbency. In addition to pain, patients frequently report paresthesias in the involved dermatome. Cauda equina syndrome with prominent bowel and bladder involvement may be the presenting syndrome with large, central disk herniations.

Often, a diagnosis of acute disk herniation may be made on clinical grounds. MRI and EMG, however, may be helpful in establishing the diagnosis and distinguishing disk pathology from other causes of lumbosacral radiculopathy. Although MRI is sensitive, lumbar disk herniations are identified in 30% to 40% of asymptomatic subjects by MRI and in an equivalent number at autopsy with CT and with myelography [7]. Initial treatment is aimed at pain control and identification of patients who require urgent surgical consideration to prevent permanent neurologic deficits.

Degenerative spondylosis

After age 50, acute disk herniation is a less common cause of lumbosacral radiculopathy, and chronic lesions related to degenerative spinal arthropathy predominate [7]. With advancing age, intervertebral disks desiccate and flatten, transferring increasing axial load to the facet joints, with resultant facet joint hypertrophy, osteophyte formation, and thickening of the ligamentum flavum [7,10]. These changes contribute to narrowing of the central spinal canal, lateral recesses, and neural foramina. L4-5 and L5-S1 levels in particular are affected [7]. Chronic radiculopathy may result from entrapment of nerve roots in the lateral recess, intervertebral foramen, or central canal, involving single or multiple nerve roots. Clinical syndromes of radicular pain involving buttock, hip, or posterior thigh and intermittent neurogenic claudication are more common than back pain [10].

MRI frequently is performed in the evaluation of these lesions, although bony pathology is demonstrated better by CT. Because degenerative changes are commonplace in older patients, electrodiagnostic studies frequently are necessary to establish the relevance of neuroimaging abnormalities. Initial management involves pain control with analgesic medications and physical therapy to strengthen supporting musculature and improve postural mechanics. Surgical decompression is considered for progressive or recalcitrant symptoms or worsening neurologic deficits.

Neoplasms

Radiculopathy may result from tumor in various locations within the spinal canal; usually, these lesions are extramedullary. Primary tumors tend to be intradural, whereas metastatic lesions are extradural. Furthermore, primary lesions tend to be solitary (neurofibromatosis type 1 being a notable exception), whereas metastatic lesions frequently are multiple.

Primary tumors

Primary nerve root tumors are a rare cause of lumbosacral radiculopathy. Most primary spinal tumors are benign and slow growing, and their clinical manifestations may be difficult to distinguish from more common causes of radiculopathy, such as disk herniation [11]. Both are characterized by back pain; however, the nature of pain related to tumor is distinctive, as it becomes increasingly severe over time and is worse when lying down, often interfering with sleep. Primary tumors producing lumbosacral radiculopathy most frequently are neurofibromas (often associated with neurofibromatosis type 1) and ependymomas; less common are schwannomas (in neurofibromatosis type 2), meningiomas, lipomas and dermoids, and lipomas [11]. Ependymomas and neurofibromas typically affect the filum terminale, producing a cauda equina syndrome [11]. Diagnosis of primary tumors is established by MRI, and their definitive treatment is surgical.

Epidural and vertebral metastases

Although metastatic tumor is the most common type of neoplasm involving the spinal canal, it is rare in the general population. In one series of 1975 patients who had low back pain, 13 (0.7%) had a malignancy to account for this problem [5]. These lesions chiefly are seen in patients who have a known malignancy and, in a small percentage, are the presenting feature. Approximately 30% of epidural metastases occur in the lumbar spine, and radicular pain is an initial symptom in approximately half [12,13]. Metastases typically invade the spinal column and extend from there into the epidural space [14]. Metastases seed the vertebrae by way of Batson's venous plexus (which drains the vertebrae and anastomoses with veins draining the viscera). Less commonly, paravertebral lesions spread directly to nerve roots through the intervertebral neural foramina [14].

The three most common cancers involving the lumbosacral spine are breast, lung, and prostate cancer, each accounting for approximately 10% to 20% of cases [14,15]. Virtually all cancers, however, may produce metastatic spinal cord compression, and in 20%, spinal cord compression is the initial feature [12]. Tumors of the pelvic region, including colon and prostate, preferably metastasize to the lumbosacral region. Back pain is the most common initial complaint and, as with primary tumors, is unremitting and characteristically worse with recumbency; radicular pain is more variable. Percussion tenderness at the site of the lesion is noteworthy. Bowel and bladder disturbances occur in a minority of patients at onset but tend to be more common as disease progresses [13,14].

Contrast-enhanced MRI is the procedure of choice in the evaluation of suspected spinal metastases [16]; as lesions frequently are multiple, scanning of the entire spine is indicated [17]. Corticosteroids and external beam radiation are the mainstays of treatment [15]. The neurologic prognosis of patients who have radiculopathy as the sole symptom of metastatic disease is good; most patients likely maintain ambulation after treatment with radiotherapy [15,18]. Prognosis is correlated closely with the degree of neurologic dysfunction at diagnosis, so early recognition is crucial.

Leptomeningeal metastases/meningeal carcinomatosis

Cancer cells may infiltrate the leptomeninges and subarachnoid space diffusely, leading to a syndrome reflecting involvement of cranial nerves, spinal nerve roots, and brain. Manifestations include radiculopathy, cranial polyneuropathy, headache, memory loss, seizures, and gait disturbances [15]. Radicular discomfort is the most common presenting symptom, usually involving lumbosacral levels resulting from involvement of the cauda equina [19]. Although all cancers have the potential to produce this condition, the most likely primary tumors to do so are leukemia, lymphoma, and breast carcinoma [15,19,20]. Other tumors that may produce leptomeningeal metastasis include melanoma, lung cancer, gastrointestinal cancers, and sarcoma [15,20,21]. Initial cerebrospinal fluid (CSF) examination reveals a mildly increased cell count in approximately half, elevated protein in a large majority, and low glucose in approximately 25% [15,20]. Positive cytologic examination is seen in half of initial lumbar punctures and 90% after three lumbar punctures [15]. MRI may reveal contrast enhancement of the meninges in a diffuse or nodular pattern [15].

Infections

Herpes zoster

Primary infection with varicella-zoster virus produces chickenpox, usually in children, after which it lies dormant in dorsal root ganglia and may be reactivated decades later, producing acute Herpes zoster (HZ) or shingles [22,23]. A common disorder, it is prevalent especially in immunocompromised and elderly populations. HZ usually affects a single dermatome and is accompanied by intense neuralgic pain reflecting the level of infection; pain often precedes the classic vesicular eruption. Ophthalmic and thoracic dermatomes are affected most commonly, whereas lumbosacral zoster accounts for approximately 20% of cases [23,24]. In the presence of rash, the diagnosis of HZ is obvious, but a minority of patients may present with zoster sine herpete, dermatomally distributed pain without rash [25]. Approximately 5% of patients may develop a local neuritis of the spinal nerve, which subsequently affects the motor axons, producing a segmental zoster paresis [26]. The pain of acute HZ, frequently overwhelming at the outset, gradually subsides as the vesicles crust over in most patients. Approximately 10% to 15% suffer from chronic pain, or postherpetic neuralgia (PHN), however, despite treatment with antiviral agents [27]. Complete resolution of motor deficits occurs in 50% to 70% of those who have segmental zoster paresis [24].

Tricyclic antidepressants, gabapentin, pregabalin, opioids, and topical lidocaine patches are effective in the treatment of acute herpetic neuralgia (grade A evidence) [28]. Amitriptyline usually is effective, in a dosage of 75 to 100 mg per day, in the treatment of pain related to PHN (grade A) [29]. Gabapentin, in doses between 1800 and 3600 per day, also is effective in relieving the symptoms of PHN (grade A) [30] and may be preferred to amitriptyline because of a lower incidence of side effects. If begun within 72 hours of development of the rash, famciclovir, valacyclovir, or acyclovir reduces the pain of acute HZ but may not be effective in the prevention of PHN (grade A) [23]. Of these antiviral agents, valacyclovir (1000 mg 3 times a day for 7 days) is preferred for its more rapid resolution of neuralgia symptoms, shorter duration of PHN, and smaller pill burden [31]. Corticosteroids by themselves do not alter the course of PHN but, in combination with an antiviral agent, may improve pain [23].

Spinal epidural abscess

Spinal epidural abscess (SEA) most commonly involves the thoracic and lumbar spine. Risk factors for development of SEA include diabetes mellitus, history of intravenous drug abuse, spinal surgery, spinal or paraspinal injection, epidural catheter placement, and immunocompromised status [32,33]. Severe back pain, often with a radicular component, is the presenting complaint [34]. Fever is a common, but not universal, sign. Leukocytosis and elevation of the erythrocyte sedimentation rate are typical and in the presence of fever and back pain, the diagnosis should be straightforward. Only 20% of patients, however, have the classical clinical triad of fever, back pain, and neurologic deficits, so a high index of suspicion should be maintained [35]. The diagnostic test of choice is contrast-enhanced MRI.

Treatment of SEA must be initiated urgently with surgical débridement generally the treatment of first choice. There is increasing evidence, however, that management with 6 to 8 weeks of intravenous antibiotics with or without oral antibiotics may result in similar outcomes (grade B) [36]. Antibiotic treatment should be directed to treat the most common infecting organisms, which include *Staphylococcus aureus*, other gram-positive cocci, gram-negative rods, and anaerobes [33]. Close monitoring is necessary, and urgent surgical decompression must be considered strongly if neurologic compromise develops.

Polyradiculopathy in HIV and AIDS

Polyradiculopathy secondary to HIV infection is uncommon, accounting for only 2% of HIV-related neurologic consultations [37]. The majority of patients have an AIDS-defining illness before the development of radiculopathy, and the CD4 count is less than 100 cells per μL in almost all patients [38,39]. Polyradiculopathy in AIDS tends to involve the lumbosacral nerve roots, producing a rapidly progressive cauda equina syndrome with severe low back pain [37–40]. Cytomegalovirus accounts for most HIV-related radiculopathy. Other causes of HIV-radiculopathy include herpes simplex virus, lymphomatous meningitis, mycobacteria, *Cryptococci*, and treponemal infection [38,39].

Examination of CSF demonstrates pleocytosis, with polymorphonuclear predominance and, in some patients, decreased glucose [38–40]. A positive CSF polymerase chain reaction for cytomegalovirus also is supportive of the diagnosis. Recommended treatment includes intravenous ganciclovir, foscarnet, or both for 3 to 6 weeks (grade B) [41]. Development of polyradiculopathy in AIDS generally portends a poor prognosis, with minimal functional recovery after treatment and a median survival time of 2.7 months [39].

Lyme radiculopathy

Lyme disease is transmitted by the bite of *Ixodes* ticks infected with the spirochete *Borrelia burgdorferi* [42]. The classic rash of erythema migrans develops in 50% to 90% of patients [43]. In addition to a flu-like illness, hematogenous dissemination may affect the heart, joints, and nervous system [42,43]. Acute Lyme radiculoneuropathy is seen most commonly in the first

2 months of infection and mimics structural disk herniation; a minority of cases affects the lumbosacral nerve roots [43]. Radicular signs and symptoms usually occur in conjunction with cranial neuropathies and lymphocytic meningitis.

The current recommendation for serologic testing is to use a two-step approach, in which a positive-screening ELISA is confirmed by a Western blot [42]. In addition to serologic analysis, lumbar puncture may be helpful in establishing a diagnosis, with CSF analysis typically showing a mildly increased protein and a lymphocytic pleocytosis of up to a few hundred white cells per mm^3 [42,43]. Recommended treatment of acute Lyme radiculopathy is ceftriaxone, 2 g daily for 14 to 28 days (grade B) [44]. Intravenous penicillin G, 18 to 24 million units daily divided every 4 hours, and cefotaxime, 2 g IV every 8 hours, are alternatives (grade B) [44]. In patients intolerant of penicillin and cephalosporins, doxycycline, 100 mg bid per day in two divided doses, is preferred (grade B) [44]. Although the prognosis of acute Lyme radiculopathy generally is excellent, axonal regeneration and resolution of neurologic symptoms may require several months [43].

Chronic Lyme radiculoneuropathy is differentiated from acute Lyme radiculopathy by its development, on average, 8 months after the symptoms of the acute illness, a milder clinical course, and the absence of CSF pleocytosis [45]. The condition can develop despite successful treatment of the acute illness [45]. Treatment regimens are similar to those used for acute Lyme radiculopathy. A small number of nonrandomized patients have been followed up; 6 months after treatment with intravenous ceftriaxone, improvement was reported in 9 of these 12 patients [45]. This improvement, however, usually was incomplete and noted weeks to months after completion of therapy, not during the course of treatment [45].

Diabetes (diabetic amyotrophy)

Diabetes may cause a syndrome of severe lower extremity pain and weakness, commonly referred to as diabetic amyotrophy. This syndrome usually involves multiple lumbosacral nerve roots but rarely presents as a monoradiculopathy [46]. Patients typically have well controlled type 2 diabetes and are middle aged or older [47]. In some patients, the neurologic impairment heralds the onset of diabetes [47]. Sudden onset, unilateral lower extremity pain variably involves the groin, anterior thigh, and lower leg; weakness follows shortly. Proximal muscles, in particular quadriceps, tend to be affected first and most conspicuously, but the majority of patients also develop distal and bilateral symptoms [48]. Weight loss is a frequent accompanying symptom [47]. The precise pathophysiology of diabetic radiculopathy is controversial, with nerve ischemia, inflammation, and metabolic causes implicated [47–50].

EMG is helpful in diagnosing diabetic amyotrophy. There is evidence of subacute polyradiculopathy with prominent denervation changes involving limbs and multiple, bilateral paraspinal regions. Underlying axonal poly-neuropathy may also be present. CSF protein is elevated without pleocytosis.

Diabetic radiculopathy is a monophasic illness that improves with time [46,47]. Improvement, however, often is incomplete and prolonged, with motor symptoms slower to resolve than sensory symptoms [47]. Pain control in the early stages can be challenging. Standard agents for neuropathic pain, such as anticonvulsants or tricyclic antidepressants, are beneficial, but narcotic analgesics also may be needed temporarily [47]. Physical therapy and orthoses should be provided as indicated [47]. Up to 20% of patients may suffer a recurrence on the same side [47,51].

Spinal cysts

Cystic lesions in the sacral spine are common, with an incidence ranging from 4.6% to 17% on imaging studies [52,53]. Most sacral meningeal cysts are dural diverticula (Tarlov cysts) produced by fluctuations in CSF pressure [52]. There is little to differentiate the presentation of meningeal sacral cysts from other causes of lumbosacral radiculopathy [52]. Radicular pain often is relieved or disappears when patients are recumbent and is aggravated by Valsalva's maneuver [52]. Because they are common and not necessarily the cause of symptoms, establishing a cyst as the cause of lumbosacral radiculopathy involves eliminating other causes first. MRI is the diagnostic procedure of choice for demonstrating lumbosacral cysts; however, clinical relevance of the imaging findings must still be established. Although analgesic medications may reduce pain, relief of symptoms with fluoroscopic-guided aspiration and surgical treatment is definitive [52].

Spinal hematomas

Hematomas are uncommon causes of lumbosacral radiculopathy. Epidural and subdural spinal hematomas occur most frequently in patients who have coagulopathies, who are taking anticoagulants, or who recently have undergone epidural injections or instrumentation of the lumbosacral spine [54–56]. Spinal subarachnoid hemorrhage is uncommon. Unlike its intracranial counterpart, spinal subarachnoid hemorrhage is caused most commonly by arteriovenous malformation rupture rather than aneurysmal rupture [57]. Hemorrhage into synovial cysts or the ligamentum flavum also may produce hematomas and lumbosacral radiculopathy [58,59].

Other uncommon causes of radiculopathy

Sarcoidosis can affect any level of the neuraxis; radiculopathy is an uncommon presentation. Cauda equina syndrome and lumbosacral polyradiculopathy are described as manifestations of sarcoid [60].

Arachnoiditis also may produce lumbosacral radiculopathy. Classically caused by a reaction to intrathecal oil-based contrast dye for myelography, other causes of arachnoiditis include neurocysticercosis and other infections, blood in the intrathecal space, surgical interventions in the spine, intrathecal corticosteroids, and trauma [61].

Tethered cord syndrome is a developmental malformation characterized by an abnormally low-lying conus medullaris tethered to an intradural abnormality [62]. Uncommonly, this syndrome presents in adulthood, most often as pain centered around the anorectal or inguinal regions, but sometimes diffusely in the legs or in a radicular distribution [63–65]. Approximately 60% to 70% of patients report an inciting traumatic event leading to presentation [65]. A mixed cauda equina and conus medullaris syndrome is seen, without other signs of spinal dysraphism, such as sacral dimples or hair tufts [63–65]. MRI has allowed earlier detection of the syndrome [63,64], with termination of the conus medullaris inferior to the inferior aspect of the L2 vertebral body being diagnostic [63].

Approach to initial diagnosis and management

An algorithm for the initial diagnosis and management of lumbosacral radiculopathy is shown in Fig. 1. First, whether or not patients have a disease process that could result in irreversible neurologic dysfunction must be determined. Indications for immediate neuroimaging and surgical evaluation include a cauda equina syndrome, rapidly progressive neurologic deficits, and risk factors for metastatic cancer or epidural abscess.

Provided that none of these indications for urgent evaluation is present, a trial of conservative therapy may be attempted for 4 to 6 weeks. Specific details of conservative and surgical management are discussed by Benzel and colleagues elsewhere in this issue of the Clinics; however, there is little difference among the outcomes of patients treated with bed rest, physical therapy, or continuation of normal activities of daily living, so treatment should be tailored to provide maximum comfort [66,67]. Analgesic medications, including nonsteroidal anti-inflammatory drugs, nonopioid analgesics (eg, tramadol), and, in some cases, narcotic analgesics should be used as indicated.

If 4 to 6 weeks of conservative therapy fails to control painful symptoms or if neurologic deficits progress, further diagnostic studies, including EMG and MRI, are warranted. Needle EMG is the preferred electrodiagnostic technique in the evaluation of radiculopathy and is performed in conjunction with nerve conduction studies to exclude alternative diagnosis, such as neuropathy or plexopathy [68]. EMG is advantageous because it assesses the physiologic integrity of the nerve roots directly and can diagnose compressive and noncompressive radiculopathies. It also provides a measure of severity of radiculopathic disease. MRI is the preferred study to view the structure of the lumbosacral spine and nerve roots. Because of the high prevalence of disk protrusions and degenerative spinal stenosis in older patients, history and physical examination remain paramount in determining the

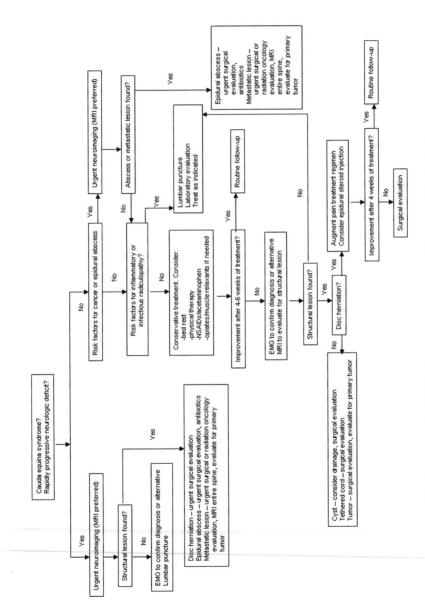

Fig. 1. Approach to initial diagnosis and treatment of lumbosacral radiculopathy.

relevance of imaging findings [69,70]. EMG also can be used to help provide confirmation of clinically suspected nerve root involvement.

In some cases, further laboratory testing is appropriate based on the history, physical examination, EMG, or imaging findings. Lumbar puncture may be indicated to investigate inflammatory or infectious causes. The direction of the evaluation is guided by patient presentation and subsequent clinical course. As discussed previously, a basic understanding of the diverse disorders producing lumbosacral radiculopathy and those who are at risk for them is the foundation for accurate diagnosis and treatment.

Summary

Lumbosacral radiculopathy is a common neurologic syndrome that is an important source of disability. Although the most common causes are disk herniation and chronic spinal arthropathy, physicians should be mindful of other causes, including neoplasm and infection. Initial evaluation should focus on localization of lumbosacral radiculopathy and exclusion of disorders that may produce irreversible neurologic compromise. Treatment is aimed at providing pain relief and preventing neurologic deficits in addition to appropriate directed therapy based on the underlying cause.

References

[1] Anderson GBJ. Epidemiology of spinal disorders. In: Frymoyer JW, editor. The adult spine: principles and practice. New York: Raven; 1991. p. 110–46.
[2] Heliovaraa M, Knekt P, Aromaa A. Incidence and risk factors of herniated lumbar intervertebral disc or sciatica leading to hospitalization. J Chronic Dis 1987;40(3):251–8.
[3] Moore KL. Clinically oriented anatomy. Baltimore (MD): Williams & Wilkins; 1992.
[4] Liang MH, Katz JN. Clinical evaluation of patients with a suspected spine problem. In: Frymoyer JW, editor. The adult spine: principles and practice. New York: Raven; 1991. p. 223–39.
[5] Deyo RA, Diehl AK. Cancer as a cause of back pain: frequency, clinical presentation, and diagnostic strategies. J Gen Intern Med 1988;3(3):230–8.
[6] Charnley J. Orthopedic signs in the diagnosis of disc protrusion with special reference to the straight leg raising test. Lancet 1951;1(4):186–92.
[7] Frymoyer JW, Moskowitz RW. Spinal degeneration. Pathogenesis and medical management. In: Frymoyer JW, editor. The adult spine: principles and practice. New York: Raven; 1991. p. 611–34.
[8] Howe JF, Loeser JD, Calvin WH. Mechanosensitivity of dorsal root ganglia and chronically injured axons: a physiological basis for the radicular pain of nerve root compression. Pain 1977;3(1):25–41.
[9] Dyck P. The femoral nerve traction test in lumbar disc protrusion. Surg Neurol 1976;6(3): 163–6.
[10] Kirkaldy-Willis WH, Yong-Hing K. Lateral recess, lateral canal, and foraminal stenosis. In: Watkins RG, Collis JS, editors. Lumbar discectomy and laminectomy. Rockville (MD): Aspen Publishers, Inc; 1987. p. 245–52.

[11] Freeman TB, Cahill DW. Tumors of the meninges, cauda equina, and spinal nerves. In: Menezes AH, Sonntag VKH, editors. Principles of spinal surgery. New York: McGraw-Hill; 1996. p. 1371–86.

[12] Schiff D, O'Neill BP, Suman VJ. Spinal epidural metastasis as the initial manifestation of malignancy: clinical features and diagnostic approach. Neurology 1997;49(2):452–6.

[13] Helweg-Larsen S, Sorensen PS. Symptoms and signs in metastatic cord compression: a study of progression from first symptom until diagnosis in 153 patients. Eur J Cancer 1994;30A(3):396–8.

[14] Schiff D. Spinal cord compression. Neurol Clin North Am 2003;21(1):67–86.

[15] Posner JB. Neurologic complications of cancer. Philadelphia: F.A. Davis Company; 1995.

[16] Sarpel S, Sarpel G, Yu E, et al. Early diagnosis of spinal-epidural metastasis by magnetic resonance imaging. Cancer 1987;59(6):1112–6.

[17] van der Sande JJ, Kroger R, Boogerd W. Multiple spinal epidural metastases; an unexpectedly frequent finding. J Neurol Neurosurg Psychiatry 1990;53(11):1001–3.

[18] Redmond J, Friedl KE, Cornett P, et al. Clinical usefulness of an algorithm for the early diagnosis of spinal metastatic disease. J Clin Oncol 1988;6(1):155–7.

[19] Kaplan JG, DeSouza TG, Farkash A, et al. Leptomeningeal metastases: comparison of clinical features and laboratory data of solid tumors, lymphomas and leukemias. J Neurooncol 1990;9(3):225–9.

[20] Little JR, Dale AJD, Okazaki H. Meningeal carcinomatosis. Arch Neurol 1974;30(2): 138–43.

[21] Fischer-Williams M, Bosanquet FD, Daniel PM. Carcinomatosis of the meninges: a report of three cases. Brain 1955;78(1):42–58.

[22] Braverman DL, Ku A, Nagler W. Herpes zoster polyradiculopathy. Arch Phys Med Rehabil 1997;78(8):880–2.

[23] Kost RG, Straus SE. Postherpetic neuralgia—pathogenesis, treatment, and prevention. N Engl J Med 1996;335(1):32–42.

[24] Thomas JE, Howard FM. Segmental zoster paresis—a disease profile. Neurology 1972; 22(5):459–66.

[25] Gilden DH, Wright RR, Schneck SA, et al. Zoster sine herpete, a clinical variant. Ann Neurol 1994;35(5):530–3.

[26] Amato AA, Dumitru D. Acquired neuropathies. In: Dumitru D, Amato AA, Zwarts MJ, editors. Electrodiagnostic medicine. 2nd edition. Philadelphia: Hanley & Belfus, Inc.; 2002. p. 937–1041.

[27] Wood MJ, Ogan PH, McKendrick MW, et al. Efficacy of oral acyclovir treatment of acute herpes zoster. Am J Med 1988;85(S2A):79–83.

[28] Dubinsky RM, Kabbani H, El-Chami Z, et al. Practice parameter: treatment of postherpetic neuralgia: an evidence-based report of the Quality Standards Subcommittee of the American Academy of Neurology. Neurology 2004;63(6):959–65.

[29] Watson CP, Evans RJ, Reed K, et al. Amitriptyline versus placebo in postherpetic neuralgia. Neurology 1982;32(6):671–3.

[30] Rowbotham MC, Harden N, Stacey B, et al. Gabapentin for the treatment of postherpetic neuralgia: a randomized controlled trial. JAMA 1998;280(21):1837–42.

[31] Beutner KR, Friedman DJ, Forszpaniak C, et al. Valaciclovir compared with acyclovir for improved therapy for herpes zoster in immunocompromised adults. Antimicrob Agents Chemother 1995;39(7):1546–53.

[32] Del Curling O, Gower DJ, McWhorter JM. Changing concepts in spinal epidural abscess: a report of 29 cases. Neurosurgery 1990;27(2):185–92.

[33] Nussbaum ES, Rigamonti D, Standiford H, et al. Spinal epidural abscess: a report of 40 cases and review. Surg Neurol 1992;38(3):225–31.

[34] Heusner AP. Nontuberculous spinal epidural infections. N Engl J Med 1948;239(23):845–54.

[35] Davis DP, Wold RM, Patel RJ, et al. The clinical presentation and impact of diagnostic delays on emergency department patients with spinal epidural abscess. J Emerg Med 2004; 26(3):285–91.

[36] Siddiq F, Chowfin A, Tight R, et al. Medical vs. surgical managment of spinal epidural abscess. Arch Intern Med 2004;164(22):2409–12.

[37] de Gans J, Portegies P, Tiessens G, et al. Therapy for cytomegalovirus polyradiculomyelitis in patients with AIDS: treatment with ganciclovir. AIDS 1990;4(5):421–5.

[38] Corral I, Quereda C, Casado JL, et al. Acute polyradiculopathies in HIV-infected patients. J Neurol 1997;244(8):499–504.

[39] So YT, Olney RK. Acute lumbosacral polyradiculopathy in Acquired Immunodeficiency Syndrome: experience in 23 patients. Ann Neurol 1994;35(1):53–8.

[40] Miller RF, Fox JD, Thomas P, et al. Acute lumbosacral polyradiculopathy due to cytomegalovirus in advanced HIV disease: CSF findings in 17 patients. J Neurol Neurosurg Psychiatry 1996;61(5):450–60.

[41] Whitley RJ, Jacobson MA, Friedberg DN, et al. Guidelines for the treatment of cytomegaolvirus diseases in patients with AIDS in the era of potent antiretroviral therapy: recommendations of an international panel. Arch Intern Med 1998;158(9):957–69.

[42] Anonymous. Guidelines for laboratory evaluation in the diagnosis of Lyme disease. Ann Intern Med 1997;127(12):1106–8.

[43] Halperin JJ. Lyme disease and the peripheral nervous system. Muscle Nerve 2003;28(2): 133–43.

[44] Wormser GP, Nadelman RB, Dattwyler RJ, et al. Practice guidelines for the treatment of Lyme disease. The Infectious Diseases Society of America. Clin Infect Dis 2000;31(Suppl 1):1–14.

[45] Logigian EL, Steere AC. Clinical and electrophysiologic findings in chronic neuropathy of Lyme disease. Neurology 1992;42(2):303–11.

[46] Naftulin S, Fast A, Thomas M. Diabetic lumbar radiculopathy: sciatica without disc herniation. Spine 1993;18(16):2419–22.

[47] Dyck PJB, Windebank AJ. Diabetic and nondiabetic lumbosacral radiculoplexus neuropathies: new insights into pathophysiology and treatment. Muscle Nerve 2002;25(4):477–91.

[48] Dyck PJB, Norell JE, Dyck PJ. Microvasculitis and ischemia in diabetic lumbosacral radiculoplexus neuropathy. Neurology 1999;53(9):2113–21.

[49] Raff MC, Sangalang V, Asbury AK. Ischemic mononeuropathy multiplex associated with diabetes mellitus. Arch Neurol 1968;18(5):487–99.

[50] Said G, Goulen-Goeau C, Lacroix C, et al. Nerve biopsy findings in different patterns of proximal diabetic neuropathy. Ann Neurol 1994;35(5):559–69.

[51] Bastron JA, Thomas JE. Diabetic polyradiculopathy: clinical and electromyographic findings in 105 patients. Mayo Clin Proc 1981;56(12):725–32.

[52] Fogel GR, Cunnigham PY, Esses SI. Surgical evaluation and management of symptomatic lumbosacral meningeal cysts. Am J Orthop 2004;33(6):278–82.

[53] Paulsen RD, Call GA, Murtagh FR. Prevalence and percutaneous drainage of cysts of the sacral nerve root sheath (Tarlov cysts). AJNR Am J Neuroradiol 1994;15(2):298–9.

[54] Kingery WS, Seibel M, Date ES, et al. The natural resolution of a lumbar spontaneous epidural hematoma and associated radiculopathy. Spine 1994;19(1):67–9.

[55] Riffaud L, Morandi X, Chabert E, et al. Spontaneous chronic spinal epidural hematoma of the lumbar spine. J Neuroradiol 1999;26(1):64–7.

[56] Domenicucci M, Ramieri A, Ciappetta P, et al. Nontraumatic acute subdural haematoma: report of five cases and review of the literature. J Neurosurg 1999;91(Suppl 1):65–73.

[57] Caplan LR. Caplan's stroke: a clinical approach. Boston: Butterworth Heinemann; 2000.

[58] Kaneko K, Inoue Y. Haemorrhagic lumbar synovial cyst. A cause of acute radiculopathy. J Bone Joint Surg Br 2000;82(4):583–4.

[59] Hirakawa K, Hanakita J, Suwa H, et al. A post-traumatic ligamentum flavum progressive hematoma. A case report. Spine 2000;25(9):1182–4.

[60] Koffman B, Junck L, Elias SB, et al. Polyradiculopathy in sarcoidosis. Muscle Nerve 1999; 22(5):608–13.

[61] Aldrete JA. Neurologic deficits and arachnoiditis following neuroaxial anesthesia. Acta Anaesthesiol Scand 2003;47(1):3–12.

[62] Marin-Padilla MD. The tethered cord syndrome: developmental considerations. In: Holtz-man RN, editor. The tethered spinal cord. New York: Thieme-Stratton Inc.; 1985. p. 3–13.

[63] Pang D, Wilberger JE. Tethered cord syndrome in adults. J Neurosurg 1982;57(1):32–47.

[64] Caruso R, Cervoni L, Fiorenz F, et al. Occult dysraphism in adulthood. A series of 24 cases. J Neurosurg Sci 1996;40(3–4):221–5.

[65] Ratliff J, Mahoney PS, Kline DG. Tethered cord syndrome in adults. South Med J 1999; 92(12):1199–203.

[66] Kofstee DJ, Gijtenbeek JM, Hoogland PH, et al. Westeinde Sciatica Trial: randomized controlled study of bed rest and physiotherapy for acute sciatica. J Neurosurg Spine 2002;96(1): 45–9.

[67] Vroomen PC, de Krom MC, Wilmink JT, et al. Lack of effectiveness of bed rest for sciatica. N Engl J Med 1999;340(6):418–23.

[68] Wilbourn AJ, Aminoff MJ. AAEE minmonograph #32: the electrophysiologic examination in patients with radiculopathies. Muscle Nerve 1988;11(11):1099–114.

[69] Boden SD, Davis DO, Dina TS, et al. Abnormal magnetic resonance scans of the lumbar spine in asymptomatic subjects: a prospective investigation. J Bone Joint Surg Am 1990; 72(3):403–8.

[70] Jensen MC, Brant-Zawadzki MN, Obuchowski N, et al. Magnetic resonance imaging of the lumbar spine in people without back pain. N Engl J Med 1994;331(2):69–73.

ELSEVIER
SAUNDERS

Neurol Clin 25 (2007) 407–418

NEUROLOGIC
CLINICS

Lumbar Spinal Stenosis

David A. Chad, MD

Department of Neurology, University of Massachusetts Memorial Health Care,
55 Lake Ave. N, Worcester, MA, 01605, USA

Lumbar spinal stenosis perhaps is understood best as a clinicopathologic disorder: narrowing of the lumbar spinal canal and the nerve root canals (causing central and lateral recess stenosis, respectively) typically is brought about by the process of osteoarthritis and leads to compression of the contents of the canals—the neural and vascular structures, causing neurologic symptoms (typically low back and leg pain and lower limb numbness and weakness) that are intermittent, characteristically triggered by ambulation (ameliorated by pausing), and generally positional (aggravated by standing and eased by trunk flexion). The emergence of spinal stenosis as a recognizable disease entity took a major step forward in 1954 with the work of the Dutch neurosurgeon, H. Verbiest [1] (described in a literature review by Javid and Hadar [2]), who coined the term, "stenosis of the vertebral canal," and defined the pathologic changes that take place in the lumbar spinal canal engendered by encroachment of the canal contents by hypertrophied articular processes. Although having a narrow lumbar spinal canal is a necessary component of the condition, alone it is not sufficient for the disorder to be expressed, because this requires a degree of narrowing that compresses canal contents and causes compromise in sensory and motor nerve function. Accordingly, there may be a poor correlation between "stenosis" demonstrated by neuroimaging methods and clinical symptoms [3]. As Haig and colleagues [4] point out, there is no criterion standard for the clinical diagnosis of lumbar spinal stenosis. Clinically, the constellation of symptoms not always is classic; radiologically, there is no clear relationship between the severity of symptoms and degree of stenosis; and electrophysiologically, there is no predictable, specific electromyographic (EMG) abnormality.

Lumbar spinal stenosis is a common problem in adult life. It is estimated to be present in 5 of every 1000 Americans over age 50 [5]. It accounts for

---

E-mail address: chadd@ummhc.org

0733-8619/07/$ - see front matter © 2007 Elsevier Inc. All rights reserved.
doi:10.1016/j.ncl.2007.01.003

5% of patients who present with persistent low back pain to a general physician and up to 14% of patients who seek the opinion of a specialist [6]. It is
the leading preoperative diagnosis for adults older than age 65 who undergo
spine surgery [7]; in the United States, rates of surgery for spinal stenosis increased eightfold from 1979 to 1992 in patients over age 65 [8]. It commonly
affects adults in their sixth and seventh decades when it most likely is a result
of acquired degenerative joint disease—lumbar spondylosis. A subset of
adults in their third and fourth decades also is affected, and these individuals
typically have congenital narrowing of the lumbosacral spine (discussed
later) [9]. Some patients who have the congenital form of spinal stenosis
have achondroplastic dwarfism and at age 38 have a relatively young
mean age of presentation, attesting to the primary nature of the stenosis
[10].

Clinical features

Patients present with the insidious onset of diffuse, often symmetric
symptoms, reflecting the bilateral nature of the underlying disease process
that often involves several vertebral levels [11]. The first symptoms of lumbar spinal stenosis frequently are low back pain and morning stiffness
relieved by activity [12]. As time passes, there frequently is low back,
buttock, thigh, and calf discomfort, often described as a cramping, burning
sensation, sometimes with associated numbness and tingling in the legs and
thighs. Weakness is not a prominent symptom but may be present, most often manifested as partial foot drop or weakness in plantar flexion, especially
after prolonged standing or walking, and pointing to the common involvement of muscles served by L5 and S1 roots [13]. A characteristic of the
symptoms produced by lumbar spinal stenosis is that they are induced or
triggered by standing and walking (activities that extend the lumbar spine)
and eased by sitting or flexing the trunk. The latency from the start of standing to the onset of pain varies from patient to patient and also changes over
time for individual patients, becoming shorter when and if the disease process evolves. A classic clinical feature of lumbar canal stenosis is neurogenic
claudication, the dynamic phenomenon of standing- and walking-related
symptoms (thigh or leg pain preceding numbness and motor weakness),
causing patients to limp and then to cease the provocative activity [14]. It
is to be distinguished from the vascular mechanism encountered more commonly underlying painful legs, induced by walking, in the context of athero-
sclerotic peripheral vascular disease. In this vascular disorder, the typical
history is that cramping develops in the calves with activity (such as walking,
cycling, or descending, and especially ascending, stairs) and that relief is obtained by sitting and resting. In neurogenic claudication, by contrast, ascending stairs typically is less likely to induce symptoms than descending,
probably because the former allows for a partially flexed trunk, whereas

in the latter, the lumbar spine straightens out, obliging patients to walk downstairs backward to adopt a forward-flexed position [5]; cycling is tolerated much more than walking. Patients who have lumbar spinal stenosis typically are fairly comfortable on shopping outings if they can lean over while pushing a grocery cart.

In the early stages of the disorder, the symptoms may be mild and provoked after an extended period of standing or walking, but as time passes, the disease seems to enter an extended plateau phase in many patients. In others, symptoms may become more pronounced and diffuse, triggered by only brief periods of standing, reaching the point where quality of life may become seriously compromised. In these advanced cases, patients barely are able to walk short distances without severe symptoms and reflexively attempt to attenuate any discomfort by using a stooped or anthropoid posture (effectively flexing the back) that presumably allows for widening of the lumbar spinal canal [15]. In approximately 10% of patients, generally those who have the most advanced degrees of lumbar spinal stenosis, there are symptoms of bladder control difficulties, manifested as recurrent urinary tract infections associated with an atonic bladder, incontinence, and, rarely, episodes of urinary retention [9].

The examination findings are muted, in contrast to the findings in lumbosacral radiculopathy (which may coexist with lumbar spinal stenosis). In lumbosacral radiculopathy, there is straight leg raising and reverse straight leg raising positivity, segmental weakness, attenuation of reflex activity, and dermatomal sensory loss. In lumbar spinal stenosis, there may be flattening of the lumbar lordosis and a decrease in lumbar extension. Positive straight leg raising—complaints of a severe sciatica-like pain in a raised leg at 30° to 40° of elevation—is uncommon in patients who have lumbar spinal stenosis [15]. Provocative measures suggestive of lumbar spinal stenosis include lying prone in lumbar hyperextension, walking, and walking with an exaggerated lumbar lordosis until symptoms appear, followed by relief of symptoms by leaning forward [7]. At rest there may be a paucity of findings [14], but with onset of symptoms after walking or extending the spine, there may be diminution in patellar and Achilles tendon reflexes, mild sensory loss in L4 to S1 dermatomes, and mild weakness in L4-, L5- and S1-innervated muscles—hence, the importance of the sage advice from Alvarez and Hardy [15] to perform a neurologic examination before and immediately after symptoms appear after a short period of ambulation.

Finally, it is important to assess patients for clinical evidence of vascular disease, which, as discussed previously, might simulate some of the symptoms of lumbar spinal stenosis, notably claudication. The examination includes the evaluation of skin color, turgor, and temperature; distal lower limb pulses; and auscultation for arterial bruits. Absence of clinical features of peripheral vascular disease should heighten confidence in a diagnosis of lumbar spinal stenosis [7].

Anatomy and pathology

The spinal cord in adults ends at the upper border of the L1 vertebral body and continues as multiple nerve roots, the cauda equina, that descend to their specific neural foramena, providing exit from the lumbosacral spinal canal. The spinal canal ranges from 15 to 23 mm in its anteroposterior diameter and is a triangular space bounded anteriorly by the dorsal surfaces of the bodies of the lumbar vertebrae and the disk spaces (covered by the posterior longitudinal ligament), medially by the pedicles that extend from the lateral margin of the vertebral body, posteriorly by the laminae of the vertebral arch and their covering, the ligamentum flavum; and the facet joints that are part of the posterior elements of each vertebral body [7,11,15]. The vertebral bodies are connected to each other by the disks anteriorly and two facet or zygoapophyseal joints posteriorly. The disks are composed of a tough outer connective tissue annulus fibrosis and a soft, jelly-like center, the nucleus pulposus.

There are two major categories of lumbar spinal stenosis: congenital and acquired. The major contributors to narrowed lumbar canals on a congenital basis are short pedicles, thickened lamina and facets, and excessive scoliotic or lordotic curves [15]. Patients who have these congenital anatomic changes have a small safety factor for the emergence of clinically significant lumbar spinal stenosis, which may be precipitated by further canal narrowing from later life–onset superimposed degenerative joint changes. Defects in cellular metabolism leading to retardation of cartilaginous growth and irregular intracartilagenous bone formation lead to congenital spinal stenosis in achondroplastic dwarfism, where there is significant narrowing of the spinal canal in all its dimensions, especially in the upper lumbar regions because of shortened pedicles, hypertrophied zygapophyseal joints, and thickened laminae [10].

The majority of cases of lumbar spinal stenosis, however, are acquired, and stem from degenerative or arthritic changes that affect the three-joint complex between lumbar vertebrae: the two zygoapophyseal (facet) joints posteriorly and the adjoining intervertebral disk anteriorly [9]. The degenerative process begins most often with the disk and affects the articular processes secondarily. Initially, there is desiccation of the disk, narrowing of the disk space, rents or fissures in the annulus, disk bulging, and frank herniation of nucleus pulposus. This soon is followed by hypertrophic degenerative changes of the facets (osteophyte formation) and thickening of the ligamentum flavum. This results in central narrowing, so that the anteroposterior diameter is attenuated (typically to less than 12 mm) [7], with compression of the cauda equina, and lateral narrowing (at the recesses), with root compression at the entrance of the intervertebral foramen. Spondylolysis (a defect in the pedicles, the pars interarticularis—congenital or acquired) may lead to spondylolisthesis, the anterior displacement of one vertebra relative to the one beneath it, further narrowing an already stenotic lumbar canal [16].

The spine is the site affected second most commonly in Paget's disease, predisposing patients to spinal stenosis, occurring in one third of those who have spinal involvement [17]. Pagetic spinal stenosis is brought about by bone remodeling of lumbar vertebrae, with bone expansion in all directions: posteriorly from the vertebral bodies, anterioromedially from the vertebral lamina, and medially from the pedicles. This leads to hypertrophic facet arthropathy and resulting spinal stenosis. Some cases of neurologic deterioration do not result from direct compression of neural elements, rather from spinal ischemia resulting from diversion of blood flow through remodeled hypervascular pagetic bone (referred to as the arterial steal phenomenon) [17].

Pathogenesis

Three explanations are advanced to explain the phenomenon of neurogenic claudication, the cardinal manifestation of lumbar spinal stenosis. They are designated the postural, the ischemic, and the venous stasis (stagnant hypoxia) theories [9]. The postural theory suggests that symptoms are explained by transient compression of the cauda equina (leading to sensory and motor axon dysfunction) by degenerated intervertebral disks and thickened ligamenta flava, when the lumbar spine is extended and lordosis is accentuated, either at rest or in the erect posture [15]. In the ischemic theory, it is proposed that the metabolic demand of the cauda equina cannot be met during activity (eg, walking), that blood flow needs of the lumbosacral nerve roots are not met by the local vasculature that is compromised by lumbar spinal stenosis. Porter [16] suggested the venous stasis theory: that the underlying mechanism of neurogenic claudication is inadequate oxygenation or the accumulation of metabolites in the cauda equina. He presented evidence from a porcine model that venous pooling of one or more nerve roots of the cauda equina between two levels of low pressure stenosis transitions to venous engorgement during exercise (walking), that in turn tends to prevent the expected arteriolar vasodilation response to activity, leading to nerve conduction failure with resulting symptoms of tiredness, weakness, and discomfort in the legs when walking.

Diagnostic testing

Standing center stage among diagnostic testing modalities in the evaluation of patients suspected of having lumbar spinal stenosis is neuroimaging with MRI. This noninvasive test with its multiplanar imaging capability provides the most complete assessment of the anatomy of the lumbosacral spine and allows adequate visualization of the spinal cord, cauda equina, and exiting nerve roots and their relationships to the various elements that comprise the spinal canal, including the ligaments, epidural fat, sub-arachnoid space, and intervertebral disks, with excellent detail [7,15]. A variety of MRI sequences with gadolinium also reveals pathology of the vertebrae, the spinal canal, and the cauda equina that might mimic the clinical features of lumbar spinal stenosis—for example, infectious or neoplastic processes (see differential diagnosis discussion). If for any reason MRI cannot be performed (eg, contraindicated because the subject has a cardiac pacemaker), CT myelography provides appropriate alternative imaging resolution and reveals spinal canal pathology clearly.

Electrodiagnostic studies are helpful in the evaluation of patients who have suspected lumbar spinal stenosis. In patients who have axon loss root disease resulting from lumbar canal stenosis, nerve conduction studies may reveal reduced amplitude of motor evoked responses recorded from the small foot muscles after stimulating the peroneal and tibial nerves, with little or no change in conduction velocities or distal latencies [13]. Sensory amplitudes recording from the superficial and sural nerves generally are expected to be unaffected, because the pathology of the nerve roots in lumbar spinal stenosis is at a preganglionic level. In rare instances, the L5 sensory ganglia have an intraspinal location and, therefore, may be involved in nerve root compressive disorders localized to the lateral recesses, causing attenuation of the superficial peroneal sensory amplitudes [18]. It also should be recalled that sensory responses in the lower extremities may be reduced or absent, because the age range of patients affected with lumbar spinal stenosis overlaps with the age when sensory responses are lost as part of normal aging. H-reflexes commonly are attenuated or absent, and, in instances when the sural response is preserved, this finding is all the more suggestive of preganglionic S1 root dysfunction [13]. Peroneal and tibial F-wave chronodispersion (the difference between the shortest and longest F latencies in a series of F waves) [19] may be increased abnormally after 3 minutes of standing [20].

The needle electrode examination is considered the single most useful diagnostic method in the electrophysiologic evaluation of patients who have suspected nerve root compromise in the setting of lumbar spinal stenosis [13]. In the older population most at risk for this condition, a painful, positive straight leg raising radiculopathy is encountered in few individuals [21], and, therefore, needle electrode examination features of single root lesions are uncommon. Patients presenting with lumbar spinal stenosis, especially those who are elderly, are much more likely to experience compressive effects on the cauda equina and, therefore, may manifest EMG changes typical of multiple root involvement [21]. Wilbourn and Aminoff [13] described bilateral, multiple lumbosacral radiculopathies in approximately half of patients who have lumbar spinal stenosis, with L5 and S1 roots involved most commonly. In many patients, especially those who have lesser degrees of lumbar spinal stenosis and accordingly less compression of the cauda equina, the needle examination may be only mildly abnormal or within normal limits. When present, needle electrode examination abnormalities typically are noted in the categories of spontaneous activity and motor unit potential morphology. Because of the chronicity of lumbar spinal stenosis, there is an opportunity for motor unit reinnervation; therefore, fibrillation potentials tend to be restricted to the distal muscles of the myotomes, and motor unit potentials have attributes of chronic neurogenic change, such as prolonged duration and increased amplitude [13].

Finally, electrodiagnostic studies also are helpful in identifying common disorders that might coexist with lumbar spinal stenosis. For example, they detect peripheral nerve involvement in the setting of diabetes (reduced or absent sensory and motor amplitudes in the lower and upper extremities, along with mild slowing of nerve conduction velocities), a condition that might lead to sensory symptoms in the legs and discomfort in the buttocks and legs. Diabetic polyneuropathy often is a complex and multifaceted disorder with features of polyneuropathy and polyradiculopathy, potentially simulating some of the clinical features of lumbar spinal stenosis [15].

The exercise treadmill test—wherein the ability of patients to walk is quantified and any difficulty in walking is characterized fully (determining if the limitation on walking is secondary to neurogenic claudication or some other cause [eg, dyspnea])—plays an important role in the diagnostic process in patients suspected of having lumbar spinal stenosis [22]. In a group of 29 patients who had mild lumbar spinal stenosis, the subset with neurogenic claudication (16/29) covered a significantly shorter distance and the time spent walking was significantly shorter than in the subset with lumbar spinal stenosis without neurogenic claudication and in two control groups (healthy controls and diabetic patients).

Differential diagnosis

The most common manifestations of lumbar spinal stenosis include low back and leg pain, numbness and tingling, and neurogenic claudication. Because low back pain typically is an initial and predominating feature of lumbar spinal stenosis, one approach to the evaluation of patients suspected of having lumbar spinal stenosis is to use back pain as the point of departure for the process of differential diagnosis and ask what other conditions present with low back pain and can mimic lumbar spinal stenosis. These conditions must be ruled out before a diagnosis of lumbar spinal stenosis can be established with certainty.

The differential diagnosis of lumbar spinal stenosis, therefore, may be viewed through the lens of the differential diagnosis of low back pain and may be divided into three major categories [11]: mechanical (97% of patients), nonmechanical (1%), and back pain stemming from visceral disease (2%). The first category includes lumbar strain or idiopathic low back pain, which makes up 70% of this group and is distinguished from lumbar spinal stenosis by the lack of neurogenic claudication, relatively normal spinal canal dimensions, and normal electrodiagnostic studies. Other conditions include age-related degenerative disease of the disk and facet joints (10%), frank disk herniations with nerve root compromise (4%), osteoporotic compression fractures (4%), and spondylolisthesis (2%), all of which may present with low back pain but have a distinctive EMG signature (in the case of radiculopathy) or defining neuroimaging characteristics. Nonmechanical spinal conditions include neoplastic and benign cystic lesions of the conus medullaris and cauda equina, infectious diseases (most importantly spinal epidural abscess), inflammatory arachnoiditis, and inflammatory arthropathies. Although not an arthropathy per se, polymyalgia rheumatica deserves mention as a related rheumatologic disorder whose presentation with bilateral aching in the buttocks associated with stiffness in the back might suggest lumbar spinal stenosis until the marked elevation of the erythrocyte sedimentation rate reveals its true character [23]. Visceral diseases include renal diseases (such as nephrolithiasis, pyelonephritis, and perinephric abscess), diseases of the pelvic organs (such as prostatitis, endometriosis, and chronic pelvic inflammatory disease), gastrointestinal diseases (such as pancreatitis, cholecystitis, and penetrating ulcer), and aortic aneurysms. Abdominal and pelvic imaging techniques in concert with routine clinical chemistry and hematologic testing are helpful in identifying nonmechanical and visceral sources of back pain.

In addition to back pain, leg numbness and tingling also are common presenting manifestations of lumbar spinal stenosis. A common cause of such sensory symptoms is polyneuropathy, often associated with diabetes.

Management

There are several prospective, long-term, observational follow-up studies that attempt to evaluate conservative versus surgical treatment outcomes for patients who have lumbar spinal stenosis. Amundsen and colleagues [24] compared conservative and surgical management in a cohort of 100 patients who had symptomatic lumbar spinal stenosis, selecting 19 patients who had severe symptoms for surgical treatment and 50 patients who had moderate symptoms for conservative treatment and randomizing 31 patients between the two treatment modalities (18, conservative; 13, surgical). After 4 years, excellent or fair results were found in half of the conservatively managed patients and 80% of the surgically treated group. Although the outcome after 10 years was most favorable for the surgically treated group, the investigators pointed out that an initial conservative approach seems advisable for many patients, because those who have initial unsatisfactory results still can be offered surgery with a good outcome at a later date.

Atlas and colleagues [25,26] reported on results of a prospective cohort study of surgical or conservative treatment of patients who had lumbar spinal stenosis recruited from the practices of orthopedic surgeons and neurosurgeons throughout Maine, designated the Maine Lumbar Spine Study. Of 148 patients enrolled initially, 4-year outcome measures (level of low back pain, leg pain, and the predominant symptom in the week immediately preceding the evaluation, rated as better, the same, or worse; and degree of patient satisfaction) were available on 119 patients (67 treated surgically and 52 treated nonsurgically) [25]. The surgically treated patients had more severe symptoms and worse functional status at baseline and better outcomes at 4-year evaluation than the nonsurgically treated group, even after adjustment for differences in baseline characteristics. The relative benefit of surgery declined over time but remained superior to nonsurgical treatment. In a second report of the Maine Lumbar Spine Study, Atlas and colleagues [26] reported on the evaluation of 105 patients still alive 10 years after enrollment. After 8 to 10 years, a similar percentage of surgical and nonsurgical patients reported that their low back pain was improved, their predominant symptom improved, and they were satisfied with their current status, although leg pain relief and back-related functional status continued to favor those treated surgically. The investigators concluded by noting that over time it is likely that symptoms of lumbar spinal stenosis will remain stable, and, therefore, for patients who have any trepidation about surgery, conservative management seems appropriate, because long-term outcomes are similar irrespective of treatment modality [26].

Deciding on the most appropriate program of management for a given patient (whether or not to treat conservatively or surgically, the timing of surgery, and which procedure to select) remains a complex decision-making process that requires factoring in the severity of a patient's symptoms, general medical condition, tolerance for anesthesia, and personal preferences for treatment options. Furthermore, lumbar spinal stenosis is a degenerative condition that does not necessarily worsen with time but has periodic exacerbations and remittances [25]. Johnsson and colleagues [27] described the clinical course of 32 untreated patients who had lumbar spinal stenosis observed over a mean of 49 years. The mean age was 60 years, all had back pain, 75% had neurogenic claudication, all had myelographically defined lumbar canal stenosis, and 30 had EMG abnormalities typical of nerve root involvement. The patients in this study had not undergone surgery because their medical conditions qualified as contraindications or because they refused surgery. At follow-up, patients were evaluated by questionnaire and asked to compare their situation before myelography with their present status, specifically with regard to their walking capacity and their level of pain. Seventy percent of the cases were unchanged, 15% showed improvement, and 15% worsened.

In light of this report and the observation that surgical intervention may be associated with significant increased morbidity, surgical complications, and mortality [8], it seems appropriate to offer conservative management to patients experiencing mild to moderate symptoms when symptoms are not progressive and when work and leisure activities are not hampered seriously. Controlled trials examining the outcome of conservative management, however, are lacking [6].

Several conservative interventions can be considered. Physical therapy can provide gentle back and leg strengthening exercises and mobility training that can reduce the risk of falling. Exercises may include use of an exercise bicycle and brief walks (encouraging walking with a rolling walker to promote a pain-alleviating flexed posture). In addition, patients should avoid lumbar extension exercises, consider the occasional use of lumbar bracing, and adopt a weight loss program if obese. Other treatments of unproved or anecdotal value include medications, such as nonsteroidal anti-inflammatory drugs and muscle relaxants, transcutaneous nerve stimulation and ultrasound therapy, and periodic courses of epidural corticosteroid injections. Delport and colleagues [28] conducted a retrospective review of 140 patients over age 55 who had lumbar spinal stenosis and who had received epidural corticosteroid injections, transforaminally or caudally and under fluoroscopic guidance. The injections provided approximately one third of patients with more than 2 months of relief and more than 50% of patients with improvement in function. Fluoroscopic guidance seems necessary to ensure proper placement of the injecting needle in the epidural space, specifically in the neighborhood of the desired nerve roots.

For some individuals, conservative measures fail to provide adequate relief from severe symptoms of neurogenic claudication that may reach the point of compromising quality of life. In such cases, it is appropriate to consider surgical intervention, even in the geriatric population, to improve walking tolerance and ease disabling leg and back pain [5,7,15]. Although widely agreed on validated indications for surgery do not exist (surgical emergencies, however, such as rapidly progressive cauda equina syndrome, are rare) [7]. Good to excellent results of surgery are reported on average in 64% of cases [29], but the range in the published literature is 24% to 100% and there is a great deal of heterogeneity among studies with regard to patient population, patient selection, and outcome measures [7]; the studies are observational and nonrandomized [26]; and surgical techniques are varied [15]. Surgical options include multilevel decompressive laminectomies (because canal stenosis occurs commonly over several levels), unilateral decompressive hemilaminectomy, and multilevel laminotomies, whereby fenestrations are created by removing portions of the lamina of adjacent involved vertebrae, preserving spinous processes, and sparing interspinous ligaments. The goals of surgical intervention are pain relief, increased mobility, preservation of neural tissue, and prevention of increasing clinical deficits [30]. Goals for successful operations include decompression of affected structures (the extent of which depends on the exact location of the stenosis: central canal or lateral recesses or both) and the maintenance of spinal stability postoperatively (usually achieved by preserving facet joint integrity and protecting the pars interarticularis). Spinal fusion becomes necessary to maintain spinal stability during multilevel procedures, when facet joint and pars integrity cannot be preserved. In a systematic review of preoperative predictors for postoperative clinical outcome (level of pain) in lumbar spinal stenosis, depression, coexisting cardiovascular comorbidity, poor walking (resulting from joint athritis, neurologic disease, cardiopulmonary disease), and scoliosis predict poorer subjective outcome (worse postoperative pain). Better subjective outcome is predicted by factors, such as better walking ability, self-rated health, higher income, less coexisting disease, and pronounced central stenosis [31].

In the special case of the management of spinal stenosis in Paget's disease, treatment of this complex metabolic bone disorder is multifaceted. Typically it begins with antipagetic medical therapy, including bisphosphonates, calcitonin, and mithramycin, which often is successful in improving or reversing the clinical symptoms of lumbar spinal stenosis [17]. Surgical decompression of spinal stenosis may be necessary should there be failure of medical treatment and is best tailored to the pathology causing neural compression.

References

[1] Verbeist H. Radicular syndrome from developmental narrowing of the lumbar vertebral canal. J Bone Joint Surg Br 1954;26:230–7.

[2] Javid MJ, Hadar EJ. Long-term follow-up review of patients who underwent laminectomy for lumbar stenosis: a prospective study. J Neurosurg 1998;89:1–7.

[3] Szpalski M, Gunzburg R. Lumbar spinal stenosis in the elderly: an overview. Eur Spine J 2003;12:S170–5.

[4] Haig AJ, Tong HC, Yamakawa KS, et al. Spinal stenosis, back pain, or no symptoms at all? A masked study comparing radiologic and electrodiagnostic diagnoses to the clinical impression. Arch Phys Med Rehabil 2006;87:897–903.

[5] Szpalski M, Gunzburg R. Lumbar spinal stenosis: clinical features and new trends in surgical treatment. Geriatric Times. July/August, 2004:vol. V(Issue 4). Available at: http://www.geriatrictimes.com/g040811.html.

[6] Treatment of Degenerative Lumbar Spinal Stenosis. Summary, Evidence Report/Technology Assesment: 32. AHRQ Publication No. 01–E047. Rockville (MD): Agency for Healthcare Research and Quality. Available at: http://www.ahrq.gov/clinic/epcsums/stenosum.htm. Accessed March 2001.

[7] Furman MB, Puttlitz KM, Pannullo R, et al. Spinal stenosis and neurogenic claudication. Available at: http://www.imedicine.com/DisplayTopic.asp?bookid=11&topic=133. Accessed March 23, 2006. The eMedicine Clinical Knowledge Base.

[8] Ciol MA, Deyo RA, Howell E, et al. An assessment of surgery for spinal stenosis: time trends, geographic variations, complications, reoperations. J Am Geriatr Soc 1996;44(3):285–90.

[9] Arbit E, Pannullo S. Lumbar stenosis. A clinical review. Clin Orthop Relat Res 2001;384:137–43.

[10] Thomeer RTWM, van Dijk JMC. Surgical treatment of lumbar stenosis in achondroplasia. J Neurosurg 2002;96(Suppl 3):292–7.

[11] Deyo RA, Weinstein JN. Low back pain. N Engl J Med 2001;344:363–70.

[12] Best JT. Understanding spinal stenosis. Orthop Nurs 2002;21:48–54.

[13] Wilbourn AJ, Aminoff MJ. AAEM minimonograph 32: the electrodiagnostic examination in patients with radiculopathies. Muscle Nerve 1998;21:1612–31.

[14] Hall S, Bartelson JD, Onofrio BM, et al. Lumbar spinal stenosis. Clinical features, diagnostic procedures, and results of surgical treatment in 68 patients. Ann Intern Med 1985;103:271–5.

[15] Alvarez JA, Hardy RH. Lumbar spine stenosis: a common cause of back and leg pain. Am Fam Physician 1998;57(8):1825–38.

[16] Porter R. Spinal stenosis and neurogenic claudication. Spine 1996;21:2046–52.

[17] Hadjipavlou AG, Gaitanis IN, Katonis PG, et al. Paget's disease of the spine and its management. Eur Spine J 2001;10:370–84.

[18] Levin KH. L5 radiculopathy with reduced superficial peroneal sensory responses: intraspinal and extraspinal causes. Muscle Nerve 1998;21:3–7.

[19] Fisher MA. Electrophysiology of radiculopathies. Clin Neurophysiol 2002;113:317–35.

[20] Tang LM, Schwartz MS, Swash M. Postural effects on F wave parameters in lumbosacral root compression and canal stenosis. Brain 1988;207:207–13.

[21] Levin KH. Electrodiagnostic approach to the patient with suspected radiculopathy. Neurol Clin 2002;20:397–421.

[22] Adamova B, Sohanka S, Dusek L. Differential diagnostics in patients with mild lumbar spinal stenosis: the contributions and limits of various tests. Eur Spine J 2003;12:190–6.

[23] Hellman DB, Stone JH. Arthritic and musculoskeletal disorders. In: Tierney LM, McPhee SJ, Papadakis MA, editors. Current medical diagnosis and treatment. 45th edition. New York: McGraw Hill; 2006. p. 815–55.

[24] Amundsen T, Weber H, Nordal HJ, et al. Lumbar spinal stenosis: conservative or surgical management? Spine 2000;11:1424–36.

[25] Atlas SJ, Keller RB, Robson D, et al. Surgical and nonsurgical management of lumbar spinal stenosis. Four-year outcomes from the Maine Lumbar Spine Study. Spine 2000;25:556–62.

[26] Atlas SJ, Keller RB, Wu YA, et al. Long-term outcomes of surgical and nonsurgical management of lumbar spinal stenosis: 8 to 10 year results from the Maine Lumbar Spine Study. Spine 2005;30:936–43.

[27] Johnsson K-E, Rosen I, Uden A. The natural history of lumbar spinal stenosis. Clin Orthop Relat Res 1992;279:82–6.

[28] Delport EG, Cucuzzella AR, Marley JK, et al. Treatment of lumbar spinal stenosis with epidural steroid injections: a retrospective outcome study. Arch Phys Med Rehabil 2004;85: 479–84.

[29] Turner JA, Ersek M, Herron L, et al. Surgery for lumbar spinal stenosis: attempted meta-analysis of the literature. Spine 1992;17:1–8.

[30] Sengupta DK, Herkowitz HN. Lumbar spinal stenosis. Treatment strategies and indications for surgery. Orthop Clin North Am 2003;34:281–95.

[31] Aalto TJ, Malmivaara A, Kovacs F, et al. Preoperative predictors for postoperative clinical outcome in lumbar spinal stenosis: systematic review. Spine 2006;31:E648–63.

Neck and Back Pain:
Musculoskeletal Disorders

Alec L. Meleger, MD*, Lisa S. Krivickas, MD

*Department of Physical Medicine and Rehabilitation, Harvard Medical School
and Spaulding Rehabilitation Hospital, 125 Nashua Street, Boston,
Massachusetts 02114, USA*

Strains and sprains

Muscle strain and ligamentous sprain are the most common causes of acute low back and neck pain seen in the general population. Acute myogenic or muscle-mediated pain can be subdivided into delayed onset muscle soreness (DOMS) and muscle contusion, which occur after direct tissue trauma. Likewise, ligamentous injury not only is limited to pathologic elongation (sprain) but also can be classified further as a partial or a complete tear. Spinal pain of myogenic or ligamentous origin typically is observed in the context of some type of physical activity, to which patients can be accustomed or unaccustomed, and the nature of this activity can be passive, active, repetitive, or occurring as a single event, frequently involving forced muscular contraction, either concentric or, more often, eccentric (a lengthening muscle contraction).

Muscle strain probably is the most common cause of neck and low back pain. Acute muscle strain typically results from a single event of macrotrauma with the severity of injury directly proportional to the amount of force applied. This type of tissue trauma usually occurs when the muscle undergoes forceful, passive elongation or, more commonly, when elongation occurs while the muscle is in the process of activation—this is seen with eccentric muscular contractions. Tearing of muscle fibers occurs primarily at the musculotendinous interface with the belly of the muscle involved less frequently [1].

All individuals who are able to engage their muscles actively experience the discomfort of DOMS at some time in their life. This typically occurs

---

* Corresponding author. Spaulding Rehabilitation Outpatient Center—Medford, Department of PMR, 101 Main St., Suite 101, Medford, MA 02155.
  E-mail address: ameleger@partners.org (A.L. Meleger).

0733-8619/07/$ - see front matter © 2007 Elsevier Inc. All rights reserved.
doi:10.1016/j.ncl.2007.01.006

after engaging in unaccustomed physical exertion. The symptoms usually appear 24 to 48 hours after such activity and abate completely within several days. The mechanism of this type of muscle injury consists of excessive eccentric muscular contraction, which leads to significant ultrastructural changes to skeletal muscle and is considered reversible [2].

When a direct and forceful compression is applied to a muscle, as occurs commonly during sports participation, muscle contusion may develop. The trauma produces local tissue necrosis, cellular death, extravasation of heme into the interstitium, and secondary inflammatory response [3]. This type of injury is not a common cause of spinal pain and more typically involves the extremities.

Ligamentous sprains are produced by forceful, passive stretching beyond the physiologic range or with strong muscular contractions and are among the most common causes of neck or back pain [4]. Any of the many spinal ligaments can be sprained, depending on the mechanism of injury and the developmental cross-sectional area of the ligament involved; thicker ligaments are less prone to injury. Traumatic micro- and macrotears of the anterior longitudinal ligament and the cervical facet joint capsule are implicated in whiplash-type injuries [4,5].

The pain of muscle strain or ligamentous sprain is described typically as aching, sharp or dull, and ranging in intensity from mild to severe, depending on the acuity and the extent of the injury. Ligamentous injury tends to be more localized and, with complete tears, less symptomatic compared with partial ligamentous tears. Active muscular contraction and having the affected tissue undergo passive stretching are the main exacerbating factors. On physical examination, patients may have an antalgic gait, postural listing, and compromised lumbosacral or cervical ranges of motion. Visual inspection and palpatory examination may reveal local tissue swelling, edema, erythema, bruising, warmth, and tenderness. When there is full thickness muscle rupture, a palpable mass may be present.

Spinal imaging usually is indicated to rule out spinal fracture, segmental instability resulting from ligamentous laxity or rupture, nerve root impingement, or intramedullary injury of the spinal cord.

Myofascial pain

Myofascial pain is a muscle-related pain disorder caused by the local formation of trigger points. It is fairly common in the general population and almost ubiquitous among chronic pain sufferers, with at least one study showing a prevalence of 85% among consecutively seen patients at a comprehensive pain center [6].

The hypothesis accepted most commonly regarding the pathophysiology of trigger point–related pain places the blame on the abnormally active motor end plate in which excessive and continuous release of acetylcholine produces a constant state of myofibril contraction. Prolonged contraction causes local tissue hypoxia with edema and, if not reversed, leads to the development of ischemic muscle pain [7]. Trigger points do not have any abnormal histologic findings, and electromyogram of muscle affected by myofascial pain is normal.

The pain of trigger points is described typically as dull, deep, and aching, with an ever-present stereotypic pain referral pattern. For example, when the trapezius muscle is involved, the pain usually is localized to the suprascapular region with a referral pattern into the upper neck and to the parietooccipital and periorbital areas. The intensity of pain can change from day to day and typically is exacerbated by maintenance of static postures, repetitive movement, stress, lack of sleep, and nutritional imbalance. Patients also complain of decreased range of motion, local tenderness, and some dysesthesias.

On physical examination, a taut and tender muscle band, which reproduces a patient's typical pattern of referred pain when an appropriate amount of pressure is applied, can be palpated locally. A local twitch response is elicited by snapping the trigger point manually. The involved region may exhibit decreased range of motion and some pain-related local muscle weakness.

Fibromyalgia pain syndrome

Fibromyalgia, a chronic and complex pain syndrome, typically presents with symptoms of diffuse body pain frequently involving the spinal region. Whereas myofascial pain may involve only one or two regions of the body, the pain of fibromyalgia is widespread and accompanied by multiple tender points, which differ from trigger points histologically and lack the typical trigger point pain referral pattern. Epidemiologic studies show that approximately 2% of United States population and 6% to 10% of patients seen in the average medical practice carry this diagnosis [8,9]. Women tend to be affected more frequently than men, with initial onset of symptoms in the second or third decade of life. Given the lack of objective clinical findings, the diagnosis of fibromyalgia can be delayed for many years, leading to unnecessary medical treatments and unfortunate desperation on a patient's part. Possible predisposing factors and triggers include physical trauma, psychologic stress, and a history of physical or sexual abuse [10]. Genetic predisposition also may play a role in the development of this condition [11]. Altered central processing of nociceptive stimuli leading to heightened pain response is believed the main pathophysiologic mechanism of fibromyalgia. Spinal fluid abnormalities, such as abnormal elevation of substance P, decreased levels of excitatory amino acids, and systemic deficiency of serotonin, also are postulated as causative factors [12–14]. Several other chronic conditions frequently are associated with fibromyalgia. These include chronic fatigue, sleep disturbance, myofascial pain, irritable bladder syndrome, irritable bowel syndrome, and cognitive dysfunction.

Patients present typically with constant, frequently debilitating, bilateral, widespread pain with an axial predisposition. The pain usually is exacerbated by physical activity, stress, lack of sleep, cold, and damp weather. Patients might complain of generalized weakness, daily fatigue, muscle and joint stiffness, and generalized tenderness. Other frequent symptoms include unrefreshed sleep, depressed mood, anxiety, urinary frequency, irritable bowel, and multiple chemical sensitivities. On physical examination, patients may have decreased spinal range of motion, pronounced pain behavior, psychomotor retardation, slowed mentation, and a relative degree of somnolence. Generalized tactile allodynia is a pathognomonic finding in fibromyalgia, and tenderness of at least 11 of 18 designated tender points tends to support the diagnosis. Breakaway weakness is observed commonly; however, neurologic examination typically is normal.

Diagnostically, imaging and laboratory studies are used to rule out other musculoskeletal conditions or systemic disorders, such as hypothyroidism, myopathy, rheumatic disease, and electrolyte or nutrient abnormalities [15]. Referral for a sleep study is recommended if a serious sleep disorder, such as sleep apnea or restless legs syndrome, is suspected.

Facet joint pain

The facet or zygapophyseal joints are true synovial, diarthrodial joints, which make up the posterior elements of the spinal column and provide stable intervertebral bridging, affording relative, but restricted, degrees of spinal mobility. The segments with the most degrees of freedom, as confirmed by the prevalence of "wear and tear" pathology, are the C5/6, C6/7, L4/5, and L5/S1 spinal segments. Each facet joint receives dual sensory, nociceptive innervation, which is carried by the medial branches of the segmentally adjacent posterior primary rami. The presence of nociceptive nerve endings and multisegmental innervation of a single facet joint implicates these structures as a possible source of back pain and explains the diffuse, nonfocal nature of their symptom production [16,17].

Traumatic capsular tears and age-related osteoarthritic changes are the most common causes of facet joint–mediated pain. Central canal and neuroforaminal narrowing secondary to facet joint hypertrophy, with or without osteophyte or synovial cyst formation, can contribute to the clinical presentation of spinal stenosis or radiculopathy.

Unfortunately, there are no known pathognomonic findings on history or physical examination that can provide a significant level of certainty in the diagnosis of facet-mediated pain. The pain is described typically as aching, deep, and dull with aggravating factors, such as standing, walking, flexion, and extension. Facet-mediated pain consists of the axial and the distal, referred component with the former producing more intense symptoms [18]. The cervical referral patterns typically involve the parietal, occipital, shoulder, upper arm, and periscapular regions. Pain produced by the lumbar facet joints can be referred to the buttocks, groin, and thigh and even distal to the knee. On physical examination, patients may have decreased spinal range of motion, localized muscle spasm, paraspinal muscle tenderness, and a normal neurologic examination unless facet joint hypertrophy or synovial cysts are causing radiculopathy or contributing to spinal stenosis. Facet joint loading achieved by spinal extension with concomitant, ipsilateral rotation can reproduce typical symptoms but is not shown to be clinically specific or sensitive.

Diagnostically, the presence of facet joint arthropathy on spinal imaging does not provide evidence that the pain experienced by a patient is facet joint mediated, because facet spondylosis is a common finding in asymptomatic individuals and in the ageing population. Fig. 1 is an axial CT image of lumbar spine showing facet joint osteophyte formation. Nevertheless, MRI provides the best overall imaging information about the degree of hypertrophy, presence or absence of intra-articular fluid, and the level of neural impingement by a facet cyst or an osteophyte. Single photon emission CT (SPECT) scanning also can provide additional information on the level of inflammatory activity within the joints; however, this study is not recommended as part of the routine diagnostic work-up. Diagnostic medial branch blockade under fluoroscopic guidance can provide a level of certainty but depends greatly on the expertise of the injectionist, the technique used, blinding of patients, and interpretation of the results with a thorough understanding of local anatomy. In addition to the facet joints, the medial branches also innervate the interspinous and supraspinous ligaments and the multifidi.

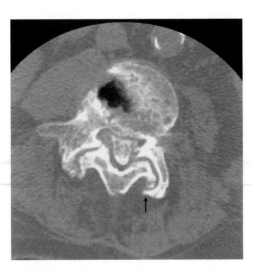

Fig. 1. CT axial image of lumbar spine. The facet joint lines appear irregular with evidence of osteophyte formation (*arrow*).

Internal disk disruption

A controversial entity, internal disk disruption (IDD), is proposed as a cause of diskogenically mediated pain limited to the internal milieu of the intervertebral disk and separate from other clinical entities that produce their pathologic effect by deformation of the disk's external contour as seen with disk protrusion, extrusion, or free disk fragments. According to one study, IDD is present in 39% of individuals suffering from chronic low back pain and most commonly affects L4/5 and L5/S1 vertebral segments [19]. IDD occurs as part of the degenerative cascade, which can be age related, post-traumatic, or influenced by genetic predisposition [20]. Progressive annular deterioration and fissuring eventually can extend to involve the outer third of the annulus fibrosis, which is populated thickly with nociceptive nerve endings [21]. Stimulation of these nociceptors, through direct extension of annular tears or via an inflammatory cascade initiated by the local release of proinflammatory cytokines, is proposed as a cause of spinal pain secondary to IDD [22].

Unfortunately, there are few symptoms and physical findings that can diagnose IDD consistently and reliably [19]. It is believed, however, that individuals who have IDD typically complain of axial spinal pain that increases with sitting and, to a lesser degree, standing. Distal and proximal referred pain also can be part of the clinical picture without direct compression of the exiting spinal nerve roots [23]. On physical examination, patients may present with a severely diminished range of motion involving the affected vertebral segment and an inability to maintain a sitting or standing position. Neurologic symptoms or findings conspicuously are absent. Severe muscle spasm and tactile hyperalgesia often can be appreciated at the involved level.

The gold standard for diagnosis of IDD is provocative diskography immediately followed by CT, which provides a better visual delineation of the location and extent of annular tears. Fig. 2 is a fluoroscopic postcontrast image from a lumbar diskogram. The L3/L4 and L4/L5 intervertebral disks appear normal. The L5/S1 disk shows extensive fissuring with significant loss in disk height. Diskographic pressurization provides more of a physiologic and dynamic examination of the disk architecture and tends to reproduce concordant pain within the symptomatic, diseased intervertebral disk. There is, however, a significant amount of controversy surrounding provocative diskography and its usefulness in directing treatment or predicting spinal fusion outcomes successfully [24,25]. Population studies fail to show good correlation between degenerative spinal pathology, as depicted on MRI, and the presence of clinically significant spinal pain [26]. Studies comparing MRI findings with the results of provocative diskography show a correlation between the presence of intradiskal high-intensity zones and positive diskographic results [27]. A high-intensity zone is believed one of the hallmarks of IDD and is believed to represent an active annular tear.

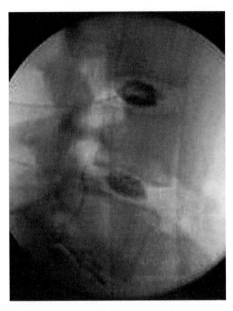

Fig. 2. Fluoroscopic postcontrast images of a lumbar diskogram. The L3/L4 and L4/L5 intervertebral disks appear normal. The L5/S1 disk shows extensive fissuring with significant loss in disk height.

Somatic dysfunction

Somatic dysfunction is an osteopathic term, defined as impaired or altered function of related components of the somatic (body framework) system; skeletal, arthrodial, and myofascial structures; and related vascular, lymphatic, and neural elements [28]. Somatic dysfunction of the vertebral column can lead to spinal pain with a proximal or distal referral pattern and clinically and functionally significant restriction of cervicothoracolumbar, occipitocervical, or sacroiliac ranges of motion. These restrictions also can lead to the development of cervicogenic headache, functional leg length discrepancy, gait abnormality, peripheral joint pain, and restricted breathing in cases involving costovertebral and sternocostal motion segments. Treatment of lumbar vertebral somatic dysfunction with osteopathic techniques is shown to relieve pain in a recent meta-analysis [29].

There are several proposed physiologic mechanisms that can lead to the development of somatic dysfunction, such as synovial meniscoid entrapment, poor tracking of the two opposing diarthrodial surfaces, physicochemical alteration of synovial fluid properties, alteration of muscle length and tone leading to asymmetric effects on the joints, and more obvious causes, such as trauma, degenerative disease, and inflammatory or neurologic conditions affecting normal physical functioning of the musculoskeletal system [28].

Diagnosis of vertebral somatic dysfunction is made by conducting a comprehensive structural examination through observation for asymmetry in posture and gait and through a detailed range-of-motion evaluation of symptomatic and distal, asymptomatic motion segments. Palpatory examination provides information on tissue texture, temperature, thickness, tone, and motion sense.

Imaging studies typically do not provide information on whether or not somatic dysfunction is present but do provide information about the possible cause of the dysfunction and can direct osteopathic treatment. In cases of acute disk herniation or osteoporosis, high-velocity low-amplitude manipulation absolutely is contraindicated.

Spinal fractures

Nonosteoporotic fractures of the spine can occur after significant spinal trauma or as a consequence of primary malignant or metastatic disease. Detailed discussion on the diagnosis and management of spinal fractures is beyond the scope of this article. In general, new-onset spinal pain after significant injury that involves axial compression, hyperextension, or flexion-type trauma should be assessed for possible fracture or fracture/dislocation. Patients who have a suspicion of post-traumatic spinal fracture need to undergo immediate clinical and radiologic assessment for fracture stability and to rule out spinal cord injury. In older individuals who have new onset of nontraumatic spinal pain or in patients who have a clinical history suspicious for primary or metastatic disease of the spine, malignant fractures need to be ruled out. Cancers that typically metastasize to the spine originate in the breast, prostate, lung, kidney, and stomach. Multiple myeloma is the most common primary spinal malignancy. Complaints of generalized malaise, deteriorating appetite, weight loss, and constant or progressive pain that is worse nocturnally are some of the typical symptoms in individuals who have malignancy.

X-ray imaging is the modality used most commonly in the diagnosis of spinal fractures. At times, when a fracture is suspected and not observed with plain radiography or if a detailed examination of a fracture is required, CT is used. MRI with intravenous contrast typically is used to assess the relative age of the fracture and the state of the neural elements and to help detect a malignant infiltrative process. Bone scintigraphy can provide information on the level of relative metabolic activity within the fracture itself.

Vertebral osteomyelitis

Bacterial osteomyelitis is the most common type of spinal vertebral infection. It is notoriously difficult to diagnose early because of its insidious nature and lack of localizing symptoms and signs. Rapid diagnosis, however, is paramount, because delay in treatment can lead to spinal deformity and instability, paralysis, sepsis, and even death. The vertebral body is the most common site of bacterial seeding, with the posterior elements, such as lamina or facet joints, rarely involved. Lumbar spine is involved most frequently, followed by the thoracic and cervical spinal regions. Hematogenous bacterial dissemination is the most common pathophysiologic mechanism for vertebral osteomyelitis. The genitourinary tract is the source of infection identified most often, followed by the respiratory tract, oral cavity, and skin ulcers or wounds [30]. Direct inoculation as a result of a spinal procedure or surgery or contiguous spread from a local soft tissue infection is another mechanism of seeding. The organism isolated most frequently in vertebral osteomyelitis is *Staphylococcus aureus*, followed by *Streptococcus* and enteric gram-negative rods *Candida*, and *Pseudomonas* are seen most commonly in intravenous drug users. Some of the well-known predisposing factors are male gender, diabetes mellitus, immunocompromised state, sickle cell anemia, hemodialysis, spinal instrumentation, and intravenous drug use [30].

In the early stages of infection, patients typically complain of axial pain, which is gradual and nontraumatic in onset, becoming constant and progressive in nature over time. Nocturnal pain, symptoms of malaise, generalized fatigue, and depressed appetite commonly are seen with fever and, surprisingly, observed rarely. Neurologic symptoms are not seen until later stages, when the infection extends directly into the epidural space and an epidural abscess begins to compress the adjacent neural tissues. On physical examination, patients may appear listless and in severe pain, unable to tolerate standing or sitting. The site of infection typically is warm to touch and sensitive to palpation, with evidence of surrounding muscle spasm. Neurologic deficits consistent with radiculopathy or spinal cord compression are seen in severe cases.

Leukocytosis notoriously is absent. Early in the disease process, elevation in sedimentation rate and C-reactive protein has high sensitivity and low specificity; blood cultures often fail to isolate the causative organisms. The results of CT-guided disk or vertebral biopsy also frequently are unsuccessful in pinpointing the bacterial cause. It can take up to several weeks for plain radiographs to show radiologic evidence of spinal infection, such as disk space narrowing and end plate destruction. In the later stages, radiographs may show vertebral collapse with or without bony sclerosis and the presence of soft tissue mass. MRI with administration of intravenous gadolinium is the imaging modality of choice for early detection of osteomyelitis. Bone scintigraphy has high sensitivity but unfortunately cannot differentiate an infection from metastasis or a degenerative, inflammatory process.

Polymyalgia rheumatica

Polymyalgia rheumatica (PMR) is a rheumatologic syndrome of unknown etiology that may produce neck and trunk pain. The disease typically develops in patients age 50 and older and tends to evolve over the course of 4 to 8 weeks. The diagnosis primarily is clinical, but suggested diagnostic criteria include (1) aching and morning stiffness lasting greater than 30 minutes and involving at least two of the following regions: neck, shoulder girdle, and pelvic girdle; (2) age greater than 50; (3) erythrocyte sedimentation rater greater than 40; (4) duration of symptoms greater than 1 month; and (5) no other disease present [31]. Patients have a normal neurologic examination without significant muscle weakness. Diseases that need to be excluded in the differential diagnosis include various forms of arthritis, viral myalgia, fibromyalgia, polymyositis, hypothyroidism, depression, and occult malignancy or infection [32]. Once a diagnosis of PMR is made, it is important to rule out temporal arteritis, which approximately 15% of patients who have PMR develop. Temporal arteritis, when untreated, can produce visual loss. PMR is treatable and responds well to low-dose oral corticosteroids (10–20 mg/day of prednisone); if it is associated with temporal arteritis, higher doses of corticosteroids are required.

Atlantoaxial instability

The transverse ligament and the two facet joints provide the majority of the stability to the C1/C2 articulation. When these structures are disrupted, pathologically excessive movement occurs, known as atlantoaxial instability. Forced rotational trauma and medical conditions, such as rheumatoid arthritis and Down syndrome, in which ligamentous laxity and inflammatory joint erosions occur, are common causes of atlantoaxial instability. Anomalies of the odontoid process, such as aplasia, hypoplasia, and os odontoideum, in which there is incomplete fusion of the odontoid to the body of the axis, also can produce atlantoaxial instability. Severe neurologic deficits can occur when the central spinal canal becomes compromised by atlantoaxial instability. Individuals who carry this diagnosis can be completely asymptomatic or present with complete tetraplegia requiring ventilator support. Early symptoms may include neck and suboccipital pain, especially with cervical flexion/extension and rotation. In more advanced cases, signs and symptoms of myelopathy become more prevalent.

Atlantoaxial instability can be diagnosed with plain radiographs by measuring the atlantodens interval with views of the cervical spine in neutral and in flexion and extension. The atlantodens interval is defined as the distance between the posterior aspect of the anterior arch of the atlas and the odontoid process. In adults, this distance should not exceed 3 mm, and in children it should not be greater than 5 mm. CT scanning and, to a better degree, MRI can assess the degree of spinal canal narrowing further and whether or not there is significant damage to the spinal cord itself.

Atlanto-occipital joint pain

Some clinical and investigational evidence points to the atlanto-occipital (C0/C1) joints as possible sources of suboccipital and occipital pain [33]. The cranium articulates with the rest of the cervical spine via these two joints which, given their sagitally oriented anatomy, allow for most of the cervical flexion and extension. This craniocervical articulation is a stable construct except when it is still underdeveloped in children or when significant trauma causes atlanto-occipital dissociation resulting in death from brain stem compression. Degenerative joint arthritis and acceleration-deceleration injury probably are the most common mechanisms leading to C0/C1 joint pain. Patients who have this type of pathology report increased pain with neck flexion and extension maneuvers.

Osteoporotic vertebral compression fracture

Osteoporosis is a systemic bone disorder characterized by pathologic decrease in the bone mass resulting from greater net bone resorption than new bone formation. Osteoporotic vertebral compression fractures can be a common cause of spinal pain in the older patient population and affect approximately 25% of postmenopausal women in the United States [34]. The prevalence of this condition shows continued progression with advancing age and, although less common, can be a source of morbidity in older males [35]. The risk factors for the development of osteoporotic fractures are the same as those for osteoporosis. They include advanced age, female gender, Caucasian and Asian races, family and personal history of prior compression fractures, susceptibility to falling, estrogen and nutritional deficiency, lack of physical activity, and low weight. Antecedent trauma not always is a prerequisite. Some compression fractures occur during quiet sleep or while performing such normal activities as sitting or bending forward [36].

The pain typically is described as having a sudden onset, axial in location, sharp, ranging from mild to severe in intensity, and exacerbated by sitting, standing, and bending forward. A percentage of these fractures, however, is clinically silent without concomitant pain. Neurologic symptoms usually are absent except when, in rare circumstances, a burst fracture causes retropulsion of bone fragments into the spinal canal. On physical examination, patients may have exaggerated thoracic kyphosis resulting form loss of anterior vertebral height at multiple levels. The area of compression fracture usually is tender to palpation with evidence of surrounding muscle spasm.

The typical radiographic appearance of an osteoporotic compression fracture includes anterior wedging of the vertebral body with sparing of elements of the middle and posterior columns. Plain radiographs, however, are not able to provide the age of the fracture, which can help with directing treatment. MRI with fat suppression and SPECT scanning can assess the relative age and the extent of metabolic activity of the compression fracture.

Scheuermann's disease (Sheuermann's kyphosis)

Scheuermann's disease is a developmental disorder of the spine, which has a familial predisposition and usually affects skeletally immature adolescent males. The initial sign is a postural deformity, specifically thoracic kyphosis, which becomes progressive over time. In the early stages of the disease, patients can be completely asymptomatic and later, with progression of the deformity and the resultant compensatory lumbar lordosis, may begin to complain of axial thoracic and lumbar discomfort. This type of kyphotic deformity does not reduce with extension, as seen in individuals who have rounded back posture. Anterior vertebral wedging of at least three adjacent vertebra with evidence of end plate abnormalities on lateral views confirms the diagnosis. MRI can depict further degenerative diskogenic changes, such as disk desiccation and formation of Schmorl's nodes, at multiple intervertebral levels.

Spondylolysis

Spondylolysis is a structural defect of pars interarticularis, which connects the superior facet articular process to its lamina. This defect can be unilateral or bilateral and is observed most commonly at the L5 vertebral level. Spondylolysis is caused by a genetic predisposition or fatigue stress injury of the neural arch, most commonly of the repetitive extension type, as seen in gymnasts, weight lifters, and football players [37]. General population studies show an overall prevalence rate of 3% to 6%, with initial occurrence in the preschool years and peaking in the early adulthood [38]. One of the major concerns with bilateral spondylolysis is progressive spondylolisthesis, when a superior vertebral body undergoes anterior slippage with respect to the inferior vertebral segment. The risk of significant slippage is low in skeletally mature individuals and occurs most frequently during the adolescent growth spurt.

Most people who have radiologically confirmed spondylolysis are clinically asymptomatic [38]. When the fatigue fracture of spondylolysis is an active or acute lesion, the pain is in the low back with intermittent radiation into the gluteal and proximal lower extremity regions. On physical examination, patients may present with a hyperlordotic lumbar spine, tight hamstrings, tenderness of the affected lumbar segment, and reproduction of pain, with maneuvers stressing lumbar extension and ipsilateral rotation. The neurologic examination should be normal unless an additional pathologic process is present.

Oblique radiographs (Scotty dog view) can demonstrate a defect in the pars, but they have low sensitivity [39]. Fig. 3 is an X-ray image showing a noticeable defect within pars interarticularis. CT scanning is the gold standard test for the presence of the spondylolytic defect. SPECT scanning is used to determine if the lesion is metabolically active, which would direct the course of treatment.

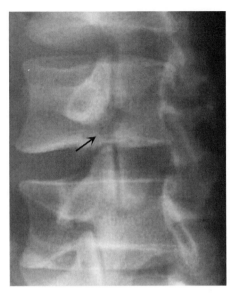

Fig. 3. Oblique X-ray image of lumbar spondylolitis. A noticeable defect within pars interarticularis (*arrow*) is present.

Spondylolisthesis

Spondylolisthesis occurs when a superior vertebra slips anteriorly with respect to the inferior vertebrae; this type of pathology is termed anterolisthesis. Retrolisthesis occurs when a posterior slip is observed. The etiology of the slippage is classified as congenital, isthmic, degenerative, pathologic, traumatic, or iatrogenic. Isthmic or spondylolytic spondylolisthesis is the most common type and is the result of bilateral defects within pars interarticularis. A congenital or dysplastic variant is seen when abnormalities in facet joint orientation or developmental abnormality of the pars occur. Pathologic slipping of degenerative spondylolisthesis occurs in the context of intervertebral disk and facet joint, age-related degeneration and is seen most often at L4-L5 vertebral level but also can be observed at other lumbar levels and the cervical spine. The spinal column also can be rendered unstable by a local or systemic disease process, by trauma, or iatrogenically, by an overzealous surgical decompression. The extent of listhesis is classified by grades ranging from I to V, with grade I associated with 25% slip, II 50%, III 75%, and IV 100%. Grade V, spondyloptosis, occurs when the superior vertebra completely "falls off" the underlying vertebra or sacral promontory, in the case of L5/S1 pathology.

Patients who have spondylolisthesis can be completely asymptomatic or present with severe neurologic compromise depending on the severity of slip. The symptoms range from mild low back pain to, in the case of high-grade slips, severe radicular pain, leg weakness, and urogenital deficits. On physical examination, a hyperlordotic posture, waddling gait, tight hamstrings, and a step off lumbar deformity can be observed. Depending on the spinal segment involved, upper or lower motor findings, sensory deficits, or an abnormal bulbocavernosus reflex can be seen on neurologic examination.

Lateral plain radiographs, CT, and MRI all are sensitive in detecting and assessing the extent of the spondylolisthetic deformity. Fig. 4 is a radiograph of L4/L5 degenerative grade II anterolisthesis. There is significant loss of intervertebral height with intraforaminal osteophyte formation emanating from the posterior border of L4 and L5 vertebral bodies. CT scanning is valuable in providing greater bone detail, and MRI provides information on the severity of neural element involvement in cases of high-grade central canal stenosis or neuroforaminal narrowing.

Pregnancy-related low back pain

Fifty percent to 90% of pregnant women experience back pain during pregnancy [40]; the lower lumbar spine and sacroiliac joints are involved most commonly. Risk factors for back pain during pregnancy are advanced maternal age, previous history of back pain, and the number of prior pregnancies. There is no demonstrated relationship between the presence of pain

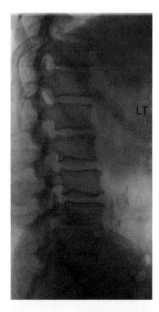

Fig. 4. X-ray image of L4/L5 degenerative grade II anterolisthesis. There is significant loss in the intervertebral disk height with presence of intraforaminal osteophyte formation emanating from the posterior borders of L4 and L5 vertebral bodies.

and the size of the baby or amount of weight gained by the mother [41,42]. Engaging in an exercise program before pregnancy reduces the risk of back pain during pregnancy [43]. The pain radiates only occasionally to the thighs and rarely has a radicular quality.

The cause of this pain is unclear and probably is multifactorial. Hormonal alterations (increased relaxin levels) produce increased ligamentous laxity, and biomechanics are altered by the anterior displacement of the center of gravity, producing an anterior pelvic tilt and increased lumbar lordosis. Some of the pain may be the result of the development of spondylolysis or progression of spondylolisthesis. Women who have had children have a higher incidence of L4-5 spondylolisthesis than those who have not had children [44]. Vascular compression by the gravid uterus when supine and disk herniation also can produce pain. If disk herniation is strongly suspected, a noncontrast MRI can be performed safely during pregnancy.

Treatment of low back pain during pregnancy should include a modified exercise program to strengthen abdominal and back muscles. A maternity support binder is helpful to some women. Acetaminophen is the pain medication of choice. Nonsteroidal anti-inflammatories are contraindicated because they can cause premature closure of the patent ductus arteriosus in the fetus. There is no evidence of risk produced by cyclobenzaprine, oxycodone, and prednisone, so they may be considered if necessary [42]. Case reports indicate that interlaminar epidural steroid injections and surgery for lumbar disk herniation can be performed safely in pregnant women if necessary (ie, surgery when neurologic deficits are progressive) [45].

Thirty percent to 45% of women continue to have low back pain in the postpartum period [46]. Risk factors for persistent pain include more severe pain during the pregnancy and failure to lose the weight gained during pregnancy. The manner in which the mother carries her infant (front pack, back pack, and so forth) may alter biomechanics of the spine and pelvis; thus, evaluation of back pain in women who have an infant should include queries along these lines. Persistent postpartum back pain should be managed as it would be in any other individual.

Kissing spines (Baastrup's disease)

An abnormality of the spine in which the spinous processes of adjacent vertebrae are in close proximity or in actual contact producing low back pain is known as Baastrup's disease, named for a Danish radiologist. Hypertrophied spinous processes, severe degenerative disk disease with significant loss in disk height, and excessive lordosis are the main contributing factors.

Patients usually complain of axial pain, which is relieved by lumbar flexion and exacerbated by standing and extension. Local palpation can elicit the typical pain, and injection of local anesthetic can relieve it, thus also serving as a diagnostic tool.

Plain radiographs or CT with sagittal reconstructions can be used to assess the extent of the spinous process hypertrophy, reactive sclerosis, and the resultant interspinous process surface flattening. Fig. 5 is a lumbar CT showing the hypertrophic spinous processes of the L4 and L5 vertebral bodies in direct contact with evident subcortical sclerosis. Lumbar MRI can evaluate further for bone edema and presence of the interspinous bursal fluid [47].

Sacroiliac joint pain

The sacroiliac joints are diarthroidial, encapsulated joints, which provide an extremely stable articulation between the sacrum and the two ilia. They are a frequent source of pain, with at least one study showing a 23% prevalence rate within a large group of patients presenting to an outpatient clinic with symptoms of low back pain [48]. These joints possess extensive, multisegmental L2-S3 sensory innervation and, thus, can present clinically with a variety of pain referral patterns. Provocation studies by intra-articular injection have produced pain in the groin, thigh, calf, and foot [49]. The idea that these joints possess a clinically relevant amount of articular translation remains controversial. Cadaveric studies show movement of 2° to 4°, and one in vivo study shows a 2° ilium on sacrum translation [50–52]. Sacroiliac

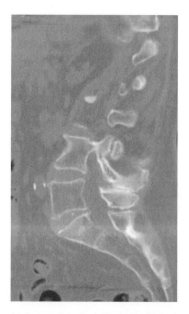

Fig. 5. Lumbar CT with sagittal reconstruction. Hypertrophic spinous processes of L4 and L5 vertebral bodies are in direct contact exhibiting significant subcortical sclerosis. Severe upper lumbar scoliosis also is evident.

joint pain often is present in individuals suffering from inflammatory conditions, such as a spondylotic arthropathy, or in a post-traumatic setting, when a capsular tear or subluxation causing somatic dysfunction occurs. In older individuals, sacroiliac joint arthropathy can produce pain.

Clinically, patients who have this source of pain complain of dull, aching, gluteal discomfort, especially with weight bearing and with ipsilateral hip and lumbosacral flexion and extension maneuvers. As discussed previously, the pain commonly is referred to other distal anatomic regions, especially the groin, but does not have proximal referral patterns, such as to the upper lumbar spine. Patients also report ipsilateral hip muscle tightness and decreased hip range of motion. On physical examination, gait antalgia on the affected side, pelvic obliquity, and leg-length discrepancy can be observed. Patients may favor their painful sacroiliac joint while sitting. Palpatory examination can exhibit sacroiliac joint line and surrounding soft tissue tenderness. Sacroiliac joint testing with the use of joint specific tests readily can reproduce a patient's usual pain, but these tests are not specific or reliably diagnostic.

Plain radiography can assess the sacroiliac joint for the presence of arthritis, but as in the case of facet joint arthropathy, arthritis is a common age-related finding with a high prevalence in asymptomatic population. MRI can detect inflammatory pathology, sacral insufficiency fractures, and ominous findings, such as tumor or abscess. Intra-articular sacroiliac joint injections performed under fluoroscopic guidance can be used for diagnostic and therapeutic purposes.

Sacral stress fracture

Stress fractures can be classified into two distinct categories: fatigue and insufficiency stress fractures. Fatigue stress fractures tend to occur in athletically active populations, when excessive and repetitive physiologic loads are applied to metabolically normal bone. Sacral insufficiency fractures occur under normal, physiologic stress in a metabolically weakened bone [53]. They are a common cause of nonspecific low back or pelvic pain in postmenopausal, osteoporotic women. Insufficiency fractures also can be part of the clinical presentation known as the female athlete triad, which consists of eating disorders, amenorrhea, and osteoporosis [54]. Some of the other known risk factors include Paget's disease, prolonged corticosteroid use, osteomalacia, rheumatoid arthritis, and local radiation treatment [55].

Typical symptoms include severe low back and gluteal or groin pain exacerbated by weight-bearing activities, such as walking and sitting. Physical examination typically reveals sacral tenderness, parasacral muscle spasm, and lack of neurologic deficits.

Plain radiographs may not detect a sacral stress fracture for up to several months after its initial occurrence and are notorious for missing these fractures altogether. MRI and bone scintigraphy are the imaging modalities of choice in terms of sensitivity and early detection. CT also can provide definitive diagnosis in cases where MRI is contraindicated or inconclusive. Insufficiency fractures also can occur in the iliac bone and within the pubic and supracetabular parts of the pelvis.

Coccygodynia

Coccygeal pain or coccygodynia is a rare disorder, observed more commonly in women and at times producing functionally limiting pain. Direct trauma to the coccyx, as seen during a fall, is a common cause. Coccygodynia also may develop when the sacrococcygeal synchondrosis is forced out of alignment during childbirth. Still, in a significant number of cases, the exact cause of coccygeal pain remains elusive.

Coccygeal pain typically is exacerbated by direct pressure on the coccyx as seen in sitting or with direct palpation. Passive internal hip rotation or straining during a bowel movement also may increase the pain.

Plain radiographs typically are ordered to rule out bone injury (such as possible dislocation) to the coccyx. In some recalcitrant cases, bone scanning might be considered to look for an ongoing inflammatory process.

References

[1] Garrett WE Jr. Muscle strain injuries: clinical and basic aspects. Med Sci Sports Exerc 1990; 22:436–43.
[2] Hesselink MK, Kuipers H, Geurten P, et al. Structural muscle damage and muscle strength after incremental number of isometric and forced lengthening contractions. J Muscle Res Cell Motil 1996;17:335–41.
[3] Fisher BD, Baracos VE, Shnitka T, et al. Ultrastructural events following acute muscle trauma. Med Sci Sports Exerc 1990;22:185–93.
[4] Ivancic PC, Pearson AM, Panjabi MM, et al. Injury of the anterior longitudinal ligament during whiplash simulation. Eur Spine J 2004;13(1):61–8.
[5] Winkelstein BA, Nightingale RW, Richardson WJ, et al. The cervical facet capsule and its role in whiplash injury: a biomechanical investigation. Spine 2000;25(10):1238–46.
[6] Fishbain DA, Goldberg M, Meagher BR, et al. Male and female chronic pain patients categorized by DSM-III psychiatric diagnostic criteria. Pain 1986;26:181–97.
[7] Mense S, Simons DG, Russell IJ. Muscle pain: understanding its nature, diagnosis, and treatment. Baltimore (MD): Lippincott Williams & Wilkins; 2001.
[8] Wolfe F, Ross K, Anderson J, et al. The prevalence and characteristics of fibromyalgia in the general population. Arthritis Rheum 1995;38:19–28.
[9] Campbell SM, Clark S, Tindall EA, et al. Clinical characteristics of fibrositis, I: a "blinded," controlled study of symptoms and tender points. Arthritis Rheum 1983;26:817–24.
[10] Wallace DJ. The fibromyalgia syndrome. Ann Med 1997;29:9–21.
[11] Offenbaecher M, Bondy B, de Jonge S, et al. Possible association of fibromyalgia with a polymorphism in the serotonin transporter gene regulatory region. Arthritis Rheum 1999;42: 2482–8.
[12] Russell IJ, Orr MD, Littman B, et al. Elevated cerebrospinal fluid levels of substance P in patients with the fibromyalgia syndrome. Arthritis Rheum 1994;37:1593–601.

[13] Russell IJ, Vaereroy H, Javors M, et al. Cerebrospinal fluid biogenic amine metabolites in fibromyalgia/fibrositis syndrome and rheumatoid arthritis. Arthritis Rheum 1992;35:550–6.

[14] Russell IJ. Neurochemical pathogenesis of fibromyalgia syndrome. Journal of Musculoskeletal Pain 1996;4:61–92.

[15] Al Faraj S, Al Mutairi K. Vitamin D deficiency and chronic low back pain in Saudi Arabia. Spine 2003;Jan 15;28(2):177–9.

[16] Ashton IK, Ashton BA, Gibson SJ, et al. Morphological basis for back pain: the demonstration of nerve fibers and neuropeptides in the lumbar facet joint capsule but not in ligamentum flavum. J Orthop Res 1992;10:72–8.

[17] Vandenabeele F, Creemers J, Lambrichts I, et al. Fine structure of vesiculated nerve profiles in the human lumbar facet joint. J Anat 1995;187:681–92.

[18] Mooney V, Robertson J. The facet syndrome. Clin Orthop Relat Res 1976;115:149–56.

[19] Schwarzer AC, Aprill CN, Derby R, et al. The prevalence and clinical features of internal disc disruption in patients with chronic low back pain. Spine 1995;20(17):1878–88.

[20] Battie MC, Videman T, Gibbons LE, et al. Volvo Award in clinical sciences. Determinants of lumbar disc degeneration: a study relating lifetime exposures and magnetic resonance imaging findings in identical twins. Spine 1995;20:2601–12.

[21] Bogduk N, Tynan W, Wilson AS, et al. The nerve supply to the human lumbar intervertebral disc. J Anat 1981;132:39–56.

[22] Burke JG, Watson RW, McCormack D, et al. Intervertebral discs which cause low back pain secrete high levels of proinflammatory mediators. J Bone Joint Surg Br 2002;84:196–201.

[23] Milette PC, Fontaine S, Lepanto L, et al. Radiating pain to the lower extremities caused by lumbar disk rupture without spinal nerve root involvement. AJNR Am J Neuroradiol 1995; 16:1605–13.

[24] Carragee EJ. 2000 Volvo Award winner in clinical studies: lumbar high-intensity zone and discography in subjects without low back problems. Spine 2000;25(23):2987–92.

[25] Carragee EJ. Low-pressure positive Discography in subjects asymptomatic of significant low back pain illness. Spine 2006;31(5):505–9.

[26] Boden SD, Davis DO, Dina TS, et al. Abnormal magnetic-resonance scans of the lumbar spine in asymptomatic subjects. J Bone Joint Surg Am 1990;72:403–8.

[27] Lam KS, Carlin D, Mulholland RC. Lumbar disc high-intensity zone: the value and significance of provocative discography in the determination of the discogenic pain source. Eur Spine J 2000;9:36–41.

[28] Greenman PE. Principles of manual medicine. 3rd edition. Philadelphia: Lippincott Williams & Wilkins; 2003. p. 65.

[29] Licciardone JC, Brimhall AK, King LN. Osteopathic manipulative treatment for low back pain: a systematic review and meta-analysis of randomized controlled trials [review]. BMC Musculoskelet Disord 2005;6:43–54.

[30] Sapico FL, Montgomerie JZ. Vertebral osteomyelitis. Infect Dis Clin North Am 1990;4: 539–50.

[31] Deal C. Polymyalgia rheumatica. In: Katirji B, Kaminski H, Preston D, et al, editors. Neuromuscular disorders in clinical practice. Boston: Butterworth Heinemann; 2002. p. 1369–75.

[32] Hunder G. Polymyalgia rheumatica: pinning down an elusive syndrome. Contemp Intern Med 1997;9:9–15.

[33] Dreyfuss P, Michaelsen M, Fletcher D. Atlanto-occipital and lateral atlanto-axial joint pain patterns. Spine 1994;19(10):1125–31.

[34] Melton LJ 3rd. Epidemiology of spinal osteoporosis. Spine 1997;22(24 Suppl):2S–11S.

[35] Resch A, Schneider B, Bernecker P, et al. Risk of vertebral fractures in men: relationship to mineral density of the vertebral body. AJR Am J Roentgenol 1995;164:1447–50.

[36] Patel U, Skingle S, Campbell GA, et al. Clinical profile of acute vertebral compression fractures in osteoporosis. Br J Rheumatol 1991;30:418–21.

[37] Rossi F. Spondylolysis, spondylolisthesis and sports. J Sports Med Phys Fitness 1978;18: 317–40.

[38] Fredrickson BE, Baker D, McHolick WJ, et al. The natural history of spondylolysis and spondylolisthesis. J Bone Joint Surg Am 1984;66:699–707.

[39] Amato M, Totty WG, Gilula LA. Spondylolysis of the lumbar spine: demonstration of defects and laminal fragmentation. Radiology 1984;153:627–9.

[40] Pivarnik JM, Chambliss HO, Clapp JF, et al. Impact of physical activity during pregnancy and postpartum on chronic disease risk. Med Sci Sports Exerc 2006;38(5):989–1006.

[41] Heckman J, Sassard R. Current concepts review: Musculoskeletal considerations in pregnancy. J Bone Joint Surg Am 1994;76:1720–30.

[42] Borg-Stein J, Dugan SA, Gruber J, et al. Musculoskeletal aspects of pregnancy. Am J Phys Med Rehabil 2005;84:180–92.

[43] Ostgaard HC, Zetherstrom G, Roos-Hansson E, et al. Reduction of back and posterior pelvic pain in pregnancy. Spine 1994;19:894–900.

[44] Sanderson P, Fraser R. The influence of pregnancy on the development of degenerative spondylolisthesis. J Bone Joint Surg Br 1996;78:951–4.

[45] Brown M, Levi A. Surgery for lumbar disc herniation during pregnancy. Spine 2001;26: 440–3.

[46] To W, Wong M. Factors associated with back pain symptoms in pregnancy and the persistence of pain 2 years after pregnancy. Acta Obstet Gynecol Scand 2003;82:1086–91.

[47] Bywaters EG, Evans S. The lumbar interspinous bursae and Baastrup's syndrome: an autopsy study. Rheumatol Int 1982;2:87–96.

[48] Bernard TN Jr, Kirkaldy-Willis WH. Recognizing specific characteristics of nonspecific low back pain. Clin Orthop Relat Res 1987;217:266–80.

[49] Fortin JD, Dwyer AP, West S, et al. Sacroiliac joint: pain referral maps upon applying a new injection/arthrography technique. Part I: asymptomatic volunteers. Spine 1994;19(13): 1475–82.

[50] Miller JAA, Schultz AB, Andersson GBJ. Load-displacement behavior of sacro-iliac joints. J Orthop Res 1987;5:92–101.

[51] Vleeming A, Van Wingerden JP, Dijkstra PF, et al. Mobility in the sacroiliac joints in the elderly: a kinematic and radiological study. Clin Biomech (Bristol, Avon) 1992;7:170–6.

[52] Sturesson B, Uden A, Vleeming A. A radiostereometric analysis of the movements of the sacroiliac joints in the reciprocal straddle position. Spine 2000;25(2):214–7.

[53] Grasland A, Pouchot J, Mathieu A, et al. Sacral insufficiency fractures: an easily overlooked cause of back pain in elderly women. Arch Intern Med 1996;156:668–74.

[54] Bennell KL, Malcolm SA, Thomas SA, et al. Risk factors for stress fractures in track and field athletes: a twelve-month prospective study. Am J Sports Med 1996;24:810–8.

[55] Blomlie V, Rofstad EK, Talle K, et al. Incidence of radiation-induced insufficiency fractures of the female pelvis: evaluation with MR imaging. AJR Am J Roentgenol 1996;167(5): 1205–10.

ELSEVIER
SAUNDERS

NEUROLOGIC
CLINICS

Neurol Clin 25 (2007) 439–471

Neck and Low Back Pain: Neuroimaging

Manzoor Ahmed, MD[a],*, Michael T. Modic, MD[b]

[a]Department of Radiology, Louis Stokes VA Medical Center, 10701 East Boulevard,
Cleveland, OH 44106-1702, USA
[b]Department of Radiology, Cleveland Clinic Foundation, 9500 Euclid Avenue,
P34, Radiology, Cleveland, OH 44195, USA

Neck and low back pain are among the most common medical disabilities in the Western world, with great economic and personal consequences [1]. According to a study by Hansson and Hansson [2], the annual total costs for back and neck problems can approximate 1% of the gross national product. Approximately 80% of the population suffers from back pain at some point in their lives [3], 80% get an imaging study, and 80% have non-specific imaging findings. A significant portion of the cost of the morbidity associated with neck and back disorders is related to diagnostic testing. A significant component of this diagnostic testing is related to medical imaging, which is used to provide accurate morphologic information. Although degenerative changes of the spine are believed to be responsible for the majority of patient symptoms, they are not the only cause, and diagnostic imaging plays an important role in providing accurate diagnostic considerations. The ability to characterize these alterations better should provide a means of stratifying patient changes more accurately, thus a more accurate understanding of etiology. Not only are morphologic changes depicted in ever-increasing anatomic detail but also additional information is emerging that may help in understanding more fundamental alterations at the cellular and biochemical level. The impact of medical imaging on therapeutic decision making and cost effectiveness, however, other than as a presurgical tool, remains untested.

What separates individuals who have dramatic morphologic findings and who have no symptoms from individuals who have identical alterations and who do have symptoms? The relationship of etiologic factors, the morphologic alterations that can be characterized by imaging, and the mechanisms of pain production and their interactions in the production of symptoms all

* Corresponding author.
E-mail address: manzoor.ahmed@med.va.gov (M. Ahmed).

0733-8619/07/$ - see front matter © 2007 Elsevier Inc. All rights reserved.
doi:10.1016/j.ncl.2007.01.007

are important and interactive factors. What follows is a review of the diagnostic imaging modalities used most commonly and their roles in patient management.

Imaging modalities

MRI

MRI currently is the test that provides the most information, albeit at a higher cost than other modalities. Using a variety of pulse sequences and paramagnetic contrast media, the extradural, intradural, and intramedullary spaces can be targeted. If the pathology is believed most likely in the extradural space, then a combination of T1, T2, and short tau inversion recovery (STIR)-weighted sequences is used. T2-weighted images provide myelographic-like display of epidural impressions by degenerative changes and sensitivity to intramedullary pathology. T1-weighted images allow a second type of contrast evaluation of the extradural structures, especially of the bone marrow and extradural soft tissue structures. STIR as a fat-suppression technique aids in the unmasking bone marrow, soft tissue edema, and infiltrative processes and provides another form of contrast for the detection of cord pathology. Gradient-echo images provide shorter scan times and sensitivity to susceptibility effects, as seen with blood by-products. Paramagnetic contrast agents are important for the detection of intramedullary disease, to assess the status of the spinal cord blood barrier. For extradural processes, such as spondylodiskitis and the postoperative spine, it can be useful in assessing epidural inflammation and fibrosis.

MR myelography generally uses a strong T2*-weighted sequence of 3-D–fast imaging with steady-state precession without intrathecal contrast injection. Although early studies have shown promise for the evaluation of nerve root compression and spinal stenosis by MR myelography [4–7], it is not used commonly in routine practice.

MR neurography uses high-resolution T1 imaging for anatomic detail, and fat-suppressed T2-weighted or STIR imaging to show abnormal nerve hyperintensity [8–10]. A wide variety of pathologies involving the sciatic nerve, such as compression, trauma, hypertrophy, neuromas, and tumor infiltration, may be seen [11,12]. MR neurography has demonstrated piriformis syndrome (piriformis muscle asymmetry and sciatic nerve hyperintensity) with a high specificity [13].

CT and other modalities

CT is an important modality in spinal imaging, with its greatest strength producing rapid, isotropic data sets, which can be post processed for evaluation of extradural disease. Without intrathecal contrast, it is insensitive to intradural and intramedullary disease. It is the most accurate modality for the evaluation of bony detail. With multidetector systems, entire regions of the spine can be examined in seconds with slices as thin as 0.6 mm, providing highly accurate bony details in the evaluation of degenerative disease and fractures and for preoperative planning. CT is also highly accurate in anatomic assessment of spinal stenosis and disk herniation [14]. Plain radiography still holds a screening role in dynamic imaging (ie, flexion and extension views to evaluate alignment for instability). Although not yet popular, dynamic CT and MRI, using flexion, extension, axial loading, or standing in open MRI systems, have been performed with positive results [15–17].

Conventional myelography has been replaced almost completely by CT myelography, particularly with the advent of multidetector scanners [18]. The use of this procedure, which requires the instillation of a contrast medium intrathecally, currently is limited to preoperative confirmation of MR findings in selected cases, inconclusive MRI scans, postoperative instrumented spine disease, and patients who have MRI contraindications. The focus of the examination is assessment of epidural impressions on the thecal sac and filling of the nerve root sleeves. Dynamic CT myelography, using flexion extension positioning or axial loading to unmask positional stenosis, can be performed but is not yet accepted widely [16]. Provocative diskography is used for the evaluation of persistent back pain that is unexplained by other less invasive tests. It also is used for pre-fusion assessment to determine the status of disk spaces above and below levels of proposed fusion. The cardinal component of diskography is disk stimulation, not the morphology of the disk at diskography [19]. The criticism of diskography is related mainly to its invasive nature, reliability of the patient response, and lack of specificity [20–22].

Several radiologic procedures are promoted as techniques that provide localizing and therapeutic value in patients who have spine disease. Diagnostic nerve root and epidural injections are reported as having a high positive predictive value but low or indeterminate negative predictive value and specificity [23,24]. Diagnostic facet and sacroiliac joint blocks involve the instillation of local anesthetic around facet joint nerves (medial branch or dorsal ramus) and are reported to be reproducible, reasonably accurate, and safe. Some reports suggest that partial to complete pain relief for 6 months to 1 year may be achieved with facet block (see the article by Levin elsewhere in this issue) [25,26].

Neck pain, cervical radiculopathy, and myelopathy

The cervical spine is more flexible and mobile than the lumbar spine. The disk spaces are thinner, the canal and foramina are narrower, and there is less epidural fat in the cervical spine. Disk herniations are less common than in the lumbar region and associated more often with concomitant bony degenerative changes. Degenerative bony changes are seen in the vertebral bodies, facet joints, and the uncinate processes, which are designed to control translational motion of the cervical vertebrae.

Disk osteophyte complex

Osteophyte formation usually develops in the setting of disk herniation in cervical spine. The majority of osteophytic spurs contains bulging or frankly herniated disk material [27]. A disk-dominated complex has a better prognosis and greater tendency to regress spontaneously [28] than an extradural defect that is predominately bony (Fig. 1A, B).

Radiculopathy

Clinical assessment is critical for tailoring cervical examinations. Cervical radiculopathy should be distinguished clinically from other causes of neck and arm pain. Spondylotic radiculopathy is most common at C5-6 and C6-7. MR or CT with intrathecal contrast (CT myelography) is the most accurate imaging test. Plain film oblique views may identify foraminal encroachment from end-plate or uncovertebral joint and facet joint spurring but is insensitive to disk disease. CT is more sensitive to bony disease (Fig. 1C). Unexplained radiculopathy should prompt the search for foraminal or far lateral disk protrusions or osteophytes.

Myelopathy

Spondylotic compressive myelopathy is the most common cause of cord dysfunction in patients over 50 years of age. Other less common causes have toxic, metabolic, or neoplastic etiologies. The term, myelitis, which also results in cervical cord dysfunction, usually is reserved for infectious or

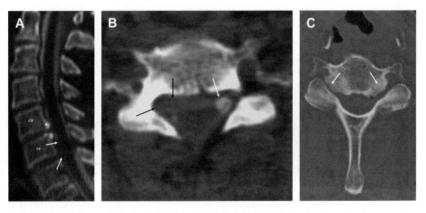

Fig. 1. Cervical degenerative disk disease. (A) Reconstructed sagittal CT myelogram—patient who had right C7 radiculopathy, anterior epidural defect dorsal to C6 body (arrows). (B) Axial CT myelogram, same patient—better shows thecal sac compression resulting from disk extrusion (dark arrows). Note intact left lateral recess thecal sac and nerve root (white arrow). Also, note bony dominant hypertrophic change at C5-6 (A) (arrowhead) with mild impression on thecal sac. (C) Axial nonmyelographic CT—different patient who had bilateral uncovertebral joint spurring (arrows) resulting in foraminal stenosis.

noninfectious inflammatory processes. MRI is the test of choice, as it can show not only cord compression but also intramedullary pathology. Sagittal T2 imaging supplemented by sagittal proton density, STIR, and axial T2 imaging is essential for diagnosis of intramedullary signal abnormality (Fig. 2).

Pyogenic cervical spondylodiskitis

Pyogenic cervical spondylodiskitis with or with out epidural abscess is more common than once believed [29]. Intravenous drug abuse is one of the most important risk factors [30]. Rarely, isolated epidural abscess is seen. There was a high incidence of multilevel involvement and epidural abscesses in a study of pyogenic cervical spine infections by Friedmand and colleagues [31]. MRI with and without contrast is the study of choice. Given the smaller cervical disk spaces and potential anatomic space in the prevertebral soft tissues, the dominant findings in cervical spondylodiskitis comprise prevertebral edema or abscess with minimal disk space or endplate marrow changes. Sagittal STIR images are the most sensitive sequence for the detection of subtle prevertebral edema and inflammation. True abscess formation usually is manifested by peripheral enhancement of a fluid collection versus confluent epidural soft tissue enhancement, which is more typical of a phlegmon (Fig. 3).

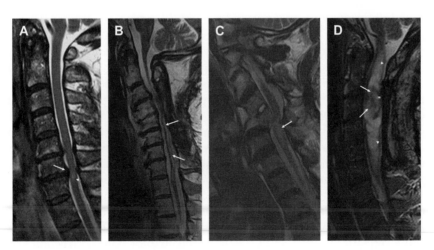

Fig. 2. Cervical melopathy: sagittal T2 images. (*A*) Posterior disk bulging or protrusion at C6-7 (*arrow*), mildly flattening the cord; associated focal signal abnormality (*arrowhead*) representing spondylotic myelomalacia. (*B*) Extensive myelomalacia (*arrows*) as a sequela of spondylosis and perioperative vascular compromise. Patient status post extensive posterior decompression at C3-7. (*C*) AS with collapsed C5 vertebra; note cord swelling and signal abnormality (*arrow*) resulting from compression by C5 retropulsion. (*D*) Ependymoma. Sagittal T2—expansile heterogenous mass (*arrows*) with marked cord edema (*arrowheads*).

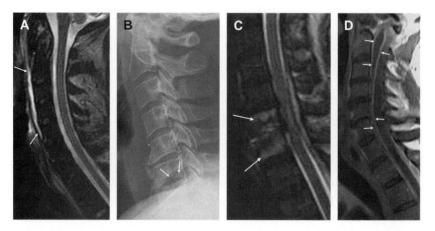

Fig. 3. Cervical spine infection. (*A*) Prevertebral abscess. Sagittal STIR with prevertebral T2 hyperintensity (*arrows*), later proved to be the result of C1-2 infection, not quite apparent on this examination. (*B, C*) DO. Lateral plain film (*C*)—focal end-plate erosion (*arrows*). Sagittal T2 (*C*)—C6-7 T2 hyperintensity in the vertebral bodies and disk space (*arrows*) resulting from DO. (*D*) Epidural abscess. Sagittal T1 post contrast—different patient who had spontaneous rim-enhancing extensive anterior epidural fluid collection (*arrows*).

Atlantodental and upper cervical spine disease

The atlantodental intervertebral level is unique as it lacks a typical disk space. It is the level most proximate to skull base. A soft tissue ligamentous complex supports the atlantodental joint. These structures give rise to the manifestations of a group of disorders. In rheumatoid arthritis, C1-2 is affected in approximately 20% to 25% of patients, resulting in neck or occipital pain, and may cause compressive myelopathy [32,33]. Typical imaging features of subluxation (usually anterior) and odontoid erosion are displayed on conventional radiographs and reformatted sagittal and coronal CT images [34]. On MRI, intermediate T1 and T2 signal intensity changes with diffuse enhancing pannus are seen, encroaching on the subarachnoid space and compressing the cord (Fig. 4A) [35,36]. Hypertrophy degeneration results from advanced osteoarthritis, calcium pyrophosphate deposition, or the sequela of chronic instability, with pseudopannus or pseudotumor formation mimicking rheumatoid arthritis [37]. Advanced age, hypertrophic bony changes, and nonenhancement of the retrodental soft tissue suggest degenerative etiology (Fig. 4B). Tuberculous spondylitis preferentially involves the craniovertebral junction and C1-2, with potential for bone destruction and large spinal or paraspinal soft tissue fluid collections and masses [38–40]. Atlantodental involvement in ankylosing spondylitis (AS) is common, with radiologic findings, including atlantodental calcification, subluxation, or ossification [41,42]. Upper cervical spine/C2 fracture in AS, although uncommon, may be seen (Fig. 4C). Spondyloarthropathy in long-term hemodialysis patients, also termed destructive spondyloarthropathy, commonly affects the

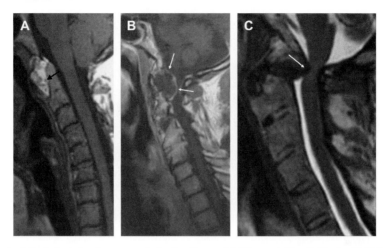

Fig. 4. Atlantodental and upper cervical spine disease. (*A*) Rheumatoid arthritis. Sagittal T1 post contrast–predental enhancing pannus (*arrow*). (*B*) Pseudopannus sagittal T1 post contrast—retrodental degenerative soft tissue hypertrophy with compression of the cord. Dorsal rim enhancement (*arrows*) likely related to epidural venous plexus. The soft issue was calcified on CT (not shown). Patient was asymptomatic. (*C*) AS. Sagittal T2 dental fracture and compromise of the foramen magnum (*arrow*).

midcervical spine with erosive end-plate changes and also causes atlantodental subluxation and pseudopannus. On MRI, there are intermediate T1 and T2 signal intensity changes secondary to amyloid deposition [43–45].

Prevertebral edema-related disorders

There are several disorders that cause acute neck pain and manifest as prevertebral soft tissue thickening and T2 hyperintensity or edema. Spondylodiskitis is discussed previously. Acute ligamentous injury resulting from flexion or extension injury may be seen without fractures. STIR-weighted sequences are the most sensitive for the detection of prevertebral or posterior paraspinal edema, indicative of ligamentous injury and neck sprain (Fig. 5A). Retropharyngeal cellulites, with or without true abscess, is a pediatric disorder related to tonsillopharyngeal pathology. It is rare in adults [46] but should be considered in immunocompromised patients who have neck pain, fever, and prevertebral edema. Calcific retropharyngeal tendonitis is a rare self-limited entity resulting from inflammation of longus colli muscles, with acute onset of severe pain localized in the back of the neck and aggravated by head movements and swallowing. Prevertebral edema with amorphous calcific deposits is characteristic (Fig. 5B, C) [47–49].

Back pain and lumbar radiculopathy

Back pain and lumbar radiculopathy are the main reasons for referral for spine imaging. Unfortunately, abnormalities on spine imaging are common

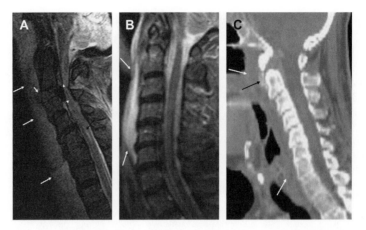

Fig. 5. Prevertebral edema. (*A*) Acute ligamentous injury. Sagittal T2—severe spinal trauma resulting from flexion extension injury with extensive prevertebral edema (*long white arrows*), anterior ligamentous disruption (*small white arrow*), posterior ligamentous disruption and epidural hematoma (*small white arrowheads*), and diffuse cord contusions (*dark arrow*). CT was negative for fractures. (*B, C*) Longus colli calcific tendonitis–extensive prevertebral edema on sagittal T2 (*A*) (*arrows*) and prevertebral focal calcification (*dark arrow*) on reconstructed sagittal CT soft tissue neck image (*B*). Note prevertebral edema on CT (*B*) (*white arrows*).

and nonspecific [50–52]. This cloud of nonspecificity superimposed on the multifactorial nature of the back pain poses a perpetual diagnostic and therapeutic challenge to clinicians and radiologists. The causes of symptoms related to the lower spine are diverse. Back pain and lumbar radiculopathy are the most common symptoms. The pain usually is attributed to (1) instability associated with disk degeneration, facet hypertrophic arthopathy; (2) mechanical compression of nerves by bone, ligament, or disk material; and (3) biochemical mediators of inflammation or pain. There is innervation of the outer layers of the intervertebral disk, which is responsible for the pain generation [53,54]. Superimposed reparative changes alter the anatomy, however, triggering pathologic nociceptive innervation and increased pain. Compression of the nerve roots, alternatively, lead to venous stasis, edema, and, ultimately, intraneural and perineural fibrosis [55]. This article's discussion on thoracolumbar spine imaging focuses on degenerative disease, followed by a brief review of other common disorders responsible for back pain.

Degenerative lumbar spine disease

Anatomic factors

Each spinal level is a three-joint complex with the anterior column (intervertebral joint between the end plates) and the two facet joints of the posterior column supported by ligaments and muscle groups. The zygoapophyseal (facet) joints and intervertebral disk joints act as an interactive functional unit, perpetually exposed to mechanical stresses, leading to degeneration of the osseomyocartilagenous complex [56], resulting in characteristic imaging manifestations. The dynamism at these joints, termed microinstability, is hypothesized to result in progressive loss of strength in the joint capsules, leading to degeneration with reactive osteocartilaginous hypertrophy and disk changes [57]. The inter-relationship of these elements is important, as evident from the ongoing transition of surgical procedures from joint fusion to joint replacement [58].

Etiology of disk degeneration

The disk is metabolically active and the metabolism is dependent on diffusion of fluid from the marrow of the vertebral bodies across the subchondral bone and cartilaginous end plate or through the annulus fibrosus from the surrounding blood vessels. Disk degeneration is linked primarily to mechanical loading with mechanical factors producing end-plate changes, considered a precursor to disk changes [59,60]. Mechanical, traumatic, and nutritional factors all play roles in the cascade of disk degeneration to variable degrees in individuals. Genetic factors play a role in disk degeneration [61–64]. Whatever the cause, by 50 years of age, more than 80% of adults show evidence of degenerative disk disease at autopsy [65]. MRI can track the evolutionary changes in disk degeneration, but the distinction between aging changes and pathologic changes remains unclear [66].

Terminology

Reports point the tendency for interobserver and intraobserver variations in spine imaging interpretation [66–69]. This is related partly to inconsistency in the terminology. In this review, the terms used follow the recommendations of Milette [68]. Spondylosis deformans refers to the consequences of normal aging affecting mainly the annulus fibrosus and adjacent apophyses with anterior and lateral osteophytosis. Intervertebral osteochondrosis, or deteriorated disk, represents a pathologic process affecting primarily the nucleus pulposus and end plates, different from fissuring of the annulus fibrosus and reactive or erosive changes in the end plates [70,71].

A transitional vertebra occurs at the junction between two types of vertebral bodies, such as at the lumbosacral junction. A transitional vertebra demonstrates characteristics of both types of vertebrae, usually involving the vertebral arch or transverse process, and usually involves a partial fusion between the two vertebrae. It has an incidence in the general population ranging from 5% to 30% [72–74]. An association with back pain is reported [75]. A transitional lumbar (L5) or sacral (S1) vertebra may be fused partially or completely with the sacrum or lumbar spine, respectively. Recognition of a transitional vertebra is crucial to appropriate localization before invasive procedures.

Degenerative disk-space changes

An intervertebral disk is composed of an inner portion, the nucleus pulposus, and a peripheral portion, the annulus fibrosus. With degeneration and aging, there is loss of the hydrostatic properties of the disk, resulting primarily from increasing type II collagen and alteration in the proteoglycans [76–78]. Although morphologic changes of the disk space readily are characterized on MRI studies, their relationship with patient symptoms cannot be interpreted. Loss of disk space T2 signal intensity is an early and common MRI sign of disk degeneration (Fig. 6A). In addition, the demarcation of hypointense outer layers of annulus fibrosus from the central zone of inner annular layers and the nucleus pulposus is blurred or lost [79]. Vacuum phenomenon and disk calcification, easily identified on plain radiographs or CT, contribute to disk space T2 signal loss. Disk space narrowing, identified readily on plain radiographs, develops as a result of progressive disk dessication.

Annular disk bulging, also described as broad-based disk protrusion, typically is visualized as a concentric bulge, sometimes with lateral or posterior asymmetry. Disk bulges and protrusions generally are incidental findings [51]. Impressions on the thecal sac or cord, however, do contribute to central canal stenosis, particularly in the presence of posterior element hypertrophy (PEH). Pseudo disk bulging is seen in the setting of anterolisthesis, as a result of uncovering of the disk at the posterior margin of the end plates.

Annular disk tear, commonly as a radial tear, is manifested by focal T2 hyperintensity in the setting of posterior disk bulging or protrusion. Such a disk signal abnormality is a strong predictor of annular tears [80,81]. Although some investigators correlate this abnormality with the presence

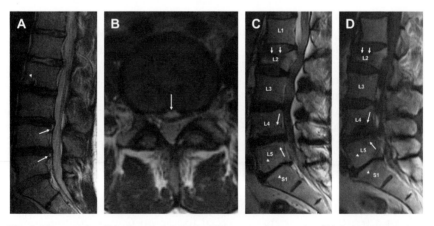

Fig. 6. Degenerative disk disease. (*A*) Sagittal T2—posterior annular disk bulges and protrusions with annular tears as T2 hyperintensities (*arrows*). Note near complete loss of T2 signal in L4-5 disk space. Arrowhead pointing to Schmorl's node. (*B*) Axial T2 broad-based disk protrusion with annular tear (*arrow*). (*C, D*) Degenerative end-plate bone-marrow changes. Sagittal T2 (*C*) and T1 (*D*) showing type I (*arrows*) and type II (*arrowhead*) changes. Note remote L2 benign compression deformity (*small arrows*).

of back pain [80,82], it has been shown to occur in up to 60% of asymptomatic patients (see Fig. 6A; Fig. 6B) [81,83].

Degenerative end-plate marrow changes

Type I changes represent granulation tissue and show decreased T1 and increased T2 end plates signal intensity. Type II changes, more common than type I changes, represent fatty marrow replacement and show increased signal on T1- and T2-weighted images. Type III changes correlate with extensive bony sclerosis on plain radiographs and show decreased signal intensity on T1- and T2-weighted images (see Fig. 6C–D) [84–86].

Degenerative facet and ligamentous changes

Disease of facet joints (including sacroiliac joints) is identified in 15% to 40% of patients who have chronic low back pain [23,87,88]. Like all diarthrodial synovium–lined joints, the lumbar facet joints are predisposed to arthropathy related to damage to articular cartilage. CT is the study of choice to detect and characterize facet arthropathy using thin axial slices generating high quality 3-D images. The typical features of arthritis include joint space narrowing, irregularity or osteophytosis, vacuum phenomenon, and sclerosis (Fig. 7A). Spondylolysis may be seen along with advanced hypertrophic arthropathy. MRI sagittal T2 images show rostrocaudal subluxation (contributing to foraminal stenosis), and axial T2 images demonstrate joint effusion and associated findings, such as synovial cysts and ligamentum flavum hypertrophy (LFH) or laxity. Synovial cysts projecting into the posterolateral spinal canal may impinge the cord, thecal sac, or nerve roots significantly. Synovial cysts demonstrate variable T1 and T2 signal depending on their proteinaceous fluid content, identified by their origin from facet joints and their rounded contours (Fig. 7B, C).

Important ligaments of the spine include the anterior longitudinal ligament, the posterior longitudinal ligament, the paired sets of ligamenta flava (connecting the laminae of adjacent vertebrae), intertransverse ligaments (extending between transverse processes), and the unpaired supraspinous ligament (along the tips of the spinous processes). LFH is a common contributor to morphologic central canal stenosis, especially when coexistent with facet.

Morphologic and functional sequelae of degenerative changes

Disk herniation

Disk herniation is a broad term encompassing different types and degrees of intervertebral disk displacement. Disk protrusion has many synonyms, such as disk prolapse or herniated nucleus pulposus. Protrusion is limited more strictly to a bulge less than or equal to 25% of disk circumference, but the

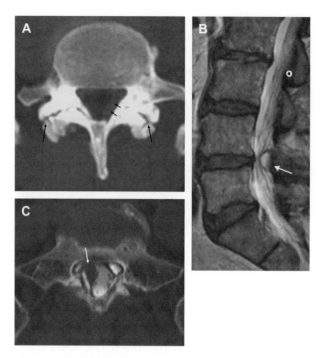

Fig. 7. Facet joints. (*A*) Facet arthropathy. Axial CT. Bilateral hypertrophic facet joint changes (*long arrows*) in an asymptomatic patient. Note faintly visualized ligamentum flavum thickening (*small arrows*). (*B, C*) Synovial cyst. Sagittal T2 (*B*)—a rounded cystic lesion (*arrow*), which on axial CT myelogram (*C*) shows right-side posterior epidural impression on thecal sac, abutting the facet joint (*arrow*).

term generally is used for any degree of focal lateral, foraminal, or posterior disk bulge with primary focus on abutment, compression, or displacement of the thecal sac and nerve roots (see Fig. 6B). Protrusion is the displacement of the nucleus pulposus and inner annular material through the annulus but not through the outer-most annular fibers. Its high prevalence in asymptomatic patients is evidence against its specific role in back pain [89].

A disk extrusion, considered a true herniated disk, extends through all the annular layers but remains connected with the primary disk material by a small isthmus or neck as the only attachment. A sequestered disk or free disk fragment is an extruded disk that has lost continuity with the primary disk. The fragment does not cross the midline because of a midline septum, but otherwise it can migrate anterior or posterior to the longitudinal ligament, lateral recess, neuroforamen, or thecal sac (intradural disk). Schmorl's nodes (herniations of the intervertebral disk through the vertebral end plates) usually are incidental findings but can been associated with back pain (see Fig. 6A) [90].

Foraminal and far lateral foraminal protrusions constitute 7% to 12% of all disk protrusions or extrusions and need more emphasis, as they can be overlooked clinically and on imaging. This subset of herniations, more common at L3-4 and L4-5, can have more severe radicular signs on clinical examination [91,92]. Look for focal herniations in the foraminal and extra-foraminal region on axial images and loss of foraminal fat on sagittal images (Figs. 8 and 9 show disk herniations).

Spinal instability

Segmental instability usually results from degenerative changes involving the intervertebral disk, vertebral bodies, or facet joints, causing impairment of the usual pattern of spinal movement and producing translational or angular motion that may be irregular, excessive, or restricted. Spondylolisthesis refers to displacement relative to the next most inferior vertebral body. Isthmic or spondylolytic spondylolisthesis is the most common type, with up to 50% to 60% of spondylolysis resulting in spondylolisthesis.

Spondylolysis refers to a defect in the pars interarticularis or isthmus and occurs with an incidence of approximately 3% to10% [93]. The majority of cases demonstrate bilateral L5 pars interarticularis defects, reflecting the uniform stress exerted by the body [94]. Lower lumbar spine spondylosis is unique to the human species because of upright posture, as spondylosis is not seen in individuals who have never walked [95,96]. Most isthmic defects appear in the first and second decades, reflecting the initial and more vigorous phases of activity in human life [93].

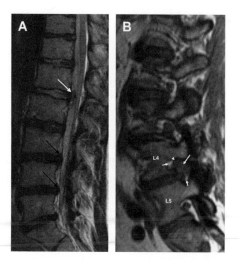

Fig. 8. Degenerative disk disease—sagittal imaging. (*A*) Postpartum 23-year-old patient who had cauda equina symptoms—sagittal T2 image showing L1-2 disc extrusion (*white arrow*) with moderate compression of thecal sac. Note diffuse disk degeneration with loss of normal T2 signal and annular disk bulges (*dark arrows*) in rest of the lumbar spine. (*B*) Sagittal T1—foraminal disk (*long arrow*) with foraminal stenosis; note L4 nerve root compression (*arrowhead*) and partial loss of hyperintense foraminal fat (*small arrows*).

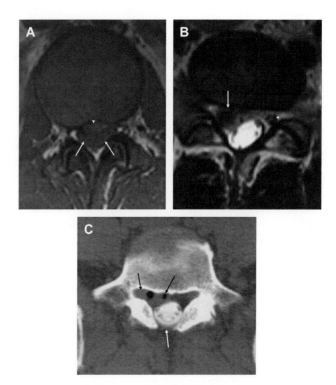

Fig. 9. Degenerative disk disease—axial imaging. (*A*) Axial T1—same patient as in Fig. 8A; disk extrusion compressing thecal sac (*arrow head*) with crowding of cauda equine nerve roots (*white arrows*). (*B*) Axial T2—a young resident physician who had acute right sciatica; note large disk extrusion (*white arrow*), compression of thecal sac and right S1 nerve root; left S1 nerve root is intact (*arrow head*). (*C*) Axial CT myelogram—different patient, mild thecal sac compression resulting from posterolateral disk protrusion with vacuum phenomenon (*dark arrows*); note decompression laminectomy (*white arrow*). Part of this epidural soft tissue impression is epidural scarring (see Fig. 19A).

Several studies address the question of the clinical significance of spondylolysis. Patients who have and who do not have back pain have a similar incidence of spondylolysis [97,98]. Approximately 25% of patients who have spondylolysis, however, eventually develop significant back pain during their lifetime [99]. Spondylolysis causes back pain in younger patients and predisposes to the development of disk and facet disorders in later life [100]. Oblique radiographs can detect defects in the pars interarticularis reliably, but thin-slice CT imaging with multiangled reformatting has improved accuracy, showing more defects compared with radiographs [101]. Single photon emission CT (SPECT) imaging is more effective in distinguishing between symptomatic and asymptomatic spondylolysis, and increased activity can aid in the localization of the source of pain [102,103]. MRI supplemented by fat saturation technique may show reversible signal abnormalities in the pars interarticularis in the absence of defects, indicating a stress reaction associated with activity-related low back pain [104,105]. Detection of spondylolytic defects on MRI is difficult [106] unless there is associated retraction and anterolisthesis. Detection is aided by assessment of sagittal and axial images [107]. Spondylolysis may be observed on imaging without associated spondylolisthesis (Fig. 10).

Degenerative spondylolisthesis usually is identified in the presence of an intact pars interarticularis and is related primarily to degenerative changes of the apophyseal joints, most commonly at the L4-5 vertebral level. Degenerative disk disease may predispose to or exacerbate this condition because of narrowing of the disk space, which can lead to malalignment of the articular processes and rostrocaudal subluxation (Fig. 11).

Spinal canal stenosis

Spinal stenosis refers to narrowing of the spinal canal, lateral recesses or nerve root canals, or intervertebral foramina [108]. Two broad groups include acquired (usually caused by degenerative changes) and congenital or developmental. Some prefer the term, clinical stenosis, reflecting the importance of symptoms in establishing the diagnosis [109]. The imaging changes in general are more extensive than expected from the clinical findings [109]. There is no strong relationship between degree of stenosis and patient symptoms. Specific imaging findings do not predict benefit from surgery [110]. Position-dependent (dynamic) stenosis that worsens in extension and improves with flexion can be distinguished from static stenosis [109,111–113].

Congenital stenosis is explained primarily by shortened stubby pedicles with flattened axial appearance of the bony canal resulting from decreased anterior-posterior diameter along with narrowing of the lateral recesses and foramina [114]. Congenital stenosis usually is asymptomatic but reduces the reserve of the spine to accommodate degenerative hypertrophic changes during aging (Fig. 12). Acquired central canal stenosis in older patients typically is associated with disk and facet disease, disk bulges, and ligamentous hypertrophy and laxity. Degenerative spondylolisthesis and scoliosis also can contribute significantly to spinal stenosis. CT myelography with axial and multiplanar reformatted images provides greater detail than routine studies. Sagittal and axial MR images with T2 weighting allow accurate assessment of thecal sac compression (Fig. 13).

Acquired lateral recess stenosis is caused by disk–end-plate or superior articular facet hypertrophic changes. Asymptomatic nerve root contact may be seen with disk bulgings, protrusions, and osteophytosis. Contact by disk extrusion, however, is a significant finding [51,115]. Axial MRI or CT myelography shows a triangular-shaped normal lateral recess [116]. Facet and disk margin hypertrophic changes cause acute angled narrowing, whereas isolated facet hypertrophic arthropathy or PEH (which alone can cause radiculopathy) results in trefoil-shaped narrowing (Fig. 14) [117].

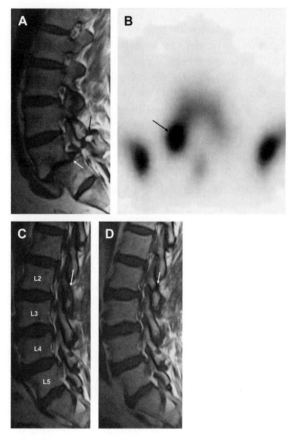

Fig. 10. Spondylolysis. (*A*) Isthmic spondylolysis.sagittal T1—grade I anterolisthesis of L5 on S1 (*arrow*) resulting from L5 pars interarticularis defect with retraction (*dark arrow*). (*B*) Bone scan. Axial SPECT—intense focal uptake right L5 pars interarticularis (*dark arrow*). (*C*, *D*) Pathologic spondylolysis. Sagittal T1—focal marrow replacement resulting from multiple myeloma (*C*) (*arrow*), transforming into pars defect on follow-up (*D*) (*arrow*); no retraction or anterolisthesis.

Acquired foraminal stenosis can be caused by lateral extension of disk bulging when associated with spondylosis, facet joint degenerative hypertrophic changes, or laxity (rostrocaudal subluxation). Loss of disk space height results in decreased vertical dimension of the foramina, whereas the sagittal dimensions are related to the sagittal dimensions of the pedicle and central canal [118]. Therefore, foraminal stenosis commonly is seen in association with canal stenosis. Sagittal MRI provides reliable assessment of the foramina [119] except in scoliosis. CT (preferably CT myelography) can complement the assessment and provide better demonstration of the bony foraminal canals.

Epidural lipomatosis is the accentuation of normal epidural fat, usually seen in the setting of endogenous or exogenous corticosteroid excess, and

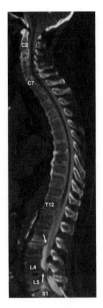

Fig. 11. Degenerative spondylolisthesis: reconstructed panaromic sagittal CT myelogram—diffuse degenerative disk disease of the spine. Note mild retrolisthesis at L2-3 and anterolisthesis at L4-5 (*arrows*). Also note moderate degenerative central canal stenosis at L4-5.

is common in obese individuals. This usually is an incidental finding, but lipomatosis in the setting of structural stenosis can add to the compromise of the central canal. Rarely, epidural lipomatosis alone can lead to radiculopathy and cauda equina (Fig. 15) [120–122].

Cauda equina syndrome is related to simultaneous compression of multiple lumbosacral nerve roots below the level of the conus medullaris, resulting in a characteristic pattern of neuromuscular and urogenital symptoms. There are many potential causes, including epidural tumors, disk herniations, and epidural hematomas. Disk herniations account for approximately 1% of cases [123–125]. Acute onset of symptoms is a medical and surgical emergency [123,125]. MRI and myelography can demonstrate compression of the thecal sac reliably, whereas MRI also can characterize the cause of compression (Figs. 8A and 9A).

Significance of imaging findings in degenerative disease

The role of spine imaging is to provide accurate morphologic information and aid therapeutic decision making. Further advancements will aid in the understanding of underlying biochemical and cellular characteristics. Therapeutic decision making, however, is confounded by the high prevalence of morphologic changes in the asymptomatic population. Up to

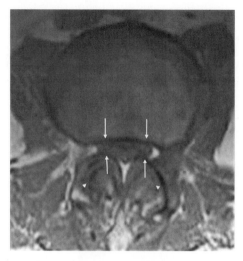

Fig. 12. Spinal stenosis: axial T1—congenital narrowing of the central canal; note decreased anteroposterior dimension of the canal (*arrows*) and stubby posterior elements (*arrowheads*).

30% of asymptomatic patients demonstrate disk herniations and most of them also have other degenerative change [51,126,127]. The MR findings do not by themselves correlate with the presence or duration of low back pain [128]. The incidence of disk herniations reaches up to 65% in patients

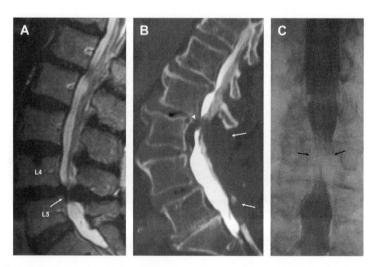

Fig. 13. Spinal stenosis. (*A*) Sagittal T2—severe central canal stenosis a result of mild disk bulging and dominant LFH at L4-L5. Note mild L4-5 anterolisthesis. (*B, C*) Acquired central canal stenosis. Sagittal CT myelogram (*B*)—severe thecal sac compression resulting from retrolisthesis and associated hypertrophic changes (*arrowhead*). Note lumbar spine decompression laminectomies (*arrows*). Corresponding conventional myelogram posterio-anterior image (*C*) showing thecal sac defect (*arrows*).

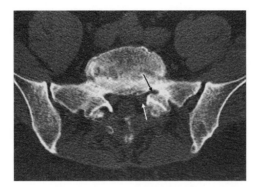

Fig. 14. Lateral recess stenosis: axial CT—left S1 lateral stenosis (*dark arrow*) resulting from facet joint hypertrophy; note the left S1 nerve is pushed medially (*white arrow*). The patient was asymptomatic.

who have back pain or radiculopathy [51,127]. Disk herniations can show dramatic reduction in size in patients undergoing conservative management [129,130]. There is no strong correlation between imaging and likelihood of clinical outcome [131]. In patients who have acute low back pain or radiculopathy, MRI does not seem to have measurable value in terms of planning conservative care [132]. The significance of bone marrow end-plate changes associated with degenerative disk disease is not clear. Type I changes, however, are shown to have a higher correlation with active low back symptoms

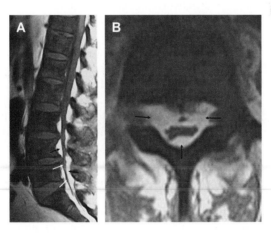

Fig. 15. Spinal epidural lipomatosis: sagittal (*A*) and axial (*B*) T1—epidural lipomatosis (*dark arrows*) with thecal sac compromise (*white arrows*) likely accounted for patient's symptoms as there was interval worsening of epidural lipomatosis after radiation therapy compared with previous examination (not shown); no epidural tumor was present. Note diffuse replacement of the normal fatty marrow resulting from prostatic metastatic disease.

[133–135]. Patients who have type I marrow changes and who undergo fusion for low back pain do better than those who do not have end-plate changes or type II patterns [133]. Furthermore, persistence of type I marrow changes after fusion is associated with significantly worse outcome [136]. Alternatively, conversion of type I marrow changes to a normal marrow signal or type II is correlated with good clinical results, successful fusion, and stabilization [133].

Diskitis osteomyelitis

Infection of the spine easily can be overlooked on clinical and imaging examinations during the early stages. Pyogenic and tuberculous spondylodiskitis have characteristic imaging features and can be differentiated to a considerable degree [137,138]. MRI is the study of choice.

Ledermann and colleagues [139] divide the imaging features of pyogenic diskitis osteomyelitis (DO) into two groups. First, disk-space changes including loss of disk space height and loss of central disk space nuclear cleft, but they are not very useful because of low sensitivity and specificity [139]. Hyperintense T2 signal in the disk space on MRI is, however, a sensitive marker of diskitis, but similar appearance in a hydrated degenerated disk is common in the authors' experience. Contrast enhancement in the disk space also is a highly sensitive marker and helpful in equivocal cases after noncontrast MRI; lack of disk space enhancement in DO is rare [137,140,141]. CT features usually are nonspecific unless there is advanced infection. DO should be suspected in cases of unusually prominent end-plate sclerosis. Look for end-plate lysis and collapse, better appreciated on sagittal reformations. The second group of imaging features is related to vertebral body and paraspinous soft tissues. MRI findings include hyperintense T2 and hypointense T1 end-plate bone marrow signal abnormality indicative of bone marrow edema and inflammation [139,142]. Partial to complete involvement of both vertebral bodies is common. Degenerative end-plate changes mimic spondylodiskitis by manifesting disk space hyperintensity and associated end-plate changes. Features favoring degenerative disease include more lateralized end-plate bone marrow signal abnormality with associated osteophytosis, lack of paraspinal soft tissue changes, or enhancement in the disk space. End-plate erosion is shown better on T1 images and may result in collapsed vertebra [142]. Paraspinal- and epidural-enhancing soft tissue thickening with or with out fluid collections is the most reliable imaging feature [142]. STIR (or other equivalent fat suppression techniques) can be helpful in unmasking the T2 hyperintensity in fat-rich paraspinal or epidural spaces and vertebral body marrow (Fig. 16). Tuberculous infection typically shows skip lesions, large paraspinal abscesses, vertebral collapse, and subligamentous spread [143,144].

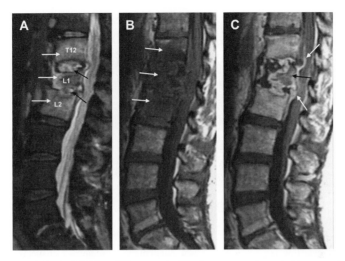

Fig. 16. DO. (*A*) Sagittal STIR—diffuse vertebral body marrow edema (*white arrows*) and disk spaces hyperintensity (*dark arrows*) at T12-L1 and L1-2; note mild compression deformity of L1. (*B*) Sagittal T1—corresponding diffuse T1 hypointensity in the vertebral bodies (*arrows*). (*C*) Sagittal post ontrast T1—diffuse rim enhancement of L1 representing osteomyelitis (*dark arrow*); note disk spaces enhancement and associated anterior epidural inflammatory enhancement/phlegmon (*white arrows*); no clear epidural abscess formation.

Compression fractures and bone marrow disease

The role of imaging in compression deformities is to determine recent versus chronic onset, compromise of the spinal canal resulting from retropulsion, and benign versus malignant etiology. Plain films have low sensitivity in detecting mild compression fracture deformities. Nuclear medicine bone scan findings are nonspecific and generally need correlation with morphologic studies. The usefulness of MRI in the evaluation of compression fractures lies in the detection of marrow edema, infiltrative changes, and associated paraspinal or epidural tumor. MRI can characterize and differentiate malignant from benign fractures in the majority of cases, facilitated by the findings of heterogeneous bone marrow signal and multilevel and multifocal marrow infiltration. Features highly in favor of malignant fractures include bulging contours, pedicle involvement, paraspinal soft tissue tumor, and marrow enhancement [145–147]. STIR sequences are helpful in identifying edema or tumor-related T2 hyperintensity (Fig. 17). Benign bone-marrow changes, such as patchy osteoporosis, reactive hematopoiesis, granulomatosis, or renal osteodystrophy, can mimic malignant infiltrative process (Fig. 18). Multidetector CT with 3-D imaging also can identify malignant fractures by identifying focal cortical or cancellous bone destruction and outlining the fracture deformities [148]. Percutaneous vertebroplasty and kyphoplasty are accepted methods of treatment of painful benign or

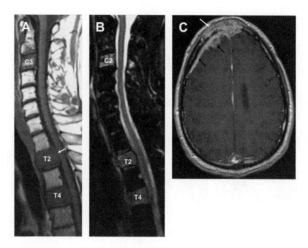

Fig. 17. Bone marrow disease: frontal sinus undifferentiated carcinoma with metastatic disease. (*A*) Sagittal T1—metastatic involvement of C3, T2, and T4. Note bulging contours at T2 and T4 and mild cord compression (*arrow*). (*B*) Sagittal STIR—corresponding hyperintense metastatic involvement. (*C*) Axial T1 postcontrast head—right frontal sinus and calvarial primary tumor (*white arrow*) with associated epidural intracranial extension (*dark arrows*).

pathologic compression fractures [149–152]; MRI and multiplanar CT are helpful in preoperative planning [153].

The postoperative spine

The United States has the highest incidence of spine surgery in the world, and it has increased over the past 2 decades [154]. There is an incidence of approximately 15% to 20% of failures, however, termed failed back syndrome [155–157]. Neuroimaging is important in this group of patients. MRI with and without contrast is the study of choice. CT myelography can be used in cases when MRI studies are inconclusive or degraded by artifact. Laminectomy is used most commonly for thecal sac decompression [158]; however, evidence of unilateral laminectomy, fenestration, or undercutting sometimes is difficult to identify on MRI. Look for attenuated ipsilateral ligamentum flavum or posterior bulge of the thecal sac into the defect. After fusion with or without instrumentation, several imaging findings can be seen. A posterolateral fusion has the appearance of clumps of corticated bone mimicking facet hypertrophic arthropathy. An interbody fusion has the appearance of partial to complete ankylosis of the disk space. Pseudoarthrosis (nonunion of the bony fusion) as assessed by MRI may be visualized poorly as a result of artifact from the cages. CT can be used to evaluate for bone formation or nonunion lucency around the cage [159]. Stabilizing fixation rods and screws are not a major limitation because of the current use of MRI-compatible metals, such as titanium. Disk

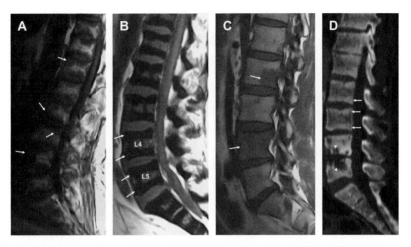

Fig. 18. Bone marrow disease. (*A*) Non-Hodgkin's lymphoma. Sagittal T1—diffuse patchy bone marrow replacement, mainly along the end plates (*arrows*). (*B*) Osteopetrosis. Sagittal T1— end-plates band-like hypointensity resulting from sclerosis (*arrows*), somewhat mimicking the appearance in (*A*). Note the uniform pattern indicating benign process. (*C*) Sarcoidosis. Sagittal T1—patchy to diffuse vertebral marrow replacement (*arrows*) with positive bone scan (not shown); biopsy showed granulomatous changes. (*D*) CT sagittal reformatted—band-like irregular sclerosis along the end plates (rugger jersey appearance) resulting from renal osteodystrophy (*arrows*). Note superimposed DO with bone erosion (*arrowheads*). Destructive spondyloarthropathy may have similar appearance.

replacement devices increasingly are used but with significant artifact degradation on MRI. Malpositioning and dislodgment of these devices can be observed on imaging (Fig. 19).

Recurrent disk herniation has an incidence of approximately 5% to 10%, generally defined as disk reherniation at the same level more than 6 months after surgery. Epidural scarring confounds imaging interpretation. In contrast to the localized bulging of a herniated disk, scarring shows a diffuse pattern with soft tissue replacement of normal epidural fat. A retractile configuration without mass effect favors epidural scarring [160]. Epidural scar typically manifests as diffuse enhancement, compared with marginal enhancement around a herniated disk, but differentiation can be difficult at times. CT myelography may be indicated as a complementary test (Fig. 20A).

A transitional phenomenon can occur as a result of a transitional level between the lower fused rigid spine and the upper flexible spine. This leads to progressive degeneration, advancing to anterior and posterior column segmental changes, termed pseudoarthrosis (distinct from nonunion of bony fusion, also referred to as pseudoarthrosis) (Fig. 20B).

Arachnoiditis is an adhesive fibrinous process involving the cauda equina. Multiple causes are described, including prior surgery, infection, intrathecal injections, and subarachnoid hemorrhage. Two patterns based on conventional myelography are described by Jorgensen and colleagues

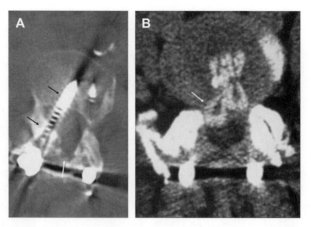

Fig. 19. Postoperative spine. (*A*) Malpositioned interpedicular screw. Axial CT—right side screw encroaching on the lateral recess of spinal canal (*dark arrows*). Note laminectomy defect (*white arrow*). (*B*) Displaced bone graft cage. Axial CT with intravenous contrast—focal compression of thecal sac by retropulsed cage (*arrow*).

[161]: type I, or featureless sac, with absence of nerve root defects, and type II, with localized or diffuse filling defects resulting from nerve roots clumping. On CT myelography or T2-weighted MRI, three patterns are described: central nerve root clumps or cords, lateral nerve root adhesions with empty

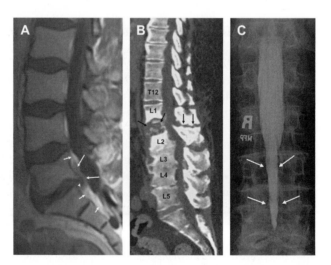

Fig. 20. Postoperative spine. (*A*) Epidural scar. Sagittal T1 post contrast—same patient as in Fig. 9C. Residual or recurrent small disk protrusion (*arrowhead*) surrounded by mildly enhancing epidural scarring (*long arrows*). Note more prominent surrounding hyperintensity resulting from epidural fat and enhancing epidural venous plexus (*small arrows*). (*B*) Pseudoarthrosis. Sagittal CT—L1-2 anterior and posterior column aligned lucency (*arrows*) resulting from abnormal motion. Note L2-3 and L3-4 anterior fusion. (*C*) Arachnoiditis. Conventional posterio-anterior myelogram—tapered lumbar myelographic block (*arrows*).

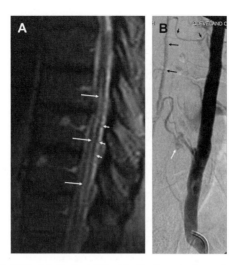

Fig. 21. Spinal dural AVF. (*A*) Sagittal T2 with distal cord edema (*long arrows*). Note surrounding prominent flow voids (*short arrows*). (*B*) Frontal view of left vertebral artery spinal angiogram. Note AVF (*white arrow*) and caudocranial flowing midline anterior spinal vein (*long dark arrows*) superimposed on anterior spinal artery fed by artery of cervical enlargement (*small dark arrows*).

thecal sac sign, and myelographic block with central mass-like appearance (Fig. 20C) [162].

Spinal arteriovenous malformations

Spinal arteriovenous malformations are rare. Clinical symptoms are believed related to venous hypertension, hemorrhage, steal phenomenon, or mass effect by varicosities. Back pain is an uncommon symptom, seen mainly in younger patients [163]. Classification focuses on the location of nidus or fistula (extradural, intradural, or intramedullary), the feeding arteries (single or multiple feeders), size of the nidus (compact or diffuse), and degree of shunting (low or high flow) [164–166]. A classification used commonly defines four types: type I (most common): dural arteriovenous fistula (AVF); type II: intramedullary glomus AVM; type III: juvenile or combined AVM; and type IV: intradural perimedullary AVF. Typical features on MRI include prominent intradural or extradural flow voids, cord edema, and perimedullary vascular and sometimes intramedullary enhancement related to venous hypertension and ischemia (Fig. 21A) [167,168]. Spinal angiography is used as confirmatory test and before endovascular treatment (Fig. 21B). Spinal MR angiography and CT angiography also are useful diagnostic tools [169–171].

References

[1] Kjellman G, Oberg B, Hensing G, et al. A 12-year follow-up of subjects initially sicklisted with neck/shoulder or low back diagnoses. Physiother Res Int 2001;6(1):52–63.

[2]   Hansson EK, Hansson TH. The costs for persons sick-listed more than one month because of low back or neck problems. A two-year prospective study of Swedish patients. Eur Spine J 2005;14(4):337–45.

[3]   Rish BL. A critique of the surgical management of lumbar disc disease in a private neuro-surgical practice. Spine 1984;9(5):500–4.

[4]   Hergan K, Amann T, Vonbank H, et al. MR-myelography: a comparison with conventional myelography. Eur J Radiol 1996;21(3):196–200.

[5]   Eberhardt KE, Hollenbach HP, Huk WJ. 3D-MR myelography in diagnosis of lumbar spinal nerve root compression syndromes. Comparative study with conventional myelography. Aktuelle Radiol 1994;4(6):313–7 [in German].

[6]   O'Connell MJ, Ryan M, Powell T, et al. The value of routine MR myelography at MRI of the lumbar spine. Acta Radiol 2003;44(6):665–72.

[7]   Kuroki H, Tajima N, Hirakawa S, et al. Comparative study of MR myelography and conventional myelography in the diagnosis of lumbar spinal diseases. J Spinal Disord 1998; 11(6):487–92.

[8]   Aagaard BD, Maravilla KR, Kliot M. Magnetic resonance neurography: magnetic resonance imaging of peripheral nerves. Neuroimaging Clin N Am 2001;11(1):viii, 131–viii, 146.

[9]   Filler AG, Maravilla KR, Tsuruda JS. MR neurography and muscle MR imaging for image diagnosis of disorders affecting the peripheral nerves and musculature. Neurol Clin 2004; 22(3):643–vii.

[10] Maravilla KR, Bowen BC. Imaging of the peripheral nervous system: evaluation of peripheral neuropathy and plexopathy. AJNR Am J Neuroradiol 1998;19(6):1011–23.

[11] Moore KR, Tsuruda JS, Dailey AT. The value of MR neurography for evaluating extraspinal neuropathic leg pain: a pictorial essay. AJNR Am J Neuroradiol 2001;22(4):786–94.

[12] Ellegala DB, Monteith SJ, Haynor D, et al. Characterization of genetically defined types of Charcot-Marie-Tooth neuropathies by using magnetic resonance neurography. J Neurosurg 2005;102(2):242–5.

[13] Filler AG, Haynes J, Jordan SE, et al. Sciatica of nondisc origin and piriformis syndrome: diagnosis by magnetic resonance neurography and interventional magnetic resonance imaging with outcome study of resulting treatment. J Neurosurg Spine 2005;2(2):99–115.

[14] Bosacco SJ, Berman AT, Garbarino JL, et al. A comparison of CT scanning and myelography in the diagnosis of lumbar disc herniation. Clin Orthop Relat Res 1984;190:124–8.

[15] Jayakumar P, Nnadi C, Saifuddin A, et al. Dynamic degenerative lumbar spondylolisthesis: diagnosis with axial loaded magnetic resonance imaging. Spine 2006;31(10):E298–301.

[16] Yamazaki T, Suzuki K, Yanaka K, et al. Dynamic computed tomography myelography for the investigation of cervical degenerative disease. Neurol Med Chir (Tokyo) 2006;46(4):210–5.

[17] Weishaupt D, Boxheimer L. Magnetic resonance imaging of the weight-bearing spine. Semin Musculoskelet Radiol 2003;7(4):277–86.

[18] Tsuchiya K, Katase S, Aoki C, et al. Application of multi-detector row helical scanning to postmyelographic CT. Eur Radiol 2003;13(6):1438–43.

[19] Shah RV, Everett CR, McKenzie-Brown AM, et al. Discography as a diagnostic test for spinal pain: a systematic and narrative review. Pain Physician 2005;8(2):187–209.

[20] Carragee EJ, Alamin TF, Miller J, et al. Provocative discography in volunteer subjects with mild persistent low back pain. Spine J 2002;2(1):25–34.

[21] Carragee EJ, Lincoln T, Parmar VS, et al. A gold standard evaluation of the "discogenic pain" diagnosis as determined by provocative discography. Spine 2006;31(18):2115–23.

[22] Manchikanti L, Singh V, Pampati V, et al. Provocative discography in low back pain patients with or without somatization disorder: a randomized prospective evaluation. Pain Physician 2001;4(3):227–39.

[23] Hildebrandt J. Relevance of nerve blocks in treating and diagnosing low back pain—is the quality decisive? Schmerz 2001;15(6):474–83 [in German].

[24] North RB, Kidd DH, Zahurak M, et al. Specificity of diagnostic nerve blocks: a prospective, randomized study of sciatica due to lumbosacral spine disease. Pain 1996;65(1):77–85.

[25] Staender M, Maerz U, Tonn JC, et al. Computerized tomography-guided kryorhizotomy in 76 patients with lumbar facet joint syndrome. J Neurosurg Spine 2005;3(6):444–9.

[26] Manchkanti L, Pampati V, Fellows B, et al. Prevalence of lumbar facet joint pain in chronic low back pain. Pain Physician 1999;2(3):59–64.

[27] Miyasaka K, Isu T, Iwasaki Y, et al. High resolution computed tomography in the diagnosis of cervical disc disease. Neuroradiology 1983;24(5):253–7.

[28] Maigne JY, Deligne L. Computed tomographic follow-up study of 21 cases of nonoperatively treated cervical intervertebral soft disc herniation. Spine 1994;19(2): 189–91.

[29] Shafaie FF, Wippold FJ, Gado M, et al. Comparison of computed tomography myelography and magnetic resonance imaging in the evaluation of cervical spondylotic myelopathy and radiculopathy. Spine 1999;24(17):1781–5.

[30] Endress C, Guyot DR, Fata J, et al. Cervical osteomyelitis due to i.v. heroin use: radiologic findings in 14 patients. AJR Am J Roentgenol 1990;155(2):333–5.

[31] Friedmand DP, Hills JR. Cervical epidural spinal infection: MR imaging characteristics. AJR Am J Roentgenol 1994;163(3):699–704.

[32] Semble EL, Elster AD, Loeser RF, et al. Magnetic resonance imaging of the craniovertebral junction in rheumatoid arthritis. J Rheumatol 1988;15(9):1367–75.

[33] Schwarz-Eywill M, Friedberg R, Stosslein F, et al. Rheumatoid arthritis at the cervical spine—an underestimated problem. Dtsch Med Wochenschr 2005;130(33):1866–70 [in German].

[34] Duan SY, Lin QC, Pang RL. Application of CT 3D reconstruction in diagnosing atlantoaxial subluxation. Chin J Traumatol 2004;7(2):118–21.

[35] Reijnierse M, Dijkmans BA, Hansen B, et al. Neurologic dysfunction in patients with rheumatoid arthritis of the cervical spine. Predictive value of clinical, radiographic and MR imaging parameters. Eur Radiol 2001;11(3):467–73.

[36] Stiskal MA, Neuhold A, Szolar DH, et al. Rheumatoid arthritis of the craniocervical region by MR imaging: detection and characterization. AJR Am J Roentgenol 1995;165(3): 585–92.

[37] Sze G, Brant-Zawadzki MN, Wilson CR, et al. Pseudotumor of the craniovertebral junction associated with chronic subluxation: MR imaging studies. Radiology 1986;161(2): 391–4.

[38] Krishnan A, Patkar D, Patankar T, et al. Craniovertebral junction tuberculosis: a review of 29 cases. J Comput Assist Tomogr 2001;25(2):171–6.

[39] Mariconda M, Lavano A, Ianno B, et al. Tuberculosis of the lower cervical spine: a description of two cases. Chir Organi Mov 1996;81(3):325–30.

[40] Wurtz R, Quader Z, Simon D, et al. Cervical tuberculous vertebral osteomyelitis: case report and discussion of the literature. Clin Infect Dis 1993;16(6):806–8.

[41] Lee JY, Kim JI, Park JY, et al. Cervical spine involvement in longstanding ankylosing spondylitis. Clin Exp Rheumatol 2005;23(3):331–8.

[42] Lee HS, Kim TH, Yun HR, et al. Radiologic changes of cervical spine in ankylosing spondylitis. Clin Rheumatol 2001;20(4):262–6.

[43] Chin M, Hase H, Miyamoto T, et al. Radiological grading of cervical destructive spondyloarthropathy in long-term hemodialysis patients. J Spinal Disord Tech 2006;19(6): 430–5.

[44] Kuntz D, Naveau B, Bardin T, et al. Destructive spondylarthropathy in hemodialyzed patients. A new syndrome. Arthritis Rheum 1984;27(4):369–75.

[45] Kiss E, Keusch G, Zanetti M, et al. Dialysis-related amyloidosis revisited. AJR Am J Roentgenol 2005;185(6):1460–7.

[46] Fogeltanz KA, Pursel KJ. Retropharyngeal abscess presenting as benign neck pain. J Manipulative Physiol Ther 2006;29(2):174–8.

[47] Karasick D, Karasick S. Calcific retropharyngeal tendinitis. Skeletal Radiol 1981;7(3): 203–5.

[48] Artenian DJ, Lipman JK, Scidmore GK, et al. Acute neck pain due to tendonitis of the longus colli: CT and MRI findings. Neuroradiology 1989;31(2):166–9.
[49] Mihmanli I, Karaarslan E, Kanberoglu K. Inflammation of vertebral bone associated with acute calcific tendinitis of the longus colli muscle. Neuroradiology 2001;43(12): 1098–101.
[50] van Tulder MW, Assendelft WJ, Koes BW, et al. Spinal radiographic findings and nonspecific low back pain. A systematic review of observational studies. Spine 1997;22(4):427–34.
[51] Jensen MC, Brant-Zawadzki MN, Obuchowski N, et al. Magnetic resonance imaging of the lumbar spine in people without back pain. N Engl J Med 1994;331(2):69–73.
[52] Videman T, Battie MC, Gibbons LE, et al. Associations between back pain history and lumbar MRI findings. Spine 2003;28(6):582–8.
[53] Edgar MA, Ghadially JA. Innervation of the lumbar spine. Clin Orthop Relat Res 1976; 115:35–41.
[54] Fagan A, Moore R, Vernon RB, et al. ISSLS prize winner: the innervation of the intervertebral disc: a quantitative analysis. Spine 2003;28(23):2570–6.
[55] Olmarker K, Rydevik B, Holm S. Edema formation in spinal nerve roots induced by experimental, graded compression. An experimental study on the pig cauda equina with special reference to differences in effects between rapid and slow onset of compression. Spine 1989; 14(6):569–73.
[56] Iida T, Abumi K, Kotani Y, et al. Effects of aging and spinal degeneration on mechanical properties of lumbar supraspinous and interspinous ligaments. Spine J 2002;2(2):95–100.
[57] Jane JA Sr, Jane JA Jr, Helm GA, et al. Acquired lumbar spinal stenosis. Clin Neurosurg 1996;43:275–99.
[58] Thalgott JS, Albert TJ, Vaccaro AR, et al. A new classification system for degenerative disc disease of the lumbar spine based on magnetic resonance imaging, provocative discography, plain radiographs and anatomic considerations. Spine J 2004;4(Suppl 6):167S–72S.
[59] Pritzker KP. Aging and degeneration in the lumbar intervertebral disc. Orthop Clin North Am 1977;8(1):66–77.
[60] Adams MA, Freeman BJ, Morrison HP, et al. Mechanical initiation of intervertebral disc degeneration. Spine 2000;25(13):1625–36.
[61] Hestbaek L, Iachine IA, Leboeuf-Yde C, et al. Heredity of low back pain in a young population: a classical twin study. Twin Res 2004;7(1):16–26.
[62] Annunen S, Paassilta P, Lohiniva J, et al. An allele of COL9A2 associated with intervertebral disc disease. Science 1999;285(5426):409–12.
[63] Marini JC. Genetic risk factors for lumbar disk disease. JAMA 2001;285(14):1886–8.
[64] Matsui H, Terahata N, Tsuji H, et al. Familial predisposition and clustering for juvenile lumbar disc herniation. Spine 1992;17(11):1323–8.
[65] Quinet RJ, Hadler NM. Diagnosis and treatment of backache. Semin Arthritis Rheum 1979;8(4):261–87.
[66] Brant-Zawadzki MN, Jensen MC, Obuchowski N, et al. Interobserver and intraobserver variability in interpretation of lumbar disc abnormalities. A comparison of two nomenclatures. Spine 1995;20(11):1257–63.
[67] Breton G. Is that a bulging disk, a small herniation or a moderate protrusion? Can Assoc Radiol J 1991;42(5):318.
[68] Milette PC. Reporting lumbar disk abnormalities: at last, consensus!. AJNR Am J Neuroradiol 2001;22(3):428–9.
[69] Raininko R, Manninen H, Battie MC, et al. Observer variability in the assessment of disc degeneration on magnetic resonance images of the lumbar and thoracic spine. Spine 1995; 20(9):1029–35.
[70] Twomey LT, Taylor JR. Age changes in lumbar vertebrae and intervertebral discs. Clin Orthop Relat Res 1987;224:97–104.
[71] Kirkaldy-Willis WH, Wedge JH, Yong-Hing K, et al. Pathology and pathogenesis of lumbar spondylosis and stenosis. Spine 1978;3(4):319–28.

[72] Elster AD. Bertolotti's syndrome revisited. Transitional vertebrae of the lumbar spine. Spine 1989;14(12):1373–7.

[73] Barzo P, Voros E, Bodosi M. Clinical significance of lumbosacral transitional vertebrae (Bertolotti syndrome). Orv Hetil 1993;134(46):2537–40 [in Hungarian].

[74] Luoma K, Vehmas T, Raininko R, et al. Lumbosacral transitional vertebra: relation to disc degeneration and low back pain. Spine 2004;29(2):200–5.

[75] Quinlan JF, Duke D, Eustace S. Bertolotti's syndrome: a cause of back pain in young people. J Bone Joint Surg Br 2006;88(9):1183–6.

[76] Adams P, Eyre DR, Muir H. Biochemical aspects of development and ageing of human lumbar intervertebral discs. Rheumatol Rehabil 1977;16(1):22–9.

[77] Brown MD. The pathophysiology of disc disease. Orthop Clin North Am 1971;2(2):359–70.

[78] Lipson SJ, Muir H. 1980 Volvo award in basic science. Proteoglycans in experimental intervertebral disc degeneration. Spine 1981;6(3):194–210.

[79] Modic MT, Pavlicek W, Weinstein MA, et al. Magnetic resonance imaging of intervertebral disk disease. Clinical and pulse sequence considerations. Radiology 1984;152(1):103–11.

[80] Peng B, Hou S, Wu W, et al. The pathogenesis and clinical significance of a high-intensity zone (HIZ) of lumbar intervertebral disc on MR imaging in the patient with discogenic low back pain. Eur Spine J 2006;15(5):583–7.

[81] Ricketson R, Simmons JW, Hauser BO. The prolapsed intervertebral disc. The high-intensity zone with discography correlation. Spine 1996;21(23):2758–62.

[82] Lam KS, Carlin D, Mulholland RC. Lumbar disc high-intensity zone: the value and significance of provocative discography in the determination of the discogenic pain source. Eur Spine J 2000;9(1):36–41.

[83] Derby R, Kim BJ, Lee SH, et al. Comparison of discographic findings in asymptomatic subject discs and the negative discs of chronic LBP patients: can discography distinguish asymptomatic discs among morphologically abnormal discs? Spine J 2005; 5(4):389–94.

[84] Modic MT, Steinberg PM, Ross JS, et al. Degenerative disk disease: assessment of changes in vertebral body marrow with MR imaging. Radiology 1988;166(1 Pt 1):193–9.

[85] de Roos A, Kressel H, Spritzer C, et al. MR imaging of marrow changes adjacent to end plates in degenerative lumbar disk disease. AJR Am J Roentgenol 1987;149(3):531–4.

[86] Chung CB, Vande Berg BC, Tavernier T, et al. End plate marrow changes in the asymptomatic lumbosacral spine: frequency, distribution and correlation with age and degenerative changes. Skeletal Radiol 2004;33(7):399–404.

[87] Manchikanti L. Facet joint pain and the role of neural blockade in its management. Curr Rev Pain 1999;3(5):348–58.

[88] Hodge JC, Bessette B. The incidence of sacroiliac joint disease in patients with low-back pain. Can Assoc Radiol J 1999;50(5):321–3.

[89] Boos N, Semmer N, Elfering A, et al. Natural history of individuals with asymptomatic disc abnormalities in magnetic resonance imaging: predictors of low back pain-related medical consultation and work incapacity. Spine 2000;25(12):1484–92.

[90] Masala S, Pipitone V, Tomassini M, et al. Percutaneous vertebroplasty in painful Schmorl nodes. Cardiovasc Intervent Radiol 2006;29(1):97–101.

[91] Lejeune JP, Hladky JP, Cotten A, et al. Foraminal lumbar disc herniation. Experience with 83 patients. Spine 1994;19(17):1905–8.

[92] Epstein NE. Foraminal and far lateral lumbar disc herniations: surgical alternatives and outcome measures. Spinal Cord 2002;40(10):491–500.

[93] Fredrickson BE, Baker D, McHolick WJ, et al. The natural history of spondylolysis and spondylolisthesis. J Bone Joint Surg Am 1984;66(5):699–707.

[94] Rothman SL, Glenn WV Jr. CT multiplanar reconstruction in 253 cases of lumbar spondylolysis. AJNR Am J Neuroradiol 1984;5(1):81–90.

[95] Kohlbach W. Spondylolysis/spondylolisthesis—a new thesis of its etiology. Rontgenblatter 1988;41(1):23–6 [in German].

[96] Rosenberg NJ, Bargar WL, Friedman B. The incidence of spondylolysis and spondylolisthesis in nonambulatory patients. Spine 1981;6(1):35–8.

[97] Porter RW, Hibbert CS. Symptoms associated with lysis of the pars interarticularis. Spine 1984;9(7):755–8.

[98] Pierce ME. Spondylolysis: what does this mean? A review. Australas Radiol 1987;31(4): 391–4.

[99] Wiltse LL. The effect of the common anomalies of the lumbar spine upon disc degeneration and low back pain. Orthop Clin North Am 1971;2(2):569–82.

[100] Cavalier R, Herman MJ, Cheung EV, et al. Spondylolysis and spondylolisthesis in children and adolescents: I. Diagnosis, natural history, and nonsurgical management. J Am Acad Orthop Surg 2006;14(7):417–24.

[101] Teplick JG, Laffey PA, Berman A, et al. Diagnosis and evaluation of spondylolisthesis and/ or spondylolysis on axial CT. AJNR Am J Neuroradiol 1986;7(3):479–91.

[102] Collier BD, Johnson RP, Carrera GF, et al. Painful spondylolysis or spondylolisthesis studied by radiography and single-photon emission computed tomography. Radiology 1985; 154(1):207–11.

[103] Papanicolaou N, Wilkinson RH, Emans JB, et al. Bone scintigraphy and radiography in young athletes with low back pain. AJR Am J Roentgenol 1985;145(5):1039–44.

[104] Hollenberg GM, Beattie PF, Meyers SP, et al. Stress reactions of the lumbar pars interarticularis: the development of a new MRI classification system. Spine 2002;27(2): 181–6.

[105] Cohen E, Stuecker RD. Magnetic resonance imaging in diagnosis and follow-up of impending spondylolysis in children and adolescents: early treatment may prevent pars defects. J Pediatr Orthop B 2005;14(2):63–7.

[106] Saifuddin A, Burnett SJ. The value of lumbar spine MRI in the assessment of the pars interarticularis. Clin Radiol 1997;52(9):666–71.

[107] Campbell RS, Grainger AJ. Optimization of MRI pulse sequences to visualize the normal pars interarticularis. Clin Radiol 1999;54(1):63–8.

[108] Arnoldi CC, Brodsky AE, Cauchoix J, et al. Lumbar spinal stenosis and nerve root entrapment syndromes. Definition and classification. Clin Orthop Relat Res 1976;115:4–5.

[109] Amundsen T, Weber H, Lilleas F, et al. Lumbar spinal stenosis. Clinical and radiologic features. Spine 1995;20(10):1178–86.

[110] Treatment of degenerative lumbar spinal stenosis. Evid Rep Technol Assess (Summ) 2001; 32:1–5.

[111] Fujiwara A, An HS, Lim TH, et al. Morphologic changes in the lumbar intervertebral foramen due to flexion-extension, lateral bending, and axial rotation: an in vitro anatomic and biomechanical study. Spine 2001;26(8):876–82.

[112] Willen J, Danielson B, Gaulitz A, et al. Dynamic effects on the lumbar spinal canal: axially loaded CT-myelography and MRI in patients with sciatica and/or neurogenic claudication. Spine 1997;22(24):2968–76.

[113] Zander DR, Lander PH. Positionally dependent spinal stenosis: correlation of upright flexion-extension myelography and computed tomographic myelography. Can Assoc Radiol J 1998;49(4):256–61.

[114] Singh K, Samartzis D, Vaccaro AR, et al. Congenital lumbar spinal stenosis: a prospective, control-matched, cohort radiographic analysis. Spine J 2005;5(6):615–22.

[115] Jarvik JG, Hollingworth W, Heagerty PJ, et al. Three-year incidence of low back pain in an initially asymptomatic cohort: clinical and imaging risk factors. Spine 2005;30(13): 1541–8.

[116] Mikhael MA, Ciric I, Tarkington JA, et al. Neuroradiological evaluation of lateral recess syndrome. Radiology 1981;140(1):97–107.

[117] Bartynski WS, Lin L. Lumbar root compression in the lateral recess: MR imaging, conventional myelography, and CT myelography comparison with surgical confirmation. AJNR Am J Neuroradiol 2003;24(3):348–60.

[118] Cinotti G, De Santis P, Nofroni I, et al. Stenosis of lumbar intervertebral foramen: anatomic study on predisposing factors. Spine 2002;27(3):223–9.

[119] Cramer GD, Cantu JA, Dorsett RD, et al. Dimensions of the lumbar intervertebral foramina as determined from the sagittal plane magnetic resonance imaging scans of 95 normal subjects. J Manipulative Physiol Ther 2003;26(3):160–70.

[120] Robertson SC, Traynelis VC, Follett KA, et al. Idiopathic spinal epidural lipomatosis. Neurosurgery 1997;41(1):68–74.

[121] Qasho R, Ramundo OE, Maraglino C, et al. Epidural lipomatosis with lumbar radiculopathy in one obese patient. Case report and review of the literature. Neurosurg Rev 1997; 20(3):206–9.

[122] Ohta Y, Hayashi T, Sasaki C, et al. Cauda equina syndrome caused by idiopathic sacral epidural lipomatosis. Intern Med 2002;41(7):593–4.

[123] Ahn UM, Ahn NU, Buchowski JM, et al. Cauda equina syndrome secondary to lumbar disc herniation: a meta-analysis of surgical outcomes. Spine 2000;25(12):1515–22.

[124] Henriques T, Olerud C, Petren-Mallmin M, et al. Cauda equina syndrome as a postoperative complication in five patients operated for lumbar disc herniation. Spine 2001;26(3):293–7.

[125] Shapiro S. Medical realities of cauda equina syndrome secondary to lumbar disc herniation. Spine 2000;25(3):348–51.

[126] Wiesel SW, Tsourmas N, Feffer HL, et al. A study of computer-assisted tomography. I. The incidence of positive CAT scans in an asymptomatic group of patients. Spine 1984;9(6): 549–51.

[127] Boden SD, Davis DO, Dina TS, et al. Abnormal magnetic-resonance scans of the lumbar spine in asymptomatic subjects. A prospective investigation. J Bone Joint Surg Am 1990; 72(3):403–8.

[128] Borenstein DG, O'Mara JW Jr, Boden SD, et al. The value of magnetic resonance imaging of the lumbar spine to predict low-back pain in asymptomatic subjects: a seven-year follow-up study. J Bone Joint Surg Am 2001;83(9):1306–11.

[129] Saal JA, Saal JS, Herzog RJ. The natural history of lumbar intervertebral disc extrusions treated nonoperatively. Spine 1990;15(7):683–6.

[130] Modic MT, Ross JS, Obuchowski NA, et al. Contrast-enhanced MR imaging in acute lumbar radiculopathy: a pilot study of the natural history. Radiology 1995;195(2):429–35.

[131] Benoist M. The natural history of lumbar degenerative spinal stenosis. Joint Bone Spine 2002;69(5):450–7.

[132] Modic MT, Obuchowski NA, Ross JS, et al. Acute low back pain and radiculopathy: MR imaging findings and their prognostic role and effect on outcome. Radiology 2005;237(2): 597–604.

[133] Vital JM, Gille O, Pointillart V, et al. Course of Modic 1 six months after lumbar posterior osteosynthesis. Spine 2003;28(7):715–20.

[134] Weishaupt D, Zanetti M, Hodler J, et al. Painful lumbar disk derangement: relevance of endplate abnormalities at MR imaging. Radiology 2001;218(2):420–7.

[135] Braithwaite I, White J, Saifuddin A, et al. Vertebral end-plate (Modic) changes on lumbar spine MRI: correlation with pain reproduction at lumbar discography. Eur Spine J 1998; 7(5):363–8.

[136] Buttermann GR, Heithoff KB, Ogilvie JW, et al. Vertebral body MRI related to lumbar fusion results. Eur Spine J 1997;6(2):115–20.

[137] Maiuri F, Iaconetta G, Gallicchio B, et al. Spondylodiscitis. Clinical and magnetic resonance diagnosis. Spine 1997;22(15):1741–6.

[138] Jung NY, Jee WH, Ha KY, et al. Discrimination of tuberculous spondylitis from pyogenic spondylitis on MRI. AJR Am J Roentgenol 2004;182(6):1405–10.

[139] Ledermann HP, Schweitzer ME, Morrison WB, et al. MR imaging findings in spinal infections: rules or myths? Radiology 2003;228(2):506–14.

[140] Post MJ, Sze G, Quencer RM, et al. Gadolinium-enhanced MR in spinal infection. J Comput Assist Tomogr 1990;14(5):721–9.

[141] Dagirmanjian A, Schils J, McHenry M, et al. MR imaging of vertebral osteomyelitis revisited. AJR Am J Roentgenol 1996;167(6):1539–43.

[142] Modic MT, Feiglin DH, Piraino DW, et al. Vertebral osteomyelitis: assessment using MR. Radiology 1985;157(1):157–66.

[143] Sharif HS, Aideyan OA, Clark DC, et al. Brucellar and tuberculous spondylitis: comparative imaging features. Radiology 1989;171(2):419–25.

[144] Sharif HS, Clark DC, Aabed MY, et al. Granulomatous spinal infections: MR imaging. Radiology 1990;177(1):101–7.

[145] Shih TT, Huang KM, Li YW. Solitary vertebral collapse: distinction between benign and malignant causes using MR patterns. J Magn Reson Imaging 1999;9(5):635–42.

[146] Yuh WT, Zachar CK, Barloon TJ, et al. Vertebral compression fractures: distinction between benign and malignant causes with MR imaging. Radiology 1989;172(1):215–8.

[147] Fu TS, Chen LH, Liao JC, et al. Magnetic resonance imaging characteristics of benign and malignant vertebral fractures. Chang Gung Med J 2004;27(11):808–15.

[148] Kubota T, Yamada K, Ito H, et al. High-resolution imaging of the spine using multidetector-row computed tomography: differentiation between benign and malignant vertebral compression fractures. J Comput Assist Tomogr 2005;29(5):712–9.

[149] Cotten A, Dewatre F, Cortet B, et al. Percutaneous vertebroplasty for osteolytic metastases and myeloma: effects of the percentage of lesion filling and the leakage of methyl methacrylate at clinical follow-up. Radiology 1996;200(2):525–30.

[150] Maynard AS, Jensen ME, Schweickert PA, et al. Value of bone scan imaging in predicting pain relief from percutaneous vertebroplasty in osteoporotic vertebral fractures. AJNR Am J Neuroradiol 2000;21(10):1807–12.

[151] Cheung G, Chow E, Holden L, et al. Percutaneous vertebroplasty in patients with intractable pain from osteoporotic or metastatic fractures: a prospective study using quality-of-life assessment. Can Assoc Radiol J 2006;57(1):13–21.

[152] Lieberman IH, Dudeney S, Reinhardt MK, et al. Initial outcome and efficacy of "kyphoplasty" in the treatment of painful osteoporotic vertebral compression fractures. Spine 2001;26(14):1631–8.

[153] Masala S, Schillaci O, Massari F, et al. MRI and bone scan imaging in the preoperative evaluation of painful vertebral fractures treated with vertebroplasty and kyphoplasty. In Vivo 2005;19(6):1055–60.

[154] Deyo RA, Mirza SK. Trends and variations in the use of spine surgery. Clin Orthop Relat Res 2006;443:139–46.

[155] Atlas SJ, Keller RB, Wu YA, et al. Long-term outcomes of surgical and nonsurgical management of lumbar spinal stenosis: 8 to 10 year results from the Maine lumbar spine study. Spine 2005;30(8):936–43.

[156] Osterman H, Sund R, Seitsalo S, et al. Risk of multiple reoperations after lumbar discectomy: a population-based study. Spine 2003;28(6):621–7.

[157] Javid MJ, Hadar EJ. Long-term follow-up review of patients who underwent laminectomy for lumbar stenosis: a prospective study. J Neurosurg 1998;89(1):1–7.

[158] Niggemeyer O, Strauss JM, Schulitz KP. Comparison of surgical procedures for degenerative lumbar spinal stenosis: a meta-analysis of the literature from 1975 to 1995. Eur Spine J 1997;6(6):423–9.

[159] Shah RR, Mohammed S, Saifuddin A, et al. Comparison of plain radiographs with CT scan to evaluate interbody fusion following the use of titanium interbody cages and transpedicular instrumentation. Eur Spine J 2003;12(4):378–85.

[160] Bundschuh CV, Modic MT, Ross JS, et al. Epidural fibrosis and recurrent disk herniation in the lumbar spine: MR imaging assessment. AJR Am J Roentgenol 1988;150(4):923–32.

[161] Jorgensen J, Hansen PH, Steenskov V, et al. A clinical and radiological study of chronic lower spinal arachnoiditis. Neuroradiology 1975;9(3):139–44.

[162] Ross JS, Masaryk TJ, Modic MT, et al. MR imaging of lumbar arachnoiditis. AJR Am J Roentgenol 1987;149(5):1025–32.

[163] Zhang H, He M, Mao B. Thoracic spine extradural arteriovenous fistula: case report and review of the literature. Surg Neurol 2006;66(Suppl 1):S18–23.

[164] Kim LJ, Spetzler RF. Classification and surgical management of spinal arteriovenous lesions: arteriovenous fistulae and arteriovenous malformations. Neurosurgery 2006; 59(5 Suppl 3):S195–201.

[165] Spetzler RF, Detwiler PW, Riina HA, et al. Modified classification of spinal cord vascular lesions. J Neurosurg 2002;96(Suppl 2):145–56.

[166] Zozulya YP, Slin'ko EI, Al Qashqish II. Spinal arteriovenous malformations: new classification and surgical treatment. Neurosurg Focus 2006;20(5):E7.

[167] Larsson EM, Desai P, Hardin CW, et al. Venous infarction of the spinal cord resulting from dural arteriovenous fistula: MR imaging findings. AJNR Am J Neuroradiol 1991;12(4): 739–43.

[168] Jones BV, Ernst RJ, Tomsick TA, et al. Spinal dural arteriovenous fistulas: recognizing the spectrum of magnetic resonance imaging findings. J Spinal Cord Med 1997;20(1):43–8.

[169] Bowen BC, Fraser K, Kochan JP, et al. Spinal dural arteriovenous fistulas: evaluation with MR angiography. AJNR Am J Neuroradiol 1995;16(10):2029–43.

[170] Lai PH, Weng MJ, Lee KW, et al. Multidetector CT angiography in diagnosing type I and type IVA spinal vascular malformations. AJNR Am J Neuroradiol 2006;27(4):813–7.

[171] Mascalchi M, Ferrito G, Quilici N, et al. Spinal vascular malformations: MR angiography after treatment. Radiology 2001;219(2):346–53.

NEUROLOGIC
CLINICS

Neurol Clin 25 (2007) 473–494

The Electrodiagnosis of Cervical and Lumbosacral Radiculopathy

Bryan Tsao, MD*

*Department of Neurology, Loma Linda University, 11175 Campus Street,
Loma Linda, CA 92354, USA*

The first clinical description of lumbosacral and cervical radiculopathy was made by Mixter and Semmes, yet the role of the electrodiagnostic (EDX) examination in the diagnosis of suspected radiculopathy was not used routinely until more than 20 years later [1–5]. Today, neck and back pain is one of the most common reasons for all office visits and for referrals to EDX laboratories. Despite many patients not having definite radiculopathy or nerve root compression, EDX consultants are faced with performing a complex test that has a potential impact on treatment.

EDX consultants need to understand the pathophysiology of radiculopathy and conduct the study in a practical manner that optimizes its diagnostic yield. Done correctly, an EDX examination serves to confirm the presence of radiculopathy, establish the involved nerve root level, determine if axon loss or conduction block is present, grade the severity of the process, estimate the age of the radiculopathy, and exclude other peripheral nerve diseases that mimic radiculopathy.

This topic has been the subject of comprehensive reviews [6–9]. The purpose of this article is to highlight the anatomy and physiology of nerve root disease, discuss the pros and cons of the various portions of the EDX examination, and review an EDX approach to the diagnosis of cervical and lumbosacral radiculopathy.

Anatomy and pathophysiology of radiculopathy

The ventral and dorsal rootlets arise from the substance of the spinal cord and enter the neural foramen (Fig. 1). Just distal to the dorsal root ganglion

* Loma Linda University, 11175 Campus St., Coleman Pavilion, #11108, Loma Linda, CA 92354.

   E-mail address: btsao@llu.edu

0733-8619/07/$ - see front matter © 2007 Elsevier Inc. All rights reserved.
doi:10.1016/j.ncl.2007.02.001   *neurologic.theclinics.com*

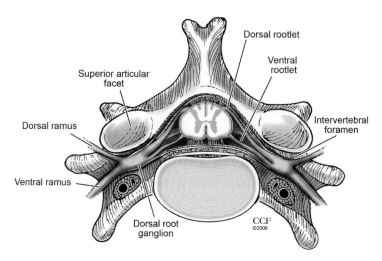

Fig. 1. The nerve root complex. The ventral (anterior) and dorsal (posterior) rootlets combine within the neural foramen to form mixed spinal nerves. The mixed spinal nerves divide into ventral and dorsal rami, which exit the intervertebral foramen and give rise to the peripheral nerves that supply the limb and paraspinal muscles, respectively. (*Courtesy of* the Cleveland Clinic Foundation, Cleveland, OH; with permission.)

(DRG), these rootlets join to form a mixed spinal nerve. On exiting the intervertebral foramen, the mixed spinal nerve divides into dorsal and ventral rami. The dorsal ramus innervates the paraspinal muscles and the skin of the neck and trunk with overlapping segmental innervation, such that the ultimate site of paraspinal muscle innervation may be anywhere from 3 to 6 segments beyond their level of spinal cord origin [10]. The ventral rami form the cervical (C2-4), brachial (C5-T1), lumbar (L2-5), and sacral (S1-5) plexi and nerves that supply the trunk, intercostal, and abdominal wall muscles.

Of the 31 pairs of spinal nerves, only the C4-C8, T1, L2-5, and S1-2 levels have limb representation that can be assessed by EDX examination. The numeric designation of nerve roots is such that the C1-C7 roots exit their neural foramen above the vertebral body of the same number (eg, the C7 root exits the spinal canal via the C6-7 neural foramina), whereas the C8 root exits between the C7 and T1 vertebrae. Below this level, all thoracic, lumbar, and sacral roots exit caudal to the vertebral body of the same number.

The spinal cord ends at approximately the L1-2 vertebral body level as the conus medullaris and continues as a loose collection of spinal nerve roots, the cauda equina. The lumbosacral nerves within the cauda equina run downward and laterally before exiting their respective foramina. Because of this arrangement, a large L4-5 disk protrusion that extends far laterally may compress the L4 nerve root at the same level of the disk, whereas a posterior disk protrusion at the same level may compress the L5 nerve root, and, if large enough, the L5 and S1 nerve roots [11]. The lumbar

DRGs vary in their location so that approximately 3% of L3-4 DRGs, 11% to 38% of L5 DRGs, and approximately 71% of S1 DRGs are within the intraspinal canal [12,13]. Although less common, the DRGs in the cervical spine also may lie proximal to the intervertebral foramina [14]. The EDX correlate of lateral disk herniation in the presence of intraspinally located DRGs is loss of sensory nerve action potential (SNAP) amplitude along the nerves of the involved segment [15].

The most common cause of compressive nerve root injury is by disk herniation or other degenerative spine elements (eg, osteophyte, facet joint hypertrophy, and ligamentous hypertrophy). Noncompressive causes include ischemia, trauma, neoplastic infiltration, spinal infections, postradiation injury, immune-mediated diseases, lipoma, and congenital conditions, such as meningomyelocele and arthrogryposis; these present with EDX patterns indistinguishable from nerve root compression [16].

Acute compression from eccentric disk herniation results in asymmetric nerve root distortion and traction, whereas spinal stenosis generally produces bilateral compression and deformity of the DRG [17,18]. The severity of nerve root injury depends on the amount and duration of compression resulting in this sequence of events: nerve distortion, intraneural edema, impaired intraneural microcirculation leading to focal nerve ischemia, localized inflammatory intraneural and connective tissue reaction, and, finally, altered nerve conduction [19]. With sufficient root compression, axon loss ensues. Prolonged vascular congestion may lead to intra- and extraneural fibrosis that perpetuates chronic compression.

Nerve conduction studies

Routine nerve conduction studies

Routine nerve conduction studies (NCS) should be performed in all patients who have suspected cervical or lumbar radiculopathy (Tables 1 and 2). Additional NCS for various levels of radiculopathy should be considered if routine NCS do not assess the appropriate levels. The technical aspects of conducting NCS are reviewed elsewhere [8,20].

Motor NCS typically are normal in patients who have radiculopathy, because only a portion of nerve fascicles within a nerve root trunk is injured. Rarely, if the radiculopathy results in sufficient motor axon loss (up to 50% of motor axons within a nerve trunk), the compound motor action potential (CMAP) amplitude may be reduced significantly, as defined by age-related norms or a 50% or greater reduction in amplitude compared with the contralateral limb. Even in the presence of severe axon loss, however, routine motor NCS may appear normal unless the CMAP is generated from a muscle that receives innervation from the injured nerve root (eg, for a suspected C5-6 radiculopathy, routine motor NCS assess only the median innervated thenar [mainly T1-derived] and ulnar innervated hypothenar [mainly

Table 1
Recommended nerve conduction studies in suspected cervical radiculopathy

Nerve (muscle)	Nerve root assessed	Parameters
General survey		
Sensory		
Median index	C6–C7	Distal amplitude, peak latency
Radial thumb	C6–C7	
Ulnar little	C8	
Motor		
Median (thenar)	T1 > C8	Distal and proximal amplitude, distal latency, conduction velocity
Ulnar (hypothenar)	C8	
Additional nerve conduction studies for suspected root level		
Sensory		
Median thumb	C6	
LABC	C6	
MABC	T1	
Motor		
Axillary (deltoid)	C5–6	
MC (biceps)	C5–6	
Ulnar (FDI)	C8	

Abbreviations: FDI, first dorsal interosseous; LABC, lateral antebrachial cutaneous; MABC, medial antebrachial cutaneous; MC, musculocutaneous.

C8-derived] muscles). In this instance, to detect motor axon loss, if present, a CMAP would have to be recorded over the biceps or deltoid muscles. In chronic axon loss radiculopathy, CMAPs may normalize if sufficient reinnervation occurs.

Table 2
Recommended nerve conduction studies in suspected lumbosacral radiculopathy

Nerve (muscle)	Nerve root	Parameters
General survey		
Sensory		
Sural	S1	Distal amplitude, peak latency
Motor		
Post tibial (AH)	S1	Distal and proximal amplitude, distal latency, conduction velocity
Peroneal (EDB)	L5	
Late response		
Posterior tibial (GM-S)	S1	H-reflex, amplitude, and motor amplitude
Additional nerve conduction studies for suspected root level		
Sensory		
Superficial peroneal	L5	
Motor		
Femoral (rectus femoris)	L2–4	

Abbreviations: AH, abductor hallucis; EDB, extensor digitorum brevis; GM-S, gastrocnemius-soleus.

The pathophysiology of radiculopathy at the root level infrequently is a focal, purely demyelinating conduction block. If this occurs, routine motor NCS remain normal even if weakness is present in corresponding myotomes.

Sensory NCS typically are normal in radiculopathy, because nerve root compression occurs proximal to the sensory DRG. The presence of a normal SNAP is useful in differentiating a radiculopathy (where they usually are present) from a plexus or peripheral neuropathy lesion (where they usually are reduced or absent) [6,7,21,22]. An exception to the normal SNAP rule in radiculopathy occurs at times in the setting of L5 radiculopathy, where the DRG can have a vulnerable intraspinal canal location in up to 40% of individuals, leading to an absent superficial peroneal sensory response [15].

Late responses

Late responses have the advantage of assessing the proximal (and intraspinal) segments of the peripheral nerve fibers, whereas routine NCS assess only the more distal portions. The two late responses used most commonly are the H-reflex and the F wave. The technical aspects of performing these studies are reviewed elsewhere [8,23].

H-reflex

The H-reflex, named after Hoffman, who first described this technique, is a monosynaptic spinal reflex that assesses an afferent 1a sensory nerve and an efferent α motor nerve. The H-reflex is recorded most commonly over the gastrocnemius-soleus muscle complex, stimulating the tibial nerve, and is considered the EDX equivalent of the Achilles or ankle stretch reflex, although discordance is frequent and the H-reflex may be absent in normal individuals [24]. In the arm, the H-reflex can be derived from the median nerve (recording the flexor carpi radialis muscle) but technically is difficult to perform and the results seldom are useful [25]. The tibial H-amplitude is a highly sensitive test, when combined with the needle electrode examination (NEE), for detecting a preganglionic S1 nerve root lesion. An abnormal amplitude is defined in the author's EDX laboratory as 1 mV or less in patients younger than 60 years or a side-to-side amplitude difference of greater than 50% on the symptomatic versus asymptomatic side [6]. An absent or asymmetrically reduced H-amplitude can be found in 80% to 89% of surgically or myelography confirmed cases of S1 radiculopathy [26,27]. The absolute normal H-reflex latency ranges from 34 to 35 milliseconds and is dependent on patient age, limb length, and height [28]. An H-amplitude ratio (defined as an abnormal H-amplitude divided by the contralateral H-amplitude) of less than 0.4 is considered abnormal, although in a study of 47 healthy adults, 2% had a ratio of 0.33 [29]. Despite its sensitivity in radiculopathy, a reduced H-reflex amplitude is not specific for etiology or precise localization, as a focal lesion anywhere along the sensory afferent, spinal synapse, or motor efferent pathways may diminish the H amplitude. Diagnosing radiculopathy based on prolonged H latency alone is insensitive, because focal slowing may be obscured by the long segment of nerve assessed and, even if present, does not localize the lesion along the nerve segment studied. Last, the H-reflex technically may be difficult to obtain in obese patients and may be absent in patients over 60 years of age.

F waves

The F wave, named for the foot muscle over which it was first recorded, is a late motor response elicited from the median or ulnar nerve in the upper extremity (recording from the thenar or hypothenar muscle, respectively) and the tibial or peroneal nerve in the lower extremity (recording from the abductor hallucis or extensor digitorum brevis muscle, respectively). Unlike the H-reflex, the F wave assesses only motor nerve fibers, first in an antidromic, then in an orthodromic, fashion. F waves have a variable latency and amplitude, are reproducible, and are approximately 5% of the CMAP size of the muscle over which they are recorded. Most authorities agree that the minimal F-wave latency, if abnormal in the face of normal routine NCS, points toward a lesion of the proximal motor nerve fibers [30]. Other F-wave measurements include F-wave duration, F-mean latency (mean of F-wave minimum and maximum latency), maximum F-wave latency, chronodispersion (maximal minus minimal F-wave response latency), and F-wave persistence (the number of F waves per number of stimulations). An F estimate, which corrects for limb length, may be performed if the F-wave latency is abnormal. With the exception of two studies that found the sensitivity of F-wave analysis comparable to the NEE in L5 or S1 radiculopathy, most authorities agree that the overall diagnostic yield (ie, 10%–20%) is low for several reasons [31,32]. The theoretic advantage that F waves evaluate the proximal segment of the motor nerve is offset by the fact that focal slowing within a short segment is diluted by normal conduction along the rest of the motor nerve pathway. The F-wave latencies are limited in that they assess only the fastest conducting fibers. Thus, a lesion that produces focal slowing has to affect all fibers equally to increase the minimal F latency, whereas most cases of radiculopathy cause partial axon loss and only rarely focal demyelination. Consequently, Aminoff [33] concludes that F waves often are normal in patients who have suspected radiculopathy, and "even when they are abnormal, their findings are inconsequential because the (needle electrode examination) findings are also abnormal and help to establish the diagnosis more definitively."

Somatosensory evoked responses

Somatosensory evoked potentials (SEPs) are cortical potentials elicited by stimulating a mixed sensory and motor nerve trunk, individual cutaneous nerves, or dermatomal distributions [34,35]. Absolute and relative latencies (ie, the interpeak latency) are obtained and adjusted to patient height and limb length. Again, although SEPs offer the theoretic advantage of assessing proximal portions of sensory nerves, their routine use is limited by a variety of factors. As with the H-reflex and F wave, SEPs record responses only from the fastest conducting nerve fibers, so that focal or partial conduction block or slowing is not apparent, masked by normally conducting afferent fibers and diluted by the long nerve segment over which the SEP travels. Furthermore, because of the normal interside and intersubject variation in amplitude of SEPs, only an absent or unelicitable response may indicate underlying pathology. Lastly, abnormal SEPs may localize a lesion to the plexus region but cannot discriminate further between plexus and root localization. The consensus of recent reviews is that SEPs by nerve trunk stimulation are unhelpful in the diagnosis of suspected radiculopathy, whereas cutaneous and dermatomal SEPs are insensitive and only support, at best, the presence of radiculopathy when the diagnosis is defined more clearly clinically or by EDX [35,36].

Thermography

Studies comparing thermography to NEE in patients who have clinical evidence of radiculopathy find that thermography may have comparable sensitivity but has no segmental localizing value and is considered of little practical use [37–39].

Motor evoked potentials

Motor evoked potentials (MEPs) are elicited by electrical or magnetic stimulation. Electrical stimulation is performed by inserting a monopolar needle electrode into the paraspinal muscles and recording from a distal limb muscle in a corresponding myotome. Normal motor amplitudes and latencies are defined by interside comparison. Using this method in 34 patients who had clinical signs of cervical radiculopathy, 40% had NEE abnormalities versus 61% by cervical root stimulation alone [40]. Thus, although cervical root stimulation had a slightly higher sensitivity for diagnosing radiculopathy, it did not add additional information to what the clinical history and NEE already provided. In 45 patients who had L5/S1 radiculopathy, the MEP latency was prolonged on the symptomatic side in 66% to 72% [41]. The downside of electrically stimulated MEPs is that they assess only motor fibers, are useful only in unilateral radiculopathy, and are tolerated poorly. Magnetic stimulation studies, reportedly less painful, demonstrate mixed results. MEP latencies were delayed and amplitudes reduced in cervical and lumbosacral radiculopathy but this has not been reproduced in subsequent studies [42–45]. Because this technique also depends on interside comparison, it is unhelpful in patients who have bilateral disease. Moreover, there is debate on the precise anatomic site of stimulation. As a result,

MEPs have no role in the routine diagnosis of radiculopathy and should be considered investigational.

Needle electrode examination

General principles

NEE is a sensitive technique to detect motor axon loss and is the single most useful diagnostic tool in radiculopathy [6,46]. The diagnosis of radiculopathy by NEE requires the identification of neurogenic abnormalities in two or more muscles that share the same nerve root innervation but differ in their peripheral nerve supply. Not all muscles within a myotome need to be affected but those innervated by adjacent root segments must be normal [6].

The timing of an EDX examination and NEE is of importance. The study generally should not be performed less than 3 weeks from the onset of symptoms, the time period necessary for most limb muscles to develop fibrillation potentials.

The diagnosis of radiculopathy by needle electrode examination

Based on clinical and EDX criteria, radiculopathy can be acute or chronic. The EDX hallmark of acute axon loss radiculopathy is the identification of fibrillation potentials in denervated muscle with normal motor unit action potentials (MUAPs). Fibrillation potentials tend to appear first in more proximal muscles, namely the paraspinals, and later in the limb muscles. Reinnervation takes place in a proximal to distal fashion so that fibrillations begin to disappear in the same sequence in which they occurred. Fibrillation potentials usually are most abundant within 6 months of symptom onset and may disappear completely in the paraspinal muscles after 6 weeks, whereas those in the distal limbs may persist for up to 1 to 2 years.

Infrequently, the pathophysiology of radiculopathy is focal, pure demyelinating conduction block manifested on a NEE with normal MUAPs firing in a reduced neurogenic recruitment rate. If this pattern is identified in sufficient muscles within a myotome, radiculopathy can be diagnosed.

The NEE definition of chronic radiculopathy largely is dependent on the identification of neurogenic recruitment and MUAP configuration changes in involved muscles with or without fibrillation potentials. These neurogenic abnormalities include MUAPs with increased duration and phases that represent reinnervation resulting from collateral sprouting. In early stages of reinnervation, these MUAPs show a moment-to-moment variation in configuration as immature motor unit junctions are established; with time, this instability is replaced with broad, large, and polyphasic MUAPs. These chronic neurogenic changes usually persist indefinitely after radiculopathy, and it is common to find such abnormalities on a NEE years after patients had their initial symptoms.

Diagnosing radiculopathy based on polyphasic MUAPs alone has several drawbacks, as up to 10% to 20% of normal limb muscles may have increased polyphasia [6,7]. Table 3 summarizes the evolution of NEE abnormalities in radiculopathy, from spontaneous activity to MUAP configuration and recruitment changes [9].

Root localization by needle electrode examination

The selection of particular muscles in myotomes examined on NEE can be based on myotomal charts derived from anatomic, clinical, electrophysiologic, or neuroimaging correlations. Each of these has its merits and limitations [27,47–60].

A general screening NEE survey should be performed in all patients who have suspected radiculopathy. In the upper limb, this should cover at least one muscle innervated by the C5, C6, C7, C8, T1 spinal roots and an appropriate cervical paraspinal muscle (Tables 4 and 5). In the lower limb, the general survey consists of at least one muscle innervated by the L2-4, L5, S1 spinal roots and an appropriate lumbosacral paraspinal muscle. Thus, the minimal NEE in any limb requires the sampling of at least five to seven muscles, including the paraspinals [6,61].

Radiculopathies often cause partial motor axon loss within a given root distribution. Thus, abnormal NEE findings within a single myotome may be variable and patchy, affecting one muscle in the myotome but not an adjacent muscle from the same myotome. Moreover, segmental nerve supply from uninvolved roots may dilute the identification of axon loss (eg, a C7 radiculopathy) further and may be associated with substantial denervation of the triceps but only partial denervation of the pronator teres. When clinical suspicion of radiculopathy is high, therefore, additional muscles within

Table 3
Findings in the needle electrode examination in affected muscles at progressive stages of axon loss radiculopathy

	Recruit	Insertion	PSP	Fib	Poly/var	Neur	MTP/CRD
<3 weeks	++	+/++	+	—	—	—	—
3–6 weeks	++	++	++	+++	—	—	—
6–26 weeks	++	+	±	++	+++	—	—
Chronic/active	++	—	±	+	++	++	—
Chronic/active	+/++	—	—	—	—	+++	+

Abbreviations: Fib, fibrillations; Insertion, abnormal insertional activity; MTP/CRD, myotonic discharge/complex repetitive discharges; Neur, neurogenic motor unit potential changes (increased duration and amplitude); Poly/var, polyphasic motor unit potential changes/motor unit potential variation; PSP, paraspinal fibrillation; Recruit, reduced neurogenic motor unit potential recruitment; +, mild amount; ++, moderate amount; +++, greatest amount; ±, equivocal amount.

Data from Levin KH. Cervical radiculopathies. In: Katirji B, Kaminski HJ, Preston DC, et al, editors. Neuromuscular disorders in clinical practice. Boston: Butterworth-Heinemann; 2002. p. 848.

Table 4
Needle electrode examination in suspected cervical radiculopathy

Muscle	Nerve root (primary)	Terminal nerve	Approximate yield in radiculopathy at specified level[a]
General screen			
Deltoid	C5–6	Axillary	86% (C5); 38% (C6)
Biceps	C5–6	Musculocutaneous	71% (C5); 44% (C6)
Pronator teres	C6–7	Median	78% (C6); 61% (C7)
Triceps	C6–7	Radial	56% (C6); 100% (C7)
First dorsal interosseous	C8	Ulnar	100%
Flexor pollicis longus	C8	Median	67%
Extensor indicis proprius	C8	Radial	100%
Cervical paraspinal	Overlap		47%
Additional high yield muscles for given level of cervical radiculopathy			
Infraspinatus	C5	Suprascapular	83%
Brachioradialis	C5	Radial	83%
Anconeus	C6	Radial	100%
Flexor carpi radialis	C6	Median	80%
Brachioradialis	C6	Radial	71%
Flexor carpi radialis	C7	Median	93%
Anconeus	C7	Radial	78%
Abductor digiti minimi	C8	Ulnar	83%

[a] Derived from 50 patients who had surgically confirmed single-level cervical radiculopathy (defined on NEE with either active motor axon loss [fibrillation potentials] or reduced MUP recruitment).

Data from Levin KH, Maggiano HJ, Wilbourn AJ. Cervical radiculopathies: comparison of surgical and EMG localization of single-root lesion. Neurology 1996;46:1023.

the suspect myotomes should be examined. Tables 4 and 5 list additional high-yield muscles that should be added to a NEE for a suspected radiculopathy level. It always is appropriate to make a comparison study on the opposite side, to exclude bilateral disease and to confirm the normal electrophysiologic appearance of asymptomatic muscles.

Even though NEE of the paraspinal muscles should be considered in all patients referred for radiculopathy, there are a few exceptions and several caveats. First, fibrillation potentials may be seen in the cervical and lumbosacral paraspinals in up to 12% and 14.5% to 42% of normal individuals, respectively [62–64]. Second, paraspinal fibrillation potentials are nonspecific for etiology (ie, present in myositis and motor neuronopathies) and yield uninterpretable results in patients who have undergone posterior cervical surgery or recent local trauma. Third, the presence of paraspinal fibrillation potentials alone (without similar evidence in the limbs) is insufficient to make a diagnosis of radiculopathy. In contrast, paraspinal fibrillation potentials may be absent in radiculopathy because they are spared, there is sampling error, or they have undergone reinnervation, at times with 6 weeks of symptom onset [54]. Finally, the extensive overlapping innervation of the paraspinal muscles prevents accurate localization of the

Table 5
Needle electrode examination in suspected lumbosacral radiculopathy

Muscle	Nerve root (primary)	Terminal nerve	Approximate yield in radiculopathy at specified level[a]
General screen			
Rectus femoris or	L3–4	Femoral	75% (L3-4)
Vastus lateralis	L3–4	Femoral	67% (L3-4)
Tibialis anterior	L4–5	Peroneal	77% (L5)
Tibialis posterior	L5	Posterior tibial	92% (L5); 18% (S1)
Extensor digitorum brevis	L5	Peroneal	38 % (L5)
Gluteus medius or	L5	Superior gluteal	50% (L5); 33% (S1)
Gluteus maximus	S1	Inferior gluteal	64% (S1); 13% (L5)
Medial gastrocnemius	S1	Posterior tibial	83% (S1)
Paraspinal	Overlap		86% (L2-4); 16% (L5); 25% (S1)
Additional high yield muscles for given level of lumbosacral radiculopathy			
Iliacus	L2–3	N. to iliacus	71%
Adductor longus	L2–4	Obdurator	100%
Vastus medialis	L2–4	Femoral	66%
Peroneus longus	L5	Peroneal	100%
Tensor fascia lata	L5	Superior gluteal	100%
Extensor hallucis longus	L5–S1	Peroneal	73% (L5); 25% (S1)
Lateral gastrocnemius	L5–S1	Tibial	13% (L5); 91% (S1)
Biceps femoris—SH	S1	Sciatic	89%
Biceps femoris—LH	S1	Sciatic	100%

Abbreviations: LH, long head; SH, short head.
[a] Derived from 45 patients who had surgically confirmed single-level lumbosacral radiculopathy (defined on NEE with either active motor axon loss [fibrillation potentials] or reduced MUP recruitment).
Data from Tsao BE, Levin KH, Bodnar RA. Comparison of surgical and electrodiagnostic findings in single root lumbosacral radiculopathies. Muscle Nerve 2003;27:61.

precise nerve root level involved. In patients who have chronic symptoms of radiculopathy and absence of active motor axon loss changes in muscles of the extremity, the diagnostic yield from examination of paraspinal muscles is low.

In summary, the presence of paraspinal fibrillation potentials supports the diagnosis of radiculopathy when corresponding abnormalities are present in the limb muscles, but the absence of such changes does not exclude a radiculopathy.

Comparative diagnostic methods

How valuable is NEE in diagnosing radiculopathy? In a consensus statement, the American Association of Neuromuscular and Electrodiagnostic Medicine conducted a critical review of the scientific literature addressing the value of EDX findings in patients who have cervical radiculopathy. The report found no gold standard against which the EDX examination could be directly compared with but concluded that NEE seems to have moderate sensitivity (50%–71%) and high specificity (65%–85%, defined as having good correlation with radiologic findings) in diagnosing cervical radiculopathy [65,66].

Several reports have compared EDX examination with imaging studies. Compared with myelography, EDX examination had a higher yield in four of five studies and was positive in 72% to 94% of cases versus myelography, which was positive in 75% to 84% [67]. Similar results were found comparing EDX examination and CT [68,69]. The correlation between MRI findings and EDX examination is uncertain, as abnormal structural MRI changes may be present in up to 19% of patients who do not have neck pain and 28% to 64% in those who do not have back pain [70–72].

Electrodiagnostic correlations

Cervical radiculopathies

Cervical radiculopathy constitutes approximately 5% to 10% of all radiculopathies and is second only to lumbosacral radiculopathy [49]. In general, C7 radiculopathy accounts for the majority of all cervical radiculopathies (up to 70%) followed by C6 (19%–25%), C8 (4%–10%), and C5 (2%) radiculopathies [5,60]. Fig. 2 shows NEE distribution of axon loss in patients who have active single-level cervical radiculopathy confirmed at surgery [60].

C5 radiculopathy

Commonly affected muscles include the deltoid, biceps, infra- and supraspinatus, brachioradialis, brachialis, and rhomboids. The rhomboid is supplied by a direct branch from the C5 nerve root; thus, involvement of this muscle confirms a C5 radiculopathy. The deltoid and biceps receive their primary innervation from the C5 root with secondary innervation from the C6 root. They are affected most often in C5 radiculopathies (86% and 71%, respectively) but may be involved, to a lesser degree, in C6 radiculopathies (38% and 44%, respectively) [60]. The brachioradialis, however, receives nearly equal innervation from the C5 and C6 nerve roots so that its involvement does not differentiate between an isolated C5 or C6 radiculopathy. The trapezius (innervated via the spinal accessory nerve with twigs from the C4 root) and pronator teres are spared in C5 radiculopathy. There is no sensory NCS that assesses the C5 nerve root reliably, but if the radiculopathy is severe enough, additional motor NCS recording the deltoid or biceps muscles may be considered.

C6 radiculopathy

Compared with other single-level cervical radiculopathies, C6 radiculopathies do not present in a stereotypic fashion but, instead, have two distinct EDX patterns; one is similar to C5 radiculopathy with additional involvement of the triceps and pronator teres, the other resembles a C7 radiculopathy.

Most myotomal charts state the triceps as supplied by the C6 through C8 roots, but it is heavily C7 weighted. The triceps is affected in approximately half the cases of C6 radiculopathy and is only rarely, if ever, abnormal in C8 radiculopathy. Sensory NCS recording the median-innervated thumb and lateral antebrachial cutaneous should be performed in suspected C6 radiculopathy. There is no reliable motor NCS method to assess the C6 nerve in isolation. If indicated, the deltoid and biceps can serve as a rough correlate of motor axon loss in the C5 and 6 nerve distributions.

C7 radiculopathy

C7 radiculopathy typically affects the triceps, anconeus, flexor carpi radialis, and pronator teres. The flexor carpi radialis is supplied equally by the C6 and C7 nerve roots, whereas the pronator teres tends to receive more innervation from the C6 than C7 nerve root (eg, the pronator teres is affected in 78% of C6 and 61% of C7 radiculopathies). The H-reflex derived from the flexor carpi radialis can be considered for further assessment of C7 in nerve root lesions but generally adds little useful information and does not separate between C6 and C7 nerve root lesions [73]. There is no reliable motor NCS to assess the C7 myotomes.

C8 radiculopathy

These produce a stereotypic pattern involving the first dorsal interosseous, abductor digiti minimi, flexor pollicis longus (rarely the abductor pollicis brevis), extensor pollicis brevis, and extensor indicis proprius. The abductor pollicis brevis is affected less in C8 radiculopathies (approximately 50% of cases) because it receives its predominant innervation from the T1 nerve root [60]. Despite the fact that routine NCS assess the C8 myotome, they usually are normal (reasons discussed previously). If the radiculopathy is severe enough, additional motor NCS, recording from the first dorsal interosseous, can be considered but generally adds little to the diagnostic impression.

T1 radiculopathy

Thoracic radiculopathies account for less than 2% of all radiculopathies and EDX assessment of the thoracic paraspinal, intercostal, and abdominal muscles is limited by inadequate relaxation, patient size, and the fear of entering the pleural or peritoneal cavity [6,8]. The first thoracic level has limb representation via the medial antebrachial cutaneous sensory NCS (usually normal in radiculopathy) and motor NCS recording from the abductor pollicis brevis. The diagnosis of a T1 radiculopathy relies on NEE of the abductor pollicis brevis and opponens pollicis. The routine assessment of multiple-level thoracic paraspinals, particularly in patients who have suspected diabetic polyradiculopathy or diabetic thoracic radiculopathy, may be considered but is limited by the aforementioned factors and the fact that abnormalities in these paraspinals, similar to those in the cervical and

NEEDLE ELECTRODE EXAMINATION RESULTS
GROUPED BY THE SURGICALLY DEFINED
ROOT LEVEL OF INVOLVEMENT

	#	SUP	INF	DEL	BRAC	BIC	PT	FCR	TRIC	ANC	EDC	EIP	FPL	APB	FDI	ADM	PSP
C5	1	●	○	○	●	○	○		○			○			○		●
	2	●		●	●	●	○		○				○		○		●
	3	○	●	◑		○	○	○	○			○	○	○	○		○
	4		●	●	○	●	○		○			○	○		○		●
	5		●	●	●	●	○		○				○		○		●
	6		●	●	●	●	○		○				○	○	○		●
	7		●	●	●	●	○	○	○			○	○	○	○		○
C6	8	●	●	●	●	●	○	○	○	●	○	○	○	○	○		●
	9	●	●	○	●	○			●		○	○	○		○		●
	10		●	●	●	●	●		●		○		○		○		●
	11	○		●	●	●	●		○		○	○	○		○		○
	12		○	○	●	●	○		○			○	○		○		●
	13		○	○	○	○	●	●	○				○		○		
	14		○	○		○	●	●	●	●		○	○		○		●
	15		○	○	○	○	●	●	●	●		○	○	○	○		○
	16					○	●	●	●	●	●	●	○	○	○	○	○
C7	17			○	○	○	●	●	●	●		○	○	○	○		○
	18			○			●	●	●	●	○		○	○	○		○
	19			○	○	○	●	●	●	●			○	○	○		●
	20		○	○	○	○	●	●	●	●	○		○	○	○		○
	21	○	○	○		○	●	●	●	●	○		○	○	○	○	●
	22		○	○	○	○	●	●	●	●	○	○	○		○		○
	23			○	○	○	●	●	●	●			○	○	○		●
	24			○	○	○	●	●	●	●			○	○	○		○
	25			○		○	●	●	●	●	●	○	○	○	○	○	●
	26		○	○		○	●	●	●	◑	◑		○	○		○	○
	27			○	○	○	●	●	●	●	○	○	○	○	○		○
	28		○	○		○	●	●	●	●	○	○	○		○		○
	29			○		○	●	●	●	●		○	○	○	○		○
	30			○	○	○	●	●	●	●	○		○	○	○		○
	31			○		○	●	●	●	●	●	○		○	○		○
	32				○	○	●		●		●			○	○		●
	33			○		○	●	●	●	●		●	○		●		●
	34			○		○	○	●	●		○	○	○	○	○		●
	35			○		○	○	●	●				○		○		○
	36		○	○		○	○	●	●	●	○	○		○	○		○
	37				○	○	●	●	●	●	○		○	○	○		○
	38		○	○	○	○	○	●	●	●		○	○	○	○		●
	39		○	○	○	○	○	●	●	●		○	○	○	○	○	○
	40			○	○	○	○	●	●	●	○	○	○	○	○		○
	41		○	○	○	○	○	●	●	◑	○		○		○		○
	42			○		○	○	●		○	●	○	○	○	○		
	43			○	○	○	○	○	●		○	○	○		○		
	44			○		○	○	○	◑	●	○	○	○		○		○
C8	45			○	○	○	○		●			●	●	●	●	●	●
	46				○	○	○		○		●	●	○	○	◑	◑	●
	47			○		○	○		○			●	○	○	●	●	○
	48	○	○	○	○	○	○		○	○		●	●	○	●	●	●
	49			○		○	○		○			●	●	●	●	●	●
	50			○		○	○		○				●	●	●	●	

● Fibrillation potentials
◑ Neurogenic recruitment changes only
○ Normal examination

lumbosacral segments, cannot differentiate between compressive, metabolic, or ischemic root lesions [6].

Lumbosacral radiculopathy

Because of the anatomic arrangement of the cauda equina, the higher incidence of bilateral and multilevel disease, and the fact that lower limb SNAPs may be absent in patients over 60 years old, the diagnosis of lumbosacral radiculopathy by NEE is less reliable compared with cervical radiculopathy. Fig. 3 shows the NEE distribution of axon loss in patients who have active single-level lumbosacral radiculopathy confirmed at surgery [27].

L2, L3, and L4 radiculopathy

Radiculopathy at the upper lumbar levels is uncommon and, even when present, it often is impossible to distinguish between those affecting individual L2, L3, or L4 nerve roots. The rectus femoris, vastus lateralis, vastus medialis, adductor longus, and iliacus are, for the most part, affected equally in L2-4 radiculopathy. Of these, the adductor longus is the only muscle innervated by the obdurator, not the femoral, nerve and its evaluation is critical for differentiation between an L2-4 radiculopathy and femoral mononeuropathy. Femoral nerve motor NCS can be considered in cases of severe radiculopathy, but a low femoral CMAP does not localize between a lesion at the lumbar root or plexus level. Likewise, NCS recording the sensory branches of the femoral nerve and lumbar plexus (the saphenous and lateral femoral cutaneous, respectively), technically are unreliable, so EDX consultants cannot rely on lower limb sensory SNAPS to distinguish between an L2-4 nerve root from an upper lumbar plexus lesion. NEE abnormalities in the paraspinal muscles may clinch the diagnosis, but such abnormalities are found more often at the lowest lumbar and sacral levels (or at least 1 to 2 levels below the affected lumbar level).

L5 radiculopathy

This is the most common single-level radiculopathy encountered in EDX laboratories. Muscles affected include the tibialis anterior, peroneus longus, tibialis posterior, tensor fascia lata, and extensor digitorum brevis. Less often, the semitendinosus, semimembranosus, and gluteus medius show

---

Fig. 2. Distribution of needle electrode findings in single-level cervical radiculopathy. Closed circle, positive waves or fibrillation potentials, with or without neurogenic recruitment and motor unit changes; half-closed circle, neurogenic recruitment changes only; open circle, normal examination. ADM, abductor digiti minimi; ANC, anconeus; APB, abductor pollicis brevis; BIC, biceps; BRAC, brachioradialis; DEL, deltoid; EDC, extensor digitorum communis; EIP, extensor indicis proprius; FDI, first dorsal interosseous; FPL, flexor pollicis longus; INF, infraspinatus; FCR, flexor carpi radialis; PSP, paraspinal muscle; PT, pronator teres; SUP, supraspinatus; TRIC, triceps. (*Data from* Levin, KH, Maggiano HJ, Wilbourn AJ. Cervical radiculopathies: comparison of surgical and EMG localization of single-root lesions. Neurology 1996;46:1023; with permission.)

NEEDLE ELECTRODE EXAMINATION RESULTS
GROUPED BY THE SURGICALLY DEFINED
ROOT LEVEL OF INVOLVEMENT

Level	#	AL	IL	VL	RF	VM	PT	TA	EDB	PL	EHL	GM ED	ST	TFL	MG	LG	AD	BF SH	BF LH	GM	AH	PSP
L2	1	●	●	●	○	○	○	○	○	○		○		○						○	○	●
L3	2	●	●	○	○	●	○	○	○		○	○		○						○	○	●
L4	3	●	●	●	●		○	○	○			○		○						○	○	●
	4	●	●	●		●	○	○	○			○		○	○							●
	5	●	○	●	●		○	○			○	○		○						○	○	●
	6	●	○	●	●		○	○			○	○		○						○	○	●
	7	●	●	○			○	○	○			○		○	○					○	○	○
L5	8			○			●	●	●	●	●	●	●	○			○					○
	9			○			●	●	●	●	●	●	○	○	●	○			○	○		○
	10			○			●	●	●	●	●	●	○	○			○				○	○
	11			○			●	●	●	●		●		○	○					○	○	●
	12			○			●	●	●	●		○		○	○		○	○				○
	13			○			●	●	●	●		○	○	○	○		○					●
	14			○			●	●	●	●		○		○	○		○	○				○
	15			○			●	●	●			●		○	○							●
	16			○			●	●	●			●		○	○					○	○	●
	17			○			●	●	●			○	○	○	○		○	○	○	○	●	●
	18			○			●	●	●			○		●	●							●
	19			○			●	●	●			●		○	○							●
	20			○			●	●		●	●	○	●	○	○		○	○	●	○		●
	21			○			●	●	○	●		●			○							●
	22			○			●	●			●	●		○	○							●
	23				○		●	●	○		○	○	○	●	○						○	○
	24			○			●	○	●	●	●	○		○	○						○	○
	25			○			●	○	●	●		●		○	○							●
	26			○			●	○	●	●		○		○	●					○		○
	27			○			●	○	●			●		○	○						○	○
	28			○			●	○	○	●	○	●	○				○				○	○
	29			○	○			○	●			●	●	○			○			○	○	○
	30	○				○		●	●	●		●		○			○				○	●
	31	○	○	○	○		○	●	○		●	●		●	○		○			○	○	○
	32						○	◐	●	●	●	○	○		○					○	○	○
	33			○			◐	◐	◐	◐	◐	○	◐	◐	○			○		○	○	○
S1	34			○			●		○		●		○		●	●	●	●	●	○	○	○
	35			○			○	○	○	○		●			●	●	●	●		●	○	○
	36			○			●	○				○			●	●	●	●		○	●	○
	37			○			○	○	○		○				●	●		●		●	○	○
	38			○				○	○		○	○			●	●	○	●	●	○	○	○
	39			○			○	○	○		○	○			●	●	○	●	●	○	○	○
	40			○			○	○				○			●	●			●	●	○	●
	41				○		○	○				○			●	●				●	○	●
	42			○			○	○	○		○				●	○	●		●	○	●	○
	43				○		○	○	○		○	○			●			●		●	●	○
	44			○			○	○	○	○		●	○		○	●	●	○		●	○	●
	45			○			○	○		○	○	●	○		○	●		●		●	○	○

● Fibrillation potentials
◐ Neurogenic recruitment changes only
○ Normal examination

abnormalities. It is important that all, or nearly all, these muscles be examined when L5 radiculopathy is suspected, because the differential diagnosis includes a common or deep peroneal neuropathy, peroneal-predominant sciatic neuropathy, or a lumbosacral trunk (the furcal nerve) lesion that involves the L5 (and to a much lesser extent the L4) contribution to the sacral plexus.

The superficial peroneal sensory NCS should be performed in all cases of suspected L5 radiculopathy and, if present, indicates a preganglionic L5 root lesion. If absent, this could result from a lesion that lies anywhere between the root level to peripheral nerve but does not exclude an L5 radiculopathy with intraforaminal DRG compression [15]. One advantage of the superficial peroneal sensory response is that tends to be spared in mild to distal polyneuropathies where the sural or medial plantar NCS generally are unelicitable.

S1 radiculopathy

S1 nerve root lesions typically affect the biceps femoris short and long head, the medial and lateral gastrocnemius, abductor digiti quinti pedis, abductor hallucis, and the gluteus maximus. The S1 root distribution also includes muscles situated in proximal and distal regions of the limb; thus, examination of multiple muscles at distal, mid, and proximal levels is necessary to provide insight into the severity and activity of radiculopathy.

Despite different opinions on the primary nerve root innervation of muscles, such as biceps femoris long and short head, the author and colleagues have found the biceps femoris short head nearly always involved in S1 radiculopathy and never in L5 radiculopathy [27]. NEE of the upper sacral paraspinal muscles is of limited use, because only lower sacral paraspinal muscles may demonstrate denervation. The H-reflex is a sensitive (but less specific) marker of S1 radiculopathy, especially when the abnormality is unilateral [26,27].

S2, S3, and S4 radiculopathy

Unfortunately, there are few muscles accessible to the NEE within the lower sacral myotomes. These are limited mainly to intrinsic foot muscles

Fig. 3. Distribution of needle electrode findings in single-level lumbosacral radiculopathy. Closed circle, positive waves or fibrillation potentials, with or without neurogenic recruitment and motor unit changes; half-closed circle, neurogenic recruitment changes only; open circle, normal examination. AD, abductor digiti quinti; AH, abductor hallucis; AL, adductor longus; BFLH, biceps femoris long head; BFSH, biceps femoris short head; EDB, extensor digitorum brevis; EHL, extensor hallucis longus; GM, gluteus maximus; GMED, gluteus medius; IL, iliacus; LG, lateral gastrocnemius; MG, medial gastrocnemius; PL, peroneus longus; PSP, paraspinal; PT, posterior tibialis; RF, rectus femoris; ST, semitendinosus; TA, tibialis anterior; TFL, tensor fascia lata; VL, vastus lateralis; VM, vastus medialis. (*From* Tsao BE, Levin KH, Bodner RA. Comparison of surgical and electrodiagnostic findings in single root lumbosacral radiculopathies. Muscle Nerve 2003;27:61; with permission.)

(abductor hallucis and abductor digiti quinti pedis), the soleus, and anal sphincter muscles.

Multiple-level lumbosacral radiculopathies and lumbar canal stenosis

Multilevel lumbosacral radiculopathies are more common than single-level radiculopathies, which reflects the frequent coexistence of multifocal spondylosis and neural foraminal stenosis. The clinical presentation of multilevel lumbosacral radiculopathy and lumbar canal stenosis (LCS) often overlap, with single- or multiple-level nerve root involvement and chronic progressive leg weakness. The patient who has classic LCS can present with exertionally related aching, numbness, or weakness in the legs that resolves with rest (neurogenic claudication). EDX findings in LCS vary widely, from essentially normal to active multilevel bilateral lumbosacral polyradiculopathies. With chronic LCS, prominent neurogenic MUAP changes typically are seen in a distal to proximal gradient (ie, in the distal foreleg and foot muscles), with more normal MUAPs in proximal muscles and, on occasion, persistent fibrillation potentials in the distal muscles. In elderly patients who have physiologically absent sural and superficial peroneal SNAPs, this constellation of findings, similar to those seen in chronic L5-S1 radiculopathy, is indistinguishable from an axon loss sensorimotor polyneuropathy.

Polyradiculoneuropathies

A wide spectrum of etiologies (immune mediated, infectious, degenerative, infiltrative, and so forth) may involve multiple root segments, unilaterally or bilaterally, and extend from the cervical, thoracic, and lumbosacral levels. Aside from the typical demyelinating polyradiculoneuropathies (such as Guillain-Barré syndrome or chronic inflammatory polyradiculoneuropathy), most of these systemic diseases result in multiple nerve root lesions, superimposed peripheral polyneuropathies and, at times, involvement of the anterior horn cells. The EDX picture in these cases, then, is dependent on the specific cause and the distribution of peripheral nerve fibers thus affected and can conform to acquired demyelinating, axon loss, or mixed disorders [74].

Summary

An EDX examination provides an important correlate to the clinical diagnosis of cervical and lumbosacral radiculopathy. EDX consultants should perform routine NCS and NEE and seek to maximize the diagnostic yield by structuring the test as guided by patients' clinical history. In this way, EDX examination can confirm the presence and severity of axon loss radiculopathy, localize which nerve root is affected, and rule out other neuromuscular disorders that may be present. Thermography, SEPs, and MEPs are not useful routinely and add little to a comprehensive EDX examination.

References

[1] Semmes RE, Murphy F. The syndrome of unilateral rupture of the sixth cervical vertebral disc with compression of the seventh cervical root: a report of four cases with symptoms simulating coronary disease. JAMA 1943;121:1209–14.

[2] Mixter W, Barr J. Rupture of the intervertebral disc with involvement of the spinal canal. N Engl J Med 1934;211:210–4.

[3] Brazier MA, Watkins AL, Michelsen JJ. Electromyography in differential diagnosis of ruptured cervical disc. Arch Neurol Psychiatry 1946;56:651–8.

[4] Shea AP, Woods WW, Werden DR. Electromyography in diagnosis of nerve root compression syndrome. Arch Neurol Psychiatry 1950;64:93–104.

[5] Marinacci AA. Clinical electromyography. Los Angeles (CA): San Lucas Press; 1955.

[6] Wilbourn AJ, Aminoff MJ. AAEM Minimonograph 23: the electrodiagnostic examination in patients with radiculopathies. Muscle Nerve 1998;21:1612–31.

[7] Aminoff MJ. Electromyography in clinical practice. 3rd edition. New York: Churchill Livingstone; 1998.

[8] Dumitru D, Zwarts MJ. Radiculopathies. In: Dumitru D, Amato AA, Zwarts M, editors. Electrodiagnostic medicine. 2nd edition. Philadelphia: Hanley & Belfus, Inc; 2002. p. 713–76.

[9] Levin KH. Electrodiagnostic approach to the patient with suspected radiculopathy. Neurol Clin N Am 2002;20:397–421.

[10] Gough JG, Koepke GH. Electromyographic determination of motor root levels in erector spinae muscles. Arch Phys Med Rehabil 1966;47:9–11.

[11] Stewart JS. Cauda equina, lumbar and sacral nerve roots, and spinal nerves. In: Stewart JS, editor. Focal peripheral neuropathies. 3rd edition. Philadelphia: Lippincott Williams & Wilkins; 2000. p. 315–20.

[12] Hamanishi C, Tanaka S. Dorsal root ganglia in the lumbosacral region observed from the axial views of MRI. Spine 1993;18:1753–6.

[13] Kikuchi S, Sato K, Konno S, et al. Anatomic and radiographic study of dorsal root ganglia. Spine 1994;19:6–11.

[14] Yabuki S, Kikuchi S. Positions of dorsal root ganglia in the cervical spine: an anatomic and clinical study. Spine 1996;21:1513–7.

[15] Levin KH. L5 radiculopathy with reduced superficial peroneal sensory responses: intraspinal and extraspinal causes. Muscle Nerve 1998;21:3–7.

[16] Eisen AA. Radiculopathies and plexopathies. In: Brown WF, Bolton CF, Aminoff MJ, editors. Neuromuscular function and disease. Philadelphia: WB Saunders; 2002. p. 781–96.

[17] Spencer DL, Miller JAA, Bertolini JE. The effect of intervertebral disc space narrowing and the contact force between the nerve root and a simulated disc protrusion. Spine 1984;9: 422–6.

[18] Garfin SR, Rydevik BL, Lind B, et al. Spinal nerve root compression. Spine 1995;20: 1810–20.

[19] Rydevik BL, Brown MD, Lundborg G. Pathoanatomy and pathophysiology of nerve root compression. Spine 1984;9:7–15.

[20] Preston DC, Shapiro BE. Electromyography and neuromuscular disorders. Boston: Butterworth-Heinemann; 1989.

[21] Benecke R, Conrad B. The distal sensory nerve action potential as a diagnostic tool for the differentiation of lesions in dorsal roots and peripheral nerves. J Neurol 1980;223: 231–9.

[22] Brandstater ME, Fullerton M. Sensory nerve conduction studies in cervical root lesions. Can J Neurol Sci 1983;10:152.

[23] Fisher MA. H-reflex and F-response studies. In: Aminoff MJ, editor. Electrodiagnosis in clinical neurology. 5th edition. New York: Churchhill Livingstone; 2005. p. 357–69.

[24] Katirji B, Weissman JD. The ankle jerk and the tibial H-reflex: a clinical and electrophysiological correlation. Electromyogr Clin Neurophysiol 1994;34:331–4.

[25] Schimsheimer RJ, Ongerboer de Visser BW, Kemp B. The flexor carpi radialis H-reflex in lesion of the sixth and seventh cervical nerve roots. J Neurol Neurosurg Psychiatry 1985; 48:445–9.

[26] Kaylan TA, Bilgic F, Ertem O. The diagnostic value of late responses in radiculopathies due to disc herniation. Electromyogr Clin Neurophysiol 1983;23:183–6.

[27] Tsao BE, Levin KH, Bodnar RA. Comparison of surgical and electrodiagnostic findings in single root lumbosacral radiculopathies. Muscle Nerve 2003;27:60–4.

[28] Braddom RI, Johnson EW. Standardization of H-reflex and diagnostic use in S1 radiculopathy. Arch Phys Med Rehabil 1974;55:161–6.

[29] Jankus WR, Robinson LR, Little JW. Normal limits of side-to-side H-reflex amplitude variability. Arch Phys Med Rehabil 1994;75:3–6.

[30] Panayiotaopoulos CP, Chroni E. F-waves in clinical neurophysiology: a review, methodogical issues and overall value in peripheral neuropathies. Electroencephalogr Clin Neurophysiol 1996;101:365–74.

[31] Berger AR, Sharma K, Lipton RB. Comparison of motor conduction abnormalities in lumbosacral radiculopathy and axonal polyneuropathy. Muscle Nerve 1999;22:1053–7.

[32] Toyokura M, Murakami K. F wave study in patients with lumbosacral radiculopathies. Electromyogr Clin Neurophysiol 1997;37:19–26.

[33] Aminoff MJ. Electrophysiological evaluation of root and spinal cord disease. Semin Neurol 2002;22:197–9.

[34] Goodin DS, Aminoff MJ. Clinical application of somatosensory evoked potentials. In: Brown WF, Bolton CF, Aminoff MJ, editors. Neuromuscular function and disease. Philadelphia: WB Saunders; 2002. p. 159–70.

[35] Aminoff MJ, Eisen A. Somatosensory evoked potentials. In: Aminoff MJ, editor. Electrodiagnosis in clinical neurology. 5th edition. New York: Churchhill Livingstone; 2005. p. 553–76.

[36] American Academy of Neurology. Assessment: dermatomal somatosensory evoked potentials. Report of the Therapeutics and Technology Assessments Subcommittee. Neurology 1997;49:1127–30.

[37] So YT, Olney RK, Aminoff MJ. A comparison of thermography and electromyography in the diagnosis of cervical radiculopathy. Muscle Nerve 1990;13:1032–6.

[38] Wilbourn AJ, Aminoff MJ. Role of the electrodiagnostic examination and thermography in the diagnosis of lumbosacral radiculopathy. In: Hardy RW, editor. 2nd edition. New York: Raven Press; 1993. p. 81–93.

[39] Harper CM, Low PA, Fealey RD, et al. Utility of thermography in the diagnosis of lumbosacral radiculopathy. Neurology 1991;41:1010–4.

[40] Berger AR, Busis NA, Logigian EL, et al. Cervical root stimulation in the diagnosis of cervical radiculopathy. Neurology 1987;37:329–32.

[41] Tabaraud F, Hugon J, Chazot F, et al. Motor evoked responses after lumbar spinal stimulation in patients with L5 or S1 radicular involvement. Electroencephalogr Clin Neurophysiol 1989;72:334–9.

[42] Chokroverty S, Sachdeo R, DiLullo J, et al. Magnetic stimulation in the diagnosis of lumbosacral radiculopathy. J Neurol Neurosurg Psychiatry 1989;52:767–72.

[43] Chokroverty S, Picone MA, Chokroverty M. Percutaneous magnetic coil stimulation of human cervical vertebral column: site of stimulation and clinical application. Electroencephalogr Clin Neurophysiol 1991;81:359–65.

[44] Linden D, Berlit P. Comparison of late responses, EMG studies and motor evoked potentials (MEPs) in acute lumbosacral radiculopathies. Muscle Nerve 1995;18:1205–7.

[45] Macdonell RAL, Cros D, Shahani BT. Lumbosacral nerve root stimulation comparing electrical with surface magnetic coil techniques. Muscle Nerve 1992;15:885–90.

[46] Weddell G, Feinstein B, Pattle RE. The electrical activity of voluntary muscle in man under normal and pathological conditions. Brain 1944;67:178–257.

[47] Sherrington CS. Notes on the arrangement of some motor fibers in the lumbo-sacral plexus. J Physiol 1892;13:621–772.

[48] Sharrard WJW. The distribution of the permanent paralysis in the lower limb in poliomyelitis. J Bone Joint Surg 1955;37:540–58.

[49] Shea PA, Woods WW. The diagnostic value of the electromyograph. Br J Phys Med 1956;19: 36–43.

[50] Yoss RE, Corbin KB, MacCarthy CS, et al. Significance of signs and symptoms in localization of involved roots in cervical disc protrusion. Neurology 1957;7:673–83.

[51] Sharrard WJW. The segmental innervation of the lower limb muscles in man. Ann R Coll Surg Engl 1964;35:106–22.

[52] Thage O. The myotomes L2-S2 in man. Acta Neurol Scand 1965;13:241–3.

[53] Brendler SJ. The human cervical myotomes: functional anatomy studied at operation. J Neurosurg 1968;28:105–11.

[54] Johnson E, Fletcher FR. Lumbosacral radiculopathy: review of 100 consecutive cases. Arch Phys Med Rehabil 1981;62:321–3.

[55] Wolf JK. Segmental anatomy. Baltimore (MD): University Park Press; 1981.

[56] Young A, Getty J, Jackson A, et al. Variations in the pattern of muscle innervation of the L5 and S1 nerve roots. Spine 1983;8:616–24.

[57] Phillips LH, Park TS. Electrophysiologic mapping of the segmental anatomy of the muscles of the lower extremity. Muscle Nerve 1991;14:1213–8.

[58] Liguori R, Krarup C, Trojaborg W. Determination of the segmental sensory and motor innervation of the lumbosacral spinal nerves. Brain 1992;115:915–34.

[59] Krarup C, Trojaborg W. Segmental innervation of lumbosacral nerves. Muscle Nerve 1994; 17:956–7.

[60] Levin KH, Maggiano HJ, Wilbourn AJ. Cervical radiculopathies: comparison of surgical and EMG localization of single-root lesion. Neurology 1996;46:1022–5.

[61] Lauder TD, Dillingham TR, Huston CW, et al. Lumbosacral root screen: optimizing the number of muscles studied. Am J Phys Med Rehabil 1994;73:394–402.

[62] Date ES, Kim BJ, Yoon JS, et al. Cervical paraspinal spontaneous activity in asympomatic subjects. Muscle Nerve 2006;21:361–4.

[63] Date ES, Mar EY, Bugola MR, et al. The prevalence of lumbar paraspinal muscle activity in asymptomatic subjects. Muscle Nerve 1996;19:350–4.

[64] Nardin R, Raynor EM, Rutkove SB. Electromyography of lumbosacral paraspinal muscles in normal subjects. Neurology 1997;48(Suppl):A147.

[65] So YT, Weber CF, Campbell WW. Practice parameter for needle electromyographic evaluation of patients with suspected cervical radiculopathy: summary statement. Muscle Nerve 1999;22(S8):S209–11.

[66] So YT, Weber CF, Campbell WW. The electrodiagnostic evaluation of patients with suspected cervical radiculopathy: literature review on the usefulness of needle electromyography. Muscle Nerve 1999;22(S8):S213–21.

[67] Wilbourn AJ. The value and limitations of electromyographic examination in the diagnosis of lumbosacral radiculopathy. In: Hardy RW, editor. Lumbar disc disease. New York: Raven Press; 1982. p. 65–109.

[68] Kharti BO, Baruah J, McQuillen MP. Correlation of electromyography and computed tomography in evaluation of lower back pain. Arch Neurol 1984;41:594–7.

[69] Schoedinger GR. Correlation of standard diagnostic studies with surgically proven lumbar disk rupture. South Med J 1987;80:44–6.

[70] Boden SA, Davis DO, Dina TS, et al. Abnormal magnetic-resonance scans of the lumbar spine in asymptomatic subjects. J Bone Joint Surg Am 1990;72:403–8.

[71] Boden SA, McCowin PR, Davis DO, et al. Abnormal magnetic-resonance scans of the cervical spine in asymptomatic subjects. A prospective investigation. J Bone Joint Surg Am 1990;72:1178–84.

[72] Jensen MC, Brant-Zawadski MN, Obuchowski N, et al. Magnetic resonance imaging of the lumbar spine in people without back pain. N Engl J Med 1994;331:69–73.

[73] Partanen J, Partanen K, Oikarinen H, et al. Preoperative electroneuromyography and myelography in cervical root compression. Electromyogr Clin Neurolophysiol 1991;31:21–6.

[74] Levin KH, et al. Cervical radiculopathies. In: Katirji B, Kaminski HJ, Preston DC, editors. Neuromuscular disorders in clinical practice. Boston: Butterworth-Heinemann; 2002. p. 855–6.

ELSEVIER
SAUNDERS

NEUROLOGIC
CLINICS

Neurol Clin 25 (2007) 495–505

Nonsurgical Interventions for Spine Pain

Kerry H. Levin, MD

*Department of Neurology, Desk S-91, Cleveland Clinic, 9500 Euclid Avenue,
Cleveland, OH 44195, USA*

Acute spine pain has a good prognosis for spontaneous recovery when it is not associated with marked neurologic deficits and when it does not develop in the setting of severe spine trauma. Sometimes spine pain with or without radiculopathy continues for more than 1 to 2 months, however, entering a subacute or chronic phase. Physical therapy and graded rehabilitation are the keys to recovery. Occasionally there are indications for surgical intervention. In addition, several nonsurgical interventions have been developed to try to alleviate pain and improve function. A summary of these interventions and available reports studying their effectiveness are reviewed in this article.

Lumbar spine disease

Subacute spine pain without radiculopathy

The precise mechanisms of subacute nonspecific spine pain are not clearly understood. Theories have been promoted to explain lumbar pain, and therapeutic strategies have been developed to try to deal with specific proposed causes. The proposed causes include nonspecific (musculoskeletal) back pain, facet joint arthritis, and internal disc disruption (discogenic back pain).

Nonspecific lumbar spine pain

In this patient group, physical therapy should be the first modality of treatment. Self-motivated individuals may consider self-taught yoga exercises and Pilates to promote stretching and flexibility. Chiropractic maneuvers, such as spinal manipulation techniques (thrust, muscle energy, counterstrain, articulation, and myofascial release), have also been used. A study by Andersson and colleagues [1] compared chiropractic spinal manipulation techniques with a medical program (analgesics,

---

E-mail address: levink@ccf.org

0733-8619/07/$ - see front matter © 2007 Elsevier Inc. All rights reserved.
doi:10.1016/j.ncl.2007.01.010 *neurologic.theclinics.com*

anti-inflammatory drugs, active physical therapy, an educational video, and therapies, such as ultrasound, hot/cold packs, and transcutaneous electrical nerve stimulation [TENS]) in a population of patients who had nonradicular lumbar spine pain of 3 to 26 weeks' duration. At 12 weeks, there was no significant difference in the degree of improvement between the two groups, although the group receiving manipulation required significantly less analgesia, anti-inflammatories, and muscle relaxants, and used less physical therapy. More than 90% of the patients in both groups were satisfied with their care.

TENS has been used in patients who have subacute and chronic spine pain, with variable results. Several factors seem to influence success, including chronicity of the pain, electrode pad placement, and prior treatments [2]. A Cochrane Database of Systematic Reviews meta-analysis published in 2004 found no scientific evidence to support the use of TENS in the treatment of chronic low back pain [3].

Epidural steroid injections are not beneficial in patients who have non-specific low back pain without features of radiculopathy [4–7]. Factors predicting poor outcome from epidural steroid injection include absence of straight leg raising sign, pain that is not medication responsive, large number of prior treatments, high-dose medication intake, pain unaffected by cough or increased activity, pain-related unemployment, and pain that does not interfere with normal activities [8].

Facet joint arthritis

Arthritis of lumbar facet joints has been proposed as a cause of subacute/chronic low back pain. The precise diagnosis of this condition is hampered by the lack of specific symptoms and signs [9,10]. A provocative test that is said to support the diagnosis involves the injection of hypertonic saline or pressurized contrast. Positive results of this test include local pain and pain referred into the proximal leg, with some reports indicating extension of pain in a sciatic pattern below the knee [11–13].

Steroid injections have been used to treat facet joint disease. A Cochrane Database of Systematic Reviews report published in 2000 evaluated existing studies of facet injection (anesthetic or corticosteroid) therapy and found three studies meeting their criteria for review [14–17]. Based on their review, evidence for the effectiveness of this procedure was still lacking.

Radiofrequency neurotomy has also been used to treat facet joint disease. Denervation of the facet joint has been proposed as an effective treatment of facet joint–related spine pain. Controlled diagnostic blocks with anesthetic have been reported to predict those individuals who are likely to respond to radiofrequency neurotomy of the medial branch of the dorsal ramus, which supplies innervation to the facet joint surface [18]. One study compared 15 patients who underwent radiofrequency neurotomy with 16 who received sham treatment [19]. Ten of 15 treated patients and 6 of 16 sham-treated patients improved. The study claimed superior pain control in the treated group at 3, 6, and 12 months posttreatment. A subsequent study with 70 patients in a double blind randomized controlled study identified no treatment effect at 4 or 12 weeks [20,21]. A Cochrane Database of Systematic Reviews report published in 2004 stated that there is insufficient information to draw conclusions on the short-term benefit of radiofrequency neurotomy in the treatment of lumbar facet disease [22].

Internal disc disruption

This condition is theorized as a discogenic cause of back pain, and is described as a degeneration of the nucleus pulposus without disruption of the annulus fibrosus or disc extrusion. There are no distinguishing clinical features of this condition aside from chronic low back pain. The anatomic findings are not clearly defined by MRI but are reported to be apparent with use of a controversial technique called discography [23,24]. Pressurized saline or contrast is instilled in the disc to reproduce the patient's pain symptoms. Intradiscal electrothermal therapy has been proposed for the treatment of internal disc disruption. The technique involves a flexible catheter that is inserted circumferentially around the periphery of the disc space internal to the annulus fibrosus. The catheter is heated with the intention of coagulating nociceptive nerve fibers in the annulus. One placebo-controlled study suggested that patients responded to electrothermal therapy and a sham procedure similarly. About 50% of the study group did not benefit, but benefit is likely in patients who are carefully selected [25]. Two other recent studies did not find favorable results from the procedure [26,27]. Several reports have described cauda equina syndrome and permanent neurologic sequelae resulting from the procedure [28,29].

Subacute radiculopathy

In general, lumbar radiculopathy has a monophasic course with eventual improvement. Patients who have at least moderate neurologic deficits may have longstanding residual deficits.

Patients who have continued spinal nerve root compression or spinal nerve root infarction are likely to have some degree of persistent pain. Drugs with particular effectiveness against neuropathic pain should be considered, including gabapentin and tricyclic antidepressants. Continuing narcotic medications should be avoided, but in individual cases may be effective at a specific dosage. Patients respond to mobilization and other physical therapy techniques, but may be limited by their neurologic deficits. Physical therapy should address issues of mobility and strengthening of weak muscles.

In postoperative patients who have continuing radicular pain, compressive root disease from residual disc fragments, hematoma, and arachnoiditis must be excluded. Neuroimaging is required to investigate treatable causes of pain. In nonoperated patients who have continued radicular pain, several nonsurgical treatment modalities can be considered.

Epidural corticosteroid injection

Few placebo-controlled, prospective studies are available to assess the value of epidural corticosteroid injections, and those that have been done have been criticized for design flaws [30]. Most of the previous studies have used a traditional interlaminar injection approach, often without fluoroscopic guidance, whereby a needle is advanced between the laminae of two adjacent vertebrae into the dorsal epidural space. One meta-analysis found no trend favoring epidural steroids [6]. Another study included patients who had radiculopathy from disc herniation and claudication from lumbar canal stenosis. It observed some effect on pain or radiculopathic findings within days to 12 weeks after treatment, but no difference in pain or deficits compared with placebo at 12 weeks [31]. A randomized double blind trial studied 158 patients who had lumbar radiculopathy of 4 to 52 weeks' duration, with evidence of radicular deficits on clinical examination and CT evidence of disc herniation [32]. Six weeks after three epidural injections of either corticosteroid or saline, patients having received corticosteroid had somewhat more improvement in leg pain, but at 3 months there was no significant difference between the two groups. In both groups 25% of patients eventually went on to lumbar spine surgery. With the interlaminar approach without fluoroscopic guidance, one study showed only about 70% of cases had successful epidural delivery of steroid [8].

Transforaminal epidural injections have been promoted as a more selective and therefore more effective treatment technique. The likelihood of steroid delivery at the root level is believed to be higher, because the needle is placed under fluoroscopic guidance in the epiradicular space just above the dorsal root ganglion in the neural foramen. One placebo-controlled study of 55 patients assessed the need for surgery for pain or neurologic deficits after treatment [33]. Of 28 treated patients, 8 ultimately underwent surgery, whereas 18 of 27 placebo-treated patients received surgery. Concerns raised with this study included a nonhomogeneous patient population (disc herniation and foraminal stenosis), atypical pain scale assessment tools, and multiple surgeons making operative decisions [34]. One prospective, randomized but non-blinded study compared transforaminal epidural steroid injection with saline trigger-point injection in 48 patients. Based on pre- and post-treatment questionnaires, 84% of epidural patients and 48% of trigger-point patients improved [35]. Difficulties with this study included lack of blinding of the single physician who performed all procedures and presumably obtained consent from and randomized all patients, lack of clear data regarding duration of symptoms before study, reliability of the clinical diagnosis of radiculopathy by inclusion criteria, and potential negative influence on the outcome among patients known to have received the nonactive treatment modality.

DePalma and colleagues [36] reviewed all studies of transforaminal epidural steroid injections and selective nerve root blocks through 2003. They identified five publications that were in the English language, prospective, and randomized [33,37–40]. These studies were judged to provide level III, or moderate, evidence to support the use of transforaminal epidural steroid injections, based on the Agency for Health Care and Policy Research (AHCPR) criteria for which level III evidence reflects evidence from well-designed trials without randomization, single group pre/post cohort, time series, or matched case-controlled studies.

All the studies reviewed by DePalma and colleagues [36] had similar limitations that diminished the conclusions of their authors. No study had a true placebo group, but rather used another intervention that could have provided therapeutic value. End points of the studies usually involved whether or not patients required surgery, bringing into question the true value of the procedure, or whether by other criteria than going on to surgery (such as pain freedom, ability to work, ability to carry out leisure activities) the procedure may not have been considered successful. These studies did not comment on the relapse rate from the procedure, and provided only limited information about outcomes beyond 1 year postprocedure.

The effect of this procedure on the natural history of lumbar radiculopathy remains unclear. The usefulness of this procedure may actually lie in its ability to lessen lumbosacral radicular pain earlier than would be the case spontaneously, without changing the overall time to complete resolution [41]. Because there is moderate evidence of the effectiveness of this procedure in the treatment of painful radicular symptoms, it seems reasonable to consider it after failure of spontaneous recovery and conservative maneuvers in the acute phase of radiculopathy [36].

Potential complications of epidural steroid injections include spinal headache, epidural or intrathecal hematoma, transient worsening of radiculopathy, and steroid effects. Bacterial discitis following this procedure has been reported [42].

Lumbar canal stenosis

With lumbar spinal stenosis (LCS), a condition characterized by narrowing of the intraspinal (central) canal, the primary symptoms include discomfort, sensory loss, and weakness in the legs, reflecting dysfunction of multiple spinal nerve roots within the lumbar spinal canal. Neurogenic claudication is the hallmark of the condition: the tendency for exacerbation of symptoms with walking, standing, and maintaining certain postures. Neurogenic claudication can be described as discomfort in the buttocks, thighs, or legs on standing or walking, which is relieved by sitting or lying.

Interventions

Physical therapy has not been proven to be effective in LCS; however, it is a mainstay of management of patients. Maneuvers, such as stretching, strengthening, and aerobic fitness, are usually recommended [43]. Techniques to reduce lumbar lordosis (and thereby decrease extension of the lumbar spine) include strengthening of abdominal muscles, using an abdominal corset, using a short cane, and losing weight.

Drug therapy for pain has included aspirin, nonsteroidal anti-inflammatory drugs, and opiates. No studies have clearly identified the superiority of one class of drugs over another, but the complication profile of each plays a role in the ultimate choice for the individual patient.

The efficacy of epidural steroid injections for LCS has not been rigorously investigated. In one study that combined patients who had lumbar radicular pain and neurogenic claudication, without fluoroscopic guidance, no statistical improvement was seen over that obtained from injection with anesthetic alone [31]. Others have demonstrated no evidence that epidural steroid injections are beneficial for nonradicular back pain [4,6]. Fukusaki and colleagues [5] identified no functional benefit over local anesthetic in patients who had LCS treated with epidural steroid injection subsequently evaluated by a treadmill exercise test. A recent retrospective review of 140 patients included patients who had central, lateral, and foraminal stenosis in whom the symptoms were either consistent with radiculopathy or neurogenic claudication [44]. Patients received fluoroscopically guided transforaminal or caudal injections. About 30% of patients described 2 months or more of pain relief, about 40% of patients described less than 2 months of pain relief, about 50% reported improvement in functional ability, and 75% were at least somewhat satisfied with their result. This study did not separately report the results for central, lateral, and foraminal sites of stenosis, however.

Chronic lumbar spine disease

A few patients who have bony disease of the lumbar spine develop chronic pain. This group of patients is difficult to treat, often because the underlying cause of pain and disability is multifactorial.

Postoperative patients who have chronic pain may have underlying structural causes for pain. These include arachnoiditis and failed back syndrome, a nonspecific condition usually associated with multiple prior lumbar surgeries. Other patients who have chronic lumbar spine pain have never had surgery; their condition may overlap with the broader disorder of chronic pain syndrome. Patients who have chronic spine pain are unlikely to respond to invasive interventions. The goal in such patients is to improve the ability to perform activities of daily living, and refocus attention away from pain perception.

Several nonmedical factors play a role in the triggering and perpetuation of pain behavior. These include psychosocial issues, such as job dissatisfaction, family stresses, and underlying psychiatric disorders. In other cases patients develop and ingrain a behavior of pain avoidance and fear of pain. Patients who have chronic pain are best treated in dedicated centers for the rehabilitation of patients who have multifactorial pain syndromes. Pain programs concentrate on the re-education of the patient to diminish fear of activities of daily living through graded exercise programs, the exploration of psychosocial stressors, and the nonnarcotic treatment of pain.

The therapeutic approach for patients who have chronic spine pain is most successful in multidisciplinary programs in which behavior modification, psychotherapy, biofeedback, relaxation techniques, physical therapy modalities, and education are used together. In one study the success rates of these programs for reduction of pain were 15% to 60%, reduction of opioid use was 70%, and increase in employment was 40% [45].

Cervical spine pain

Subacute cervical radiculopathy and chronic neck pain

When symptoms of radiculopathy extend beyond 4 weeks, in the presence of neurologic deficits that are fixed or worsening, it is necessary to re-evaluate for structural causes that could respond to surgical intervention. In the absence of surgical indications, several nonsurgical therapeutic options are available, although their efficacy has not been proven. Physical therapy evaluation and the use of exercises to promote ideal posture, the use of TENS units, and cervical traction all have their advocates, and some patients seem to respond to one or more of these maneuvers.

Epidural injections

Epidural corticosteroid injections at the cervical levels have been performed for several decades, but not to the extent of epidural injections at the lumbar levels. Epidural injection of a combination of corticosteroid and anesthetic can lead to temporary reduction of pain in some patients. The few trials that have been performed have not been well controlled and have lacked homogeneous study populations. One study involving injections performed at the C5-6 and C6-7 interspaces produced pain relief for one month or longer in 38% of patients [46].

One retrospective study of 100 patients attempted to identify a patient profile that predicted response to cervical epidural injection of a combination of corticosteroid and anesthetic [47]. Based on clinical outcomes determined by subjective reports of pain relief and return to activities of daily living, only the presence of radicular pain predicted a better outcome from epidural injection. Other measured predictors, including age, abnormal sensory examination, change in muscle stretch reflexes, motor changes on examination, and abnormal electromyographic findings, were not found to be significant. Predictors of a poor outcome included normal radiologic examination findings and the presence of a herniated disc. In those whose pain relief amounted to 50% or more, the response occurred irrespective of the cervical level involved. In patients who had symptoms and neurologic signs of true radiculopathy, whether or not a structural abnormality was seen radiographically, the probability of at least 50% improvement was 62%, whereas the probability was only 35% for patients who had only radicular pain symptoms and radiologic structural changes. The poorest probability was seen in patients who had radicular pain symptoms without structural changes, and in patients who had nonspecific axial pain symptoms. Another study described a 76% success rate for paravertebral transforaminal epidural steroid injections [48].

Although reported complications of cervical injections are rare, they can be severe, including myelopathy from spinal cord penetration and brainstem infarction [49–51].

These procedures were performed through an interlaminar injection approach, and it is likely that more recently advanced transforaminal selective nerve root injections are somewhat less likely to result in these injuries.

Facet joint treatment

Short-term benefits have been reported for steroid injections into facet joints in the setting of chronic neck pain believed to arise from those structures. Systematic review of facet joint injection at the cervical level is lacking. For the lumbosacral level, a Cochrane Database of Systematic Reviews report published in 2000 found insufficient evidence to support its effectiveness [17]. Facet coagulation has been in use as a permanent method of denervating facet joints at the lumbar level [52].

A small subset of patients who have chronic pain from whiplash injury is believed to have the condition based on facet joint injury [53]. This chronic pain disorder does not seem to have specific clinical or radiologic hallmarks, but it responds to local anesthetic block to the nerves supplying the painful joint. Although a controlled trial showed that intra-articular injections of corticosteroids offered no particular benefit, percutaneous radiofrequency neurotomy of the medial branch of the cervical dorsal ramus that innervates the joint provided pain relief for up to 263 days, compared with 8 days in the placebo group [54]. Patient selection was based on double blind controlled trials of local anesthetic to the medial branches of the cervical dorsal rami at the levels of clinical involvement. Return of pain after a successful radiofrequency procedure was believed to represent regeneration of nerve branches to the joint and was treated with repeat neurotomy, with variable results.

Remaining treatment options

A small number of patients fail to respond to all the above-mentioned therapeutic interventions. Some of these patients have chronic spine pain without evidence of structural intraspinal pathology, others have had previously treated structural lesions, and some have had multiple previous surgical interventions, a condition described as the failed spine syndrome. The goal in such patients is to improve the ability to perform activities of daily living and refocus attention away from pain perception.

Several nonmedical factors play a role in the triggering and perpetuation of pain behavior. These include psychosocial issues, such as job dissatisfaction, family stresses, and underlying psychiatric disorders. In other cases patients develop and ingrain a behavior of pain avoidance and fear of pain. Patients who have chronic pain are best treated in dedicated centers for the rehabilitation of patients who have multifactorial pain syndromes. Pain programs concentrate on the re-education of the patient to diminish fear of activities of daily living through graded exercise programs, the exploration of psychosocial stressors, and the nonnarcotic treatment of pain.

References

[1] Andersson GBJ, Lucente R, Davis AM, et al. A comparison of osteopathic spinal manipulation with standard care for patients with low back pain. N Engl J Med 1999;341:1426–31.

[2] Deyo RA, Walsh NE, Martin DC, et al. A controlled trial of transcutaneous electrical nerve stimulation (TENS) and exercise for chronic low back pain. N Engl J Med 1990;322:1627–34.

[3] Milne S, Welch V, Brosseau L, et al. Transcutaneous electrical nerve stimulation (TENS) for chronic low-back pain. Cochrane Database of Systematic Reviews 2001;2:CD003008.

[4] Cannon D, Aprill C. Lumbosacral epidural steroid injections. Arch Phys Med Rehabil 2000; 81:S81–98.

[5] Fukusaki M, Kobayashi I, Hara T, et al. Symptoms of spinal stenosis do not improve after epidural steroid injection. Clin J Pain 1998;14:148–51.

[6] Koes B, Scholten R, Mens J, et al. Efficacy of epidural steroid injections for low back pain and sciatica: a systematic review of randomized clinical trials. Pain 1995;63:279–88.

[7] Serrao J, Marks R, Morley S, et al. Intrathecal midazolam for the treatment of chronic mechanical low back pain: a controlled comparison with the epidural steroid in a pilot study. Pain 1992;48:5–12.

[8] Karasek ME. Epidural steroid injections: pro. American Academy of Neurology Course Syllabus 2DS.009: controversies in the use of spine injections for the treatment of spine disease; 2001. p. 29–36.

[9] Schwarzer AC, Aprill CN, Derby R, et al. Clinical features of patients with pain stemming from the lumbar zygapophyseal joints: is the lumbar facet syndrome a clinical entity? Spine 1994;19:1132–7.

[10] Schwarzer AC, Aprill CN, Derby R, et al. The false-positive rate of uncontrolled diagnostic blocks of the lumbar zygapophyseal joints. Pain 1994;58:195–200.

[11] Fukui S, Ohseto K, Shiotani M, et al. Distribution of referred pain from the lumbar zygapophyseal joints and dorsal rami. Clin J Pain 1997;13:303–7.

[12] Kaplan M, Dreyfuss P, Halbrook B, et al. The ability of lumbar medial branch blocks to anesthetize the zygapophysial joint. A physiologic challenge. Spine 1998;23:1847–52.

[13] Mooney V, Robertson J. The facet syndrome. Clin Orthop 1976;115:149–56.

[14] Carette S, Marcoux S, Truchon R, et al. A controlled trial of corticosteroid injections into facet joints for chronic low back pain. N Engl J Med 1991;325:1002–7.

[15] Lilius G, Harilainnen A, Laasonen EM, et al. Chronic unilateral low back pain—predictors of outcome of facet joint injections. Spine 1990;15:780–2.

[16] Marks RC, Houston T, Thulbourne T. Facet joint injection and facet nerve block: a randomized comparison in 86 patients with chronic low back pain. Pain 1992;49:325–8.

[17] Nelemens PJ, Bie RA, de Vet HCW, et al. Injection therapy for subacute and chronic benign low back pain. Cochrane Database Syst Rev 2000;2:CD001824.

[18] Dreyfuss P, Halbrook B, Pauza K, et al. Efficacy and validity of radio frequency neurotomy for chronic lumbar zygapophyseal joint pain. Spine 2000;25:1270–7.

[19] Van Kleef M, Barendse GA, Kessles A, et al. Randomized trial of radiofrequency lumbar facet denervation for chronic low back pain. Spine 1999;24:1937–42.

[20] Leclaire R, Fortin L, Lambert R, et al. Radiofrequency facet joint denervation in the treatment of low back pain: a placebo-controlled clinical trial to assess efficacy. Spine 2001;26: 1411–6.

[21] Deyo RA. Point of view. Spine 2001;26:1417.

[22] Niemisto L, Kalso E, Malmivaara A, et al. Cochrane Collaboration Back Review Group. Radiofrequency denervation for neck and back pain: a systematic review within the framework of the cochrane collaboration back review group. Spine 2003;28(16):1877–88.

[23] Bogduk N, Modic MT. Controversy: lumbar discography. Spine 1990;21:402–4.

[24] Guyer RD, Ohnmeiss DD. Contemporary concepts in spine care—lumbar discography. Spine 1995;20:2048–59.

[25] Pauza KJ, Howell S, Dreyfuss P, et al. A randomized, placebo-controlled trial of intradiscal electrothermal therapy for the treatment of discogenic low back pain. Spine J 2004;4:27–35.

[26] Davis TT, Delamarter RB, Sra P, et al. The IDET procedure for chronic discogenic low back pain. Spine 2004;29:752–6.

[27] Freeman BJC, Fraser RD, Cain CMJ, et al. A randomized, double blind, controlled trial: intradiscal electrothermal therapy versus placebo for the treatment of chronic discogenic low back pain. Spine 2005;30:2369–77.

[28] Hsia AW, Isaac K, Katz JS. Cauda equina syndrome from intradiscal electrothermal therapy. Neurology 2000;55:320.

[29] Ackerman WE III. Cauda equina syndrome after intradiscal electrothermal therapy. Reg Anesth Pain Med 2002;27:622.

[30] Malanga GA, Nadler SF. Nonoperative treatment of low back pain. Mayo Clin Proc 1999; 74:1135–48.

[31] Cuckler JM, Bernini PA, Wiesel SW, et al. The use of epidural steroids in the treatment of lumbar radicular pain. J Bone Joint Surg Am 1985;67:63–6.

[32] Carette S, Leclaire R, Marcoux S, et al. Epidural corticosteroid injections for sciatica due to herniated nucleus pulposus. N Engl J Med 1997;336:1634–40.

[33] Riew KD, Yin Y, Gilula L, et al. The effect of nerve root injections on the need for operative treatment of lumbar radicular pain. J Bone Joint Surg Am 2000;82:1589–93.

[34] Joelson E. Epidural steroid injections: con. American Academy of Neurology Course Syllabus 2DS.009: controversies in the use of spine injections for the treatment of spine disease; 2001. p. 37–41.

[35] Vad VB, Bhatt AT, Lutz GE, et al. Transforaminal epidural steroid injections in lumbosacral radiculopathy: a prospective randomized study. Spine 2002;27:11–6.

[36] DePalma MJ, Bhargava A, Slipman CW. A critical appraisal of the evidence for selective nerve root injection in the treatment of lumbosacral radiculopathy. Arch Phys Med Rehabil 2005;86:1477–83.

[37] Kraemer J, Ludwig J, Bickert U, et al. Lumbar epidural perineural injection: a new technique. Eur Spine J 1997;6:357–61.

[38] Kolsi I, Delecrin J, Berthelot JM, et al. Efficacy of nerve root versus interspinous injections of glucocorticoids in the treatment of disc-related sciatica. A pilot, prospective, randomized, double blind study. Joint Bone Spine 2000;67:113–8.

[39] Karppinen J, Malmivaara A, Kurunlahti M, et al. Periradicular infiltration for sciatica: a randomized controlled trial. Spine 2001;26:1059–67.

[40] Bogduk N. Epidural spinal injections. Pain Dig 1999;9:226–7.

[41] Saal JA, Saal JA, Herzog RJ. The natural history of lumbar intervertebral disc extrusions treated nonoperatively. Spine 1990;15:683–6.

[42] Hooten WM, Mizerak A, Carns PE, et al. Discitis after lumbar epidural corticosteroid injection: a case report and analysis of the case report literature. Pain Med 2006;7:46–51.

[43] Mazanec DJ, Podichetty VK, Hsia A. Lumbar canal stenosis: start with nonsurgical therapy. Cleve Clin J Med 2002;69:909–17.

[44] Delport EG, Cucuzzella AR, Marley JK, et al. Treatment of lumbar spinal stenosis with epidural steroid injections: a retrospective outcome study. Arch Phys Med Rehabil 2004; 85:479–84.

[45] Turk DC. Clinical effectiveness and cost-effectiveness of treatments for patients with chronic pain (Critical Review). Clinical Journal of Pain 2002;18(6):355–65.

[46] Shulman M. Treatment of neck pain with cervical epidural steroid injection. Reg Anesth 1986;11:92–4.

[47] Ferrante FM, Wilson SP, Iacobo C, et al. Clinical classification as a predictor of therapeutic outcome after cervical epidural steroid injection. Spine 1993;18:730–6.

[48] Bush K, Hillier S. Outcome of cervical radiculopathy treated with periradicular/epidural corticosteroid injections: a prospective study with independent clinical review. Eur Spine J 1996;5:319–25.

[49] Rathmell JP, Aprill C, Bogduk N. Cervical transforaminal injection of steroids. Anesthesiology 2004;100:1595–600.

[50] Williams KN, Jackowski A, Evans PJD. Epidural haematoma requiring surgical decompression following repeated cervical epidural steroid injections for chronic pain. Pain 1990;42: 197–9.

[51] Hodges SD, Castleberg RL, Miller T, et al. Cervical epidural steroid injection with intrinsic spinal cord damage, two case reports. Spine 1998;23:2137–42.

[52] Jerosch J, Castro WH, Liljenqist U. Percutaneous facet coagulation—indication, technique, results, and complications. In: Fessler RG, editor. Neurosurgery clinics of North America. Philadelphia: WB Saunders Co; 1996. p. 119–34.

[53] Lord SM, Barnsley L, Wallis BJ, et al. Chronic cervical zygapophysial joint pain after whiplash: a placebo-controlled prevalence study. Spine 1996;21:1737–45.

[54] Lord SM, Barnsley L, Wallis BJ, et al. Percutaneous radio-frequency neurotomy for chronic cervical zygapophyseal-joint pain. N Engl J Med 1996;335:1721–6.

NEUROLOGIC
CLINICS

Neurol Clin 25 (2007) 507–522

ELSEVIER
SAUNDERS

Surgical Management of Neck and Low Back Pain

Ajit A. Krishnaney, MD, John Park, MD,
Edward C. Benzel, MD*

*Cleveland Clinic Center for Spine Health and Department of Neurosurgery,
Cleveland Clinic Neurological Institute, Cleveland Clinic, 9500 Euclid Ave.,
S-80, Cleveland, OH 44195-001, USA*

Neck and low back pain can have a variety of causes. In the majority of cases, neck or back pain is amenable to nonoperative therapy. In select cases, when there is a clearly identifiable structural pathology (eg, fracture or tumor), a neurologic dysfunction resulting from spinal cord or nerve root compression, or nonoperative therapy has failed, surgical intervention should be considered. The choice to proceed with surgery is complex and involves several factors, including patient history and pain pattern, a thorough physical examination, and an evaluation of radiologic and neurophysiologic studies. Paramount to the success of any operation is the ability of a surgeon to identify an anatomic structure that likely is the cause of a patient's pain. In the cases of fracture or spinal tumor, the pathologic anatomic structure often is obvious. In the more common scenario associated with advanced degenerative changes, it often is impossible to identify a single offending pathologic structure. This often is associated with a suboptimal success rate.

Neck pain

Preoperative evaluation

Degenerative changes in the cervical spine can be described as anatomic adaptations of the involved structures to the continued "wear and tear" of the spine. Structural changes, including thickening and calcification of ligaments, the formation of appositional bone, and facet hypertrophy, can occur. This process may be associated with pain. Pain associated with the

---

* Corresponding author.
  E-mail address: benzele@ccf.org (E.C. Benzel).

0733-8619/07/$ - see front matter © 2007 Elsevier Inc. All rights reserved.
doi:10.1016/j.ncl.2007.01.005
neurologic.theclinics.com

degenerated cervical spine may result from compression of neurologic structures (myelopathy or radiculopathy), mechanical pain, or myofascial elements secondary to cervical deformity. An understanding of the location, quality, and mitigating and exacerbating factors often can help identify the offending structure. When a patient's symptoms are attributable to a specific anatomic structure, surgical intervention may be considered.

In patients who do not have neurologic deficits, it is important to determine if the pain predominately is radicular or axial in nature. Often a patient complains of neck and upper extremity pain. In these cases, a clinician must treat the symptom of greatest clinical significance. In general, it is reasonable to treat patients conservatively and defer imaging for a period of 6 to 8 weeks. Certain symptoms, however, should raise red flags. These include unrelenting pain, night pain, weight loss, night sweats, fevers, and chills. The presence of any of these red flags should trigger a more urgent imaging evaluation and referral to a spine surgeon. Such findings are suggestive of the presence of an infectious or neoplastic process. Moreover, patients who have neck pain and a recent history of trauma are at risk for occult pathology, such as subluxation or fracture, and should be imaged immediately.

For patients who have radicular pain and no neurologic deficit and who have failed a trial of conservative therapy, plain radiographs and MRI are indicated. Patients who have only axial neck pain and no neurologic deficit are evaluated best with plain radiographs only. MRI may be helpful, however, in the early identification of infection.

Patients who have a neurologic deficit at the time of initial evaluation should be imaged with MRI or CT myelography. The presence of myelopathy or radiculopathy with motor weakness or sensory loss constitutes reason to refer to a spine surgeon.

Surgical intervention

Most cervical spine surgical procedures involve neural decompression, stabilization (fusion), or deformity correction. Decompression is indicated in cases in which degenerative changes cause direct compression of neural structures, resulting in neurologic deficits (eg, radiculopathy or myelopathy). Bony compression can result from osteophyte formation ventrally or uncovertebral and facet joints dorsolaterally. Soft tissue compression may result from extruded disk material, ligamentous buckling, or facet joint capsule hypertrophy.

Fusion is indicated in the setting of spinal instability. Instability may result from the degenerative process or may be iatrogenic (ie, post decompression). Some suggest that fusion alone may improve radicular symptoms by eliminating mechanical irritation in cases of foraminal stenosis. In addition, if the normal anatomic height and alignment of the spine are restored, the foramina may be decompressed indirectly.

Deformity correction may improve neck pain by restoring the normal mechanical advantage that lordosis affords the cervical musculature. Kyphosis is the most common cervical deformity. This may result in postural neck pain that is related to reflex compensatory mechanisms. The combination of decompression, traction, and fusion may be used to restore anatomic alignment in cases of severe kyphosis or to prevent progression in milder cases.

Radiculopathy

The goal of surgical intervention for radiculopathy is decompression of the affected nerve root. Effective decompression may be achieved through a dorsal or ventral approach. Ventral decompression usually involves complete diskectomy and osteophytectomy, followed by interbody fusion. Dorsally, the nerve root may be decompressed via a laminotomy and foraminotomy. Although either approach is efficacious, both have advantages and drawbacks. The ventral approach provides excellent exposure with little blood loss. Ventral surgery usually is achieved, however, via a complete diskectomy and fusion (Fig. 1). Dorsal decompression does not necessitate fusion. It requires, however, more extensive muscle dissection.

Myelopathy

The goal of surgery in myelopathic patients is decompression of the spinal cord. As with radiculopathy, this may be accomplished vial a dorsal or ventral approach. Laminoplasty also may be considered for multilevel compression in patients who have preserved lordosis. With laminoplasty,

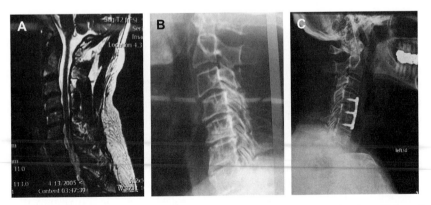

Fig. 1. A 59-year-old man presented with a 1-year history of mechanical neck pain and bilateral shoulder pain. Preoperative imaging revealed cervical spondylosis with effacent of the thecal sac at C4-5 and C5-6 (A). Lateral radiographs exhibited local kyphosis at C4-5 and C5-6 with moderate spondylosis (B, C). C4-5 and C5-6 anterior cervical discectomies and fusion with structural allograft bone grafts and anterior cervical plate fixation was performed with improvement in the patient's neck pain and resolution of his shoulder pain.

the lamina is unhinged via a variety of techniques, thereby expanding the diameter of the central canal. Laminoplasty facilitates decompression over multiple segments while obviating fusion.

Suboccipital pain

Osteoarthritis of the atlantoaxial and atlanto-occipital joints has a prevalence of 4.8% [1]. Degenerative changes in this region present most commonly as unilateral suboccipital pain. The pain usually responds to external immobilization. In patients who have failed conservative therapy, surgical immobilization can provide relief in selected cases.

Surgical immobilization of the atlantoaxial segment can be achieved via a variety of fusion techniques. All of these techniques use a dorsal midline approach to the upper cervical spine and achieve immobilization via fusion. Currently available fixation strategies include segmental fixation with C2 pars or translaminar screws and C1 lateral mass screws, transarticular screw fixation, or a variety of wire or cable fixation techniques.

The literature regarding osteoarthritis of the C0-C1 facet joints is sparse. If degeneration of the atlanto-occipital facet joint or atlanto-occipital instability is believed the source of a patient's pain, however, atlanto-occipital fixation may be indicated. Stabilization and fusion of the atlanto-occipital segment is achieved via a midline dorsal approach. In this case, the suboccipital bone and the dorsal arch of C1 are exposed. Rods may be affixed to the skull via a plate screwed into the occipital keel or via wires threaded through burr holes. The caudal end of the construct then is affixed to the upper cervical spine via screws or wires (Fig. 2).

Subaxial cervical spine pain

In patients who have neck pain refractory to conservative therapy, including neck strengthening and flexibility exercises, epidural steroid and facet injections, and anti-inflammatory medications, surgical intervention may be indicated. In cases in which surgical intervention is considered, a focal single level cause of the pain should be identified.

Precise localization of the painful level often is difficult. Surgery, therefore, should be considered carefully. The mainstay of evaluation is the history and physical examination. Radiologic evaluation consists of plain radiographs, CT, and MRI. Often these studies reveal degenerative changes, including disk desiccation, loss of disk space height, and osteophyte formation at multiple levels. Moreover, as many as 85% of asymptomatic individuals over 60 years of age exhibit degenerative changes in their cervical disks on MRI [2,3]. This further diminishes the indication for surgical intervention.

Treatment of acute axial neck pain includes rest, anti-inflammatory agents, muscle relaxants, analgesics, and physical therapy. Therapy of neck pain in the chronic phase includes physical therapy with muscle

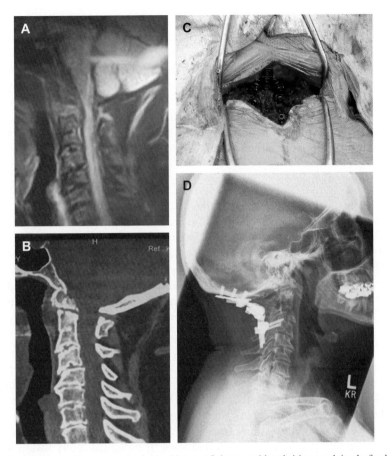

Fig. 2. A 73-year-old woman who had a history of rheumatoid arthritis complained of suboc-cipital and upper cervical pain with movement. Preoperative MRI (*A*) and CT (*B*) revealed autofusion of occiput to C3 with a chronic fracture of the dens. Occiput to C3 fusion with in-strumentation was performed with resolution of suboccipital and cervical pain. Intraoperative photograph (*C*) and postoperative lateral radiograph (*D*) show the construct consisting of an occipital plate and C3 lateral mass screw fixation.

strengthening, flexibility, and range-of-motion exercises. Epidural steroid injections also may be helpful in the chronic phase, although the risk asso-ciated with such injections precludes their routine use. Surgical intervention for neck pain in the absence of radicular pain should be considered only after all conservative measures are exhausted. When considering fusion for neck pain, selection of the levels to be included in the fusion is crucial. This decision is based on the available clinical and radiographic data, including subluxation or spinal instability that is manifested by excessive segmental motion.

Neck pain is treated surgically most effectively with cervical fusion. Cervical fusion may be accomplished via a dorsal or ventral approach.

The choice of approach is a complex one and depends on several factors, including the number of levels to be fused, cervical sagittal alignment, history of prior surgery, patient comorbidities and body habitus. The ventral approach is preferred for correction of kyphotic segments and in cases where a degenerative disk is the suspected cause of the pain. Dorsal fusion may be considered when multiple levels are involved and sagittal alignment is acceptable. Combined ventral and dorsal fusion may be required when correcting severe kyphosis or in cases where anatomic considerations prevent adequate fixation from either approach alone.

Ventral approach

The ventral cervical spine is approached via a corridor medial to the ventral border of the steroncleidomastoid muscle and medial to the carotid sheath. Once the appropriate level is identified, a diskectomy is performed. If further decompression or deformity correction is required, a corpectomy may be performed. Once decompression is complete, a graft is placed in the evacuated space. A variety of graft materials currently is available, including iliac crest autograft, cadaveric allograft, and synthetic spacers. A plate then may be affixed across the fused segments with screws (Fig. 1).

Dorsal fusion

The dorsal cervical spine is exposed via a midline incision. Dissection proceeds deep to the posterior cervical fascia via the midline rafe to minimize muscle bleeding. Subperiostial dissection is used to expose the cervical lamina and lateral masses. Once the appropriate levels are identified, decompression may be performed via a laminotomy for radiculopathy or laminectomy for spinal cord compression at the affected level. If indicated, bony fusion may be achieved by placing a bone graft across the exposed facet joints. Internal fixation can be achieved through a variety of wiring and cabling techniques or with any of several commercially available screw-hook-rod systems.

Low back pain

Seventy percent to 85% of people have back pain at some point in their life. In the United States, back pain is the second most common reason for a visit to a physician, the fifth most common cause of admission to a hospital, and the third most common indication for surgery [4]. Back pain can be characterized by its duration: acute back pain typically lasts 0 to 4 weeks, subacute back pain lasts 4 to 12 weeks, and chronic back pain is greater than 12 weeks in duration [5]. For the most part, back pain is a benign and self-limited entity, with 60% to 70% of patients recovering by 6 weeks and 80% to 90% recovering by 12 weeks. Recovery after this period, however, often is slow and uncertain, and such patients are a major source of disability and lost workdays. Many nonsurgical therapies exist for nonspecific low back pain, including exercise therapy, cognitive behavioral therapy, manipulation, and medications. A combination program involving exercise and cognitive therapy may be particularly efficacious for those who have chronic low back pain [5]. Patients who have back pain refractory to such measures, however, may be candidates for surgical intervention, provided a thorough assessment to establish candidacy for surgery is performed.

Preoperative evaluation

Various terms are used to characterize back pain and its associated symptoms. Radiculopathy arises from compression of an exiting nerve root. This may be caused by a bulging or herniated disk, degenerative stenosis of the intervertebral foramen, a synovial cyst, or other pathologic entities. Pain often is shock-like, radiating along a dermatomal distribution, and occasionally may be accompanied by motor weakness and a decreased muscle stretch reflex, corresponding to the affected nerve root. Radiculopathy pain can be elicited by tests, such as a straight leg raise, where a positive test consists of leg pain or parasthesia in the distribution of the affected nerve after less than 60° of leg elevation [6].

Neurogenic claudication secondary to lumbar canal stenosis consists of numbness, fatigue, weakness, or cramping leg pain (occasionally without back pain) that is aggravated by walking and lumbar extension and relieved by sitting. Patients tend to stoop when walking, often bending over carts while shopping. They tolerate bicycling better than walking, because of the flexed posture assumed during cycling [7]. Lumbar flexion opens the neuroforamina and provides greater room for exiting nerve roots. This, in turn, decreases exiting nerve root compression and associated symptoms.

Diskogenic pain, a somewhat controversial diagnosis, is axial spine pain without sciatica secondary to a degenerative disk [8]. Degenerative tears of the annulus fibrosus stimulate sinuvertebral nerve endings that innervate the annulus fibrosus and posterior longitudinal ligament [9]. Diskogenic pain also is believed to correlate with the increased nociceptive innervation that develops within symptomatic degenerative disks [10]. Nevertheless, diskogenic pain is defined poorly and should be considered suspect as an indication, in and of itself, for surgery.

The facet syndrome refers to back pain generated within the facet joints. Lumbar extension generally is believed to worsen this pain. The existence of the facet syndrome as a definitive clinical entity is questioned [11].

Mechanical back pain is a deep, dull, agonizing pain worsened when load is placed on the spine. It is exacerbated by an upright posture and by activity in general. Bed rest and inactivity diminish the pain by removing load from the spine. Muscle pain may be present in the same patient but is not a component of mechanical pain. Unlike mechanical pain, muscle pain tends to be sharp, to be associated with palpable tenderness, and to respond poorly to rest. Mechanical back pain often is associated with degenerative disease of the spine, which can give rise to dysfunctional motion within the spine [12].

An initial assessment should seek neurologic symptoms that may require urgent attention, such as weakness and signs of cauda equina syndrome (saddle anesthesia, urinary incontinence, or motor deficit). The initial examination also should screen for other potentially serious conditions, such as fracture, infection, or cancer [6]. Physical examination findings also may point to other pathologies unlikely to benefit from spinal surgery, such as hip or sacroiliac joint pain syndromes.

Before considering surgical options, it is prudent to evaluate patients for psychosocial factors that may complicate the outcome of spinal surgery. Because pain is a subjective experience, a patient's personality and emotional character may affect the perception of pain and the pain response to surgery. Higher levels of hysteria, hypochondriasis, and depression, as measured by the Minnesota Multiphasic Personality Inventory, and poor pain coping skills are predictive of suboptimal outcomes after spine surgery [13]. Physical examination may uncover nonphysiologic findings (Waddell [14] signs,, such as superficial tenderness, lumbar pain with axial loading or simulated rotation, and diminished pain when distracting patients during straight leg raising). The presence of several of these signs suggests a pain behavior pattern that is predictive of a poor surgical outcome. Social factors also could affect the probability of satisfactory outcome from spinal surgery negatively, including involvement in disability pension claims and workers' compensation claims, long preoperative sick leave, litigation, and the reinforcement of pain behavior by family members [15]. Patients who have such negative predictors of satisfactory surgical outcome may be served best by chronic pain programs and rigorous physical and cognitive therapy before surgery is undertaken. Cessation of smoking is another behavioral modification strategy that should be pursued before surgery, particularly if patients are considered for spinal fusion [16]. Smoking is associated with a markedly decreased fusion rate and a suboptimal response to surgery.

Diagnostic studies

Several imaging studies can be used to evaluate patients considered surgical candidates. If patients present with back pain for the first time, plain radiography is not recommended unless they present with symptoms suggestive of systemic disease or trauma. Such symptoms include fever, weight loss, a history of cancer, neurologic deficit, alcohol or intravenous drug abuse, age greater than 50, and trauma [17]. Plain radiographs are appropriate initial imaging studies in patients not improving after a 1-month course of conservative therapy [18]. Plain radiographs can reveal gross bony abnormalities, such as fractures and osteopenia. They also can be used to diagnose spinal imbalance, spondylolisthesis (displacement of one vertebra over the one beneath it), or scoliosis. Anteroposterior and lateral views may be supplemented by flexion and extension views aimed at detecting abnormal motion and instability. Such findings may provide sufficient indication for a fusion. Plain radiographs also are useful for detecting anatomic variations that could confuse a surgeon intraoperatively, such as the presence of six lumbar vertebrae or a sacralized fifth lumbar vertebra.

More advanced studies include CT and MRI. MRI provides better soft tissue resolution and a superior ability to detect malignant or vascular abnormalities. It facilitates the detection of stenosis of the spinal canal or foramina caused by ligamentous hypertrophy and inflammatory changes within disks, vertebral bodies, and facet joints. With gadolinium enhancement, it is for detecting paravertebral soft tissue abnormalities, osteomyelitis, and intradural pathology [18]. Noncontrast CT facilitates delineation of bony anatomy and bone abnormalities. It is suitable if MRI is contraindicated, as may be the case in patients who have cardiac pacemakers and claustrophobia. CT myelography could delineate central canal stenosis and nerve root compression further, especially in those unable to undergo MRI or in postsurgical patients in whom instrumentation may result in excessive MRI artifacts. The use of imaging studies should be judicious because of the high incidence of imaging abnormalities in asymptomatic individuals [18]. Degenerative disk changes and stenosis of the lumbar spine canal and foramen are found in a high percentage of asymptomatic individuals [19,20]. Hence, radiographic findings should be correlated with a patient's symptoms before deciding to treat the patient through surgery.

More invasive studies to evaluate surgical candidates are available. Diskography involves injection of contrast into the disk interspace of a radiographically abnormal disk. Pain that is concordant with a patient's usual back pain, combined with lack of pain or pain that is not concordant at adjacent disks, is believed to implicate the abnormal disk as a source of diskogenic pain. Radiographically normal disks are not considered candidates for surgical intervention, even if diskography is positive [21]. Diskography can be used to evaluate the extent of disk abnormality, to correlate the abnormal disk with clinical symptoms, and to investigate an abnormal disk when other tests fail to provide clear proof that the disk is the source of pain [22]. The test carries a risk of infection, however, albeit low, and remains controversial with respect to reliability. Production of pain in asymptomatic postdiskectomy patients is not significantly different from postdiskectomy patients suffering from pain, and patients who have abnormal psychologic profiles have significantly higher pain responses overall to diskography [23]. In addition, chronic cervical pain sufferers who do not have back pain and patients who have somatization disorders but do not have back pain also are highly likely to develop pain with lumbar diskography, again showing the confounding influence of psychologic background in evaluating diskogenic pain via diskography [24].

In patients who have radicular pain in whom the source of the pain is unclear because of multiple radiographic abnormalities, a selective nerve root block can be useful in determining the cause of the pain [25]. This test is helpful primarily as a negative predictor for the presence of nerve compression if the result of the block is negative, because it has great sensitivity in demonstrating symptomatic nerve root compression but only moderate specificity [26]. Similarly, a facet block can be used to evaluate a facet joint as a source of pain.

Surgical options

Surgery should be tailored to a patient's symptoms and diagnostic study findings. Radicular pain from disk herniation that fails to respond to a trial of conservative therapy can be treated with a unilateral diskectomy (Fig. 3). The approach depends on the side of the patient's symptoms and the laterality of the disk herniation on imaging [27,28]. Fusion typically is not necessary for such cases. Newer techniques using minimally invasive access techniques facilitate the performance of the procedure using tube dilators or expandable retractors. These techniques allow for a smaller incision and decrease stripping of muscle off its bony attachment [29].

The efficacy of lumbar diskectomy over nonoperative treatment of radicular pain remains somewhat controversial. A recent randomized control trial by the Spine Patient Outcomes Research Trial (SPORT) group compared lumbar diskectomy versus nonoperative care over a period of 2 years for patients who had radicular pain [30]. It found that surgical and nonsurgical patients experienced significant improvements in primary and secondary outcome measures. Examination of primary outcome measures did show that surgical patients had slightly better outcomes in every stage of follow-up than did nonsurgical patients, but this difference was not statistically significant. Conclusions about the superiority of operative therapy or

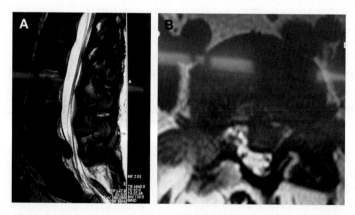

Fig. 3. A 28-year-old man who had a 6-week history of left L5 radicular pain who had failed conservative management. MRI (*A*, *B*) revealed a large left sided L4-5 extruded disc fragment. He underwent a left L4-5 microdiscectomy with immediate relief of his symptoms.

conservative management could not be made because of the large number of patients crossing over between the two groups [30]. The SPORT group also ran a concurrent observational cohort study looking at patients eligible for the randomized study who declined randomization [31]. In this study, surgical patients demonstrated a significant improvement in primary outcome measures compared with nonsurgical patients. This study looked at subjective results among an unmasked, nonrandomized pool of patients, however, making it vulnerable to confounding factors, such as expectations of treatment success and differences in perception of care.

Severe neurogenic claudication secondary to degenerative spinal canal stenosis may require decompression of the thecal sac and nerve roots. Anatomic factors contributing to stenosis include short pedicles, osteophytes, hypertrophy of the facet joints, thickening of the ligamentum flavum, and bulging degenerated disks. Laminectomy involves partial removal of the lamina and removal of the spinous processes and ligamentum flavum, thus removing dorsal compression. It may be accompanied by partial resection of the medial portions of the facet joints, foraminotomies to enlarge the intervertebral foramen and decompress exiting nerve roots, and diskectomies to relieve ventral compression. Care must be taken to avoid dural tears and nerve root injuries. Overly aggressive decompression also may destabilize the spine if too much of the facet is removed or if an excessive lateral removal of the lamina results in fracture of the pars interarticularis (which would result in the disconnection of the superior and inferior articular processes of the affected vertebrae). In the absence of spinal instability, surgical fusion or instrumentation generally is unnecessary [32].

Preoperative radiographic evaluation may reveal anatomic factors that could predispose the spine to instability after dorsal decompression. Dorsal decompression in the presence of significant degenerative scoliosis could lead to progressively worsening deformity after surgery as a result of loss of stabilization provided by the dorsal spinal arch complex. Surgeons may wish to consider a less extensive hemilaminectomy or laminotomy, with limited bony removal, followed by undercutting and removal of compressive pathology via the smaller exposure. Preoperative flexion-extension films also may demonstrate instability, with slippage of 3 mm or more of one vertebral body over the next or the development of 10° or more of angulation [32]. In cases of radiologic instability or in cases where the risk of iatrogenic destabilization is significant, surgeons may wish to consider fusion while remaining mindful of its risks, which include increased operative time and increased operative blood loss. The decision for fusion usually requires smoking cessation (typically for several weeks before the surgery) and the avoidance of steroids and nonsteroidal anti-inflammatory medications to decrease the risk of fusion failure.

Fusion, either instrumented or noninstrumented, involves the laying of bone graft or bone graft substitute between adjacent vertebral structures (such as along the pars interarticularis or transverse processes or within the facet joints), with the goal of creating a motion-limiting bony mass over time. Instrumentation can involve dorsal placement of pedicle screws, which serve as an internal fixator while the fusion mass solidifies, thereby decreasing the risk of fusion failure. Pedicle screws are shown to lead to a higher radiographic fusion rate, although there was no long-term clinical advantage over noninstrumented fusion with respect to back or leg pain [33].

Surgeons also may choose to perform interbody fusion, which involves placement of a bony graft or a synthetic cage (filled with bone or bone substitute, such as recombinant human bone morphogenic protein) [34] between the vertebral bodies after a diskectomy. Lumbar lordosis can be maintained or improved by placing an appropriately fashioned interbody graft. In addition, the distraction between the vertebral bodies provided by an interbody graft can open up the intervertebral foramen, decreasing pressure on exiting nerve roots. Performing an interbody fusion can be accomplished through a ventral or dorsal approach. The dorsal approach can be performed via a direct dorsal route into the gap left by the diskectomy (posterior lumbar interbody fusion) (Fig. 4). Alternatively, the diskectomy and the insertion of the graft can be performed slightly more laterally in the area of the spinal foramen (transforaminal lumbar interbody fusion). Anterior lumbar interbody fusion (ALIF), which can be performed via a retroperitoneal or transperitoneal approach, allows surgeons to avoid the neural elements and is believed by some investigators to be biomechanically superior to a dorsally placed graft [27]. Performing an ALIF, however, does not permit direct decompression of the neural elements and carries with it risks, such as bowel or vascular injury, thrombosis caused by retraction of major vessels, and retrograde ejaculation in males. Convincing evidence that any method of

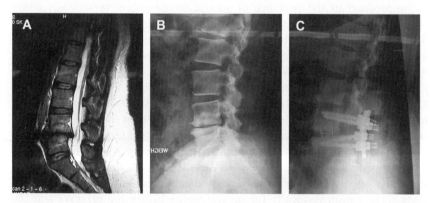

Fig. 4. A 47-year-old woman who had mechanical low back pain and right L4 radiculopathy who had failed 3 months of conservative therapy. Preoperative MRI and plain radiographs (*A*, *B*) reveal an L4-5 degenrerative disc with a grade 1 spondylolisthesis and narrowing of the L4-5 foramen. An L4-5 decompression and interbody fusion with instrumentation was performed, resulting in restored intervertebral height and resolution of radicular and low back pain (*C*).

interbody fusion technique is superior with regards to radiographic fusion and clinical outcome is lacking [35]. The decision for instrumentation or interbody fusion requires evaluation of the patient's overall health status because of the additional operative time and blood loss. Other mitigating factors include osteoporosis, the risk to neural and adjacent structures during instrumentation, and the additional cost of instrumentation. In addition, the preservation of lumbar lordosis with any fusion procedure should be a primary objective. The loss of lordosis can result in a flattened back that makes proper posture difficult, leading to tightness and pain in the low back and hamstrings [12].

Lumbar fusion often is performed to treat intractable back pain secondary to degenerative disk disease without stenosis or spondylolisthesis. This indication is controversial, however, and concern is raised about the appropriateness of the rapid rise in the number of spinal fusion operations, especially considering the risks and expense of spinal fusion [8]. A large multicenter randomized control trial evaluated whether or not lumbar fusion could reduce pain and disability in 289 patients using multiple outcome measures and found significant improvement in the fusion group compared with those treated with standard conservative measures [36]. Alternatively, a later and smaller randomized trial compared instrumented fusion versus an intensive course of cognitive therapy and exercise and found equal improvement in both groups along with an 18% early complication rate in the surgical group [37]. Lumbar fusion has, henceforth, been recommended for carefully selected patients who have disabling pain as a result of one- or two-level degenerative disease without stenosis or spondylolisthesis, whereas intensive physical and cognitive therapy is recommended as a treatment option for patients with multi-level degenerative changes [38].

Postoperatively, patients are encouraged to mobilize, and standing films can be taken to evaluate instrumentation. The use of a brace postoperatively after fusion is of unknown benefit [39] and often a matter of surgeon preference.

A possible long-term complication of spinal fusion is the development of degenerative changes in levels adjacent to the fused vertebrae [40]. These problems include spondylolisthesis, worsening spinal canal stenosis, and scoliosis. The theory that preserving motion in the disk space decreases the risk of so-called "adjacent segment disease" has led to interest in total disk replacement to treat pain resulting from degenerative disk disease. Disk arthroplasty is performed via a ventral approach. Two-year follow-up demonstrates clinical improvement comparable to that of lumbar fusion [41]. Long-term data examining clinical outcome, preservation of motion, and prevention of adjacent segment degeneration, however, are scant [42] and at times contradictory. Some investigators report good clinical outcomes comparable to results for lumbar fusion [43], whereas others suggest a high rate of spontaneous ankylosis and motion impairment at long-term follow-up [44].

Other surgical procedures are of limited application in the treatment of back pain. Spinal cord stimulation can be used for treatment of failed back syndrome, a persistent or recurrent pain that affects predominantly the lower back and legs despite anatomically successful spinal surgery. Spinal cord stimulation produces a sustained 50% or more reduction in pain in a large portion of patients who have failed back syndrome, especially when used early in the course of treatment [45]. An implantable drug delivery system to administer intrathecal narcotic medication also can be used for patients who have failed back syndrome or back pain resistant to other types of therapy [46]. Intradiskal electrothermal therapy uses controlled thermal energy delivered via an intradiskal catheter to treat diskogenic back pain, theoretically by coagulating nociceptors in the disk annulus and by causing collagen contraction. Although it is considered safe, its efficacy has not been demonstrated in several studies [47,48]. Patients suspected of having facet syndrome can undergo facet blocks; those who have a positive response to the block can undergo radiofrequency facet joint denervation (facet ablation). Evidence regarding facet ablation is conflicting, with prospective double-blind randomized trials supporting [49] and refuting [50] the efficacy of this procedure.

Summary

The surgical management of neck and low back pain can be challenging and often is met with mixed results. It should be considered a last resort. In patients who have failed nonsurgical therapy with a discrete anatomic lesion that correlates with the level of the pain, surgical intervention should be considered. Currently, the mainstay of surgical therapy is fusion through a ventral or dorsal approach. Recently introduced procedures, such as disk arthroplasty, hold great promise, but as yet have not shown improved outcomes over spinal fusion.

References

[1] Zapleat J, Valois JC. Radiologic prevalence of advanced C1-2 osteoarthritis. Spine 1997;21: 2511–3.
[2] Boden S, McCowin P, Davis DO, et al. Abnormal magnetic resonance scans of the cervical spine in asymptomatic subjects. J Bone Joint Surg Am 1990;72:1178–83.
[3] Matsumoto M, Fujimura Y, Suzuki N, et al. MRI of cervical intervertebral discs in asymptomatic subjects. J Bone Joint Surg Br 1998;80:19–24.
[4] Andersson GB. Epidemiological features of chronic low-back pain. Lancet 1999;354(9178): 581–5.
[5] Nordin M, Balague F, Cedraschi C. Nonspecific lower-back pain: surgical versus nonsurgical treatment. Clin Orthop Relat Res 2006;443:156–67.
[6] Greenberg MS. Handbook of neurosurgery. 5th edition. New York: Thieme; 2001.
[7] Binder DK, Schmidt MH, Weinstein PR. Lumbar spinal stenosis. Semin Neurol 2002;22(2): 157–66.

[8] Deyo RA, Nachemson A, Mirza SK. Spinal-fusion surgery—the case for restraint. N Engl J Med 2004;350(7):722–6.

[9] Roh JS, Teng AL, Yoo JU, et al. Degenerative disorders of the lumbar and cervical spine. Orthop Clin North Am 2005;36(3):255–62.

[10] Coppes MH, Marani E, Thomeer RT, et al. Innervation of "painful" lumbar discs. Spine 1997;22(20):2342–9 [discussion: 2349–50].

[11] Schwarzer AC, Aprill CN, Derby R, et al. Clinical features of patients with pain stemming from the lumbar zygapophysial joints. Is the lumbar facet syndrome a clinical entity? Spine 1994;19(10):1132–7.

[12] Benzel EC. Biomechanics of spine stabilization. New York: Thieme; 2001.

[13] Epker J, Block AR. Presurgical psychological screening in back pain patients: a review. Clin J Pain 2001;17(3):200–5.

[14] Waddell G, McCulloch JA, Kummel E, et al. Nonorganic physical signs in low-back pain. Spine 1980;5(2):117–25.

[15] Mannion AF, Elfering A. Predictors of surgical outcome and their assessment. Eur Spine J 2006;15(Suppl 1):S93–108.

[16] Andersen T, Christensen FB, Laursen M, et al. Smoking as a predictor of negative outcome in lumbar spinal fusion. Spine 2001;26(23):2623–8.

[17] Deyo RA, Weinstein JN. Low back pain. N Engl J Med 2001;344(5):363–70.

[18] Atlas SJ, Nardin RA. Evaluation and treatment of low back pain: an evidence-based approach to clinical care. Muscle Nerve 2003;27(3):265–84.

[19] Powell MC, Wilson M, Szypryt P, et al. Prevalence of lumbar disc degeneration observed by magnetic resonance in symptomless women. Lancet 1986;2(8520):1366–7.

[20] Jensen MC, Brant-Zawadzki MN, Obuchowski N, et al. Magnetic resonance imaging of the lumbar spine in people without back pain. N Engl J Med 1994;331(2):69–73.

[21] Resnick DK, Choudhri TF, Dailey AT, et al, American Association of Neurological Surgeons/Congress of Neurological Surgeons. Guidelines for the performance of fusion procedures for degenerative disease of the lumbar spine. Part 6: magnetic resonance imaging and discography for patient selection for lumbar fusion. J Neurosurg Spine 2005;2(6):662–9.

[22] Guyer RD, Ohnmeiss DD, NASS. Lumbar discography. Spine J 2003;3(3 Suppl):11S–27S.

[23] Carragee EJ, Chen Y, Tanner CM, et al. Provocative discography in patients after limited lumbar discectomy: a controlled, randomized study of pain response in symptomatic and asymptomatic subjects. Spine 2000;25(23):3065–71.

[24] Carragee EJ, Tanner CM, Khurana S, et al. The rates of false-positive lumbar discography in select patients without low back symptoms. Spine 2000;25(11):1373–80 [discussion: 1381].

[25] Slipman CW, Issac Z. The role of diagnostic selective nerve root blocks in the management of spinal pain. Pain Physician 2001;4(3):214–26.

[26] Saal JS. General principles of diagnostic testing as related to painful lumbar spine disorders: a critical appraisal of current diagnostic techniques. Spine 2002;27(22):2538–45 [discussion: 2546].

[27] Benzel EC. Spine surgery: techniques, complication avoidance, and management. 2nd edition. Philadelphia: Elsevier Churchill Livingstone; 2005.

[28] Fessler RG, Sekhar L. Atlas of neurosurgical techniques: spine and peripheral nerves. New York: Thieme; 2006.

[29] Lehman RA Jr, Vaccaro AR, Bertagnoli R, et al. Standard and minimally invasive approaches to the spine. Orthop Clin North Am 2005;36(3):281–92.

[30] Weinstein JN, Tosteson TD, Lurie JD, et al. Surgical vs nonoperative treatment for lumbar disk herniation: the Spine Patient Outcomes Research Trial (SPORT): a randomized trial. JAMA 2006;296(20):2441–50.

[31] Weinstein JN, Lurie JD, Tosteson TD, et al. Surgical vs nonoperative treatment for lumbar disk herniation: the Spine Patient Outcomes Research Trial (SPORT) observational cohort. JAMA 2006;296(20):2451–9.

[32] Bambakidis NC, Feiz-Erfan I, Klopfenstein JD, et al. Indications for surgical fusion of the cervical and lumbar motion segment. Spine 2005;30(16 Suppl):S2–6.

[33] Fischgrund JS, Mackay M, Herkowitz HN, et al. 1997 Volvo award winner in clinical studies. Degenerative lumbar spondylolisthesis with spinal stenosis: a prospective, randomized study comparing decompressive laminectomy and arthrodesis with and without spinal instrumentation. Spine 1997;22(24):2807–12.

[34] Burkus JK, Gornet MF, Dickman CA, et al. Anterior lumbar interbody fusion using rhBMP-2 with tapered interbody cages. J Spinal Disord Tech 2002;15(5):337–49.

[35] Resnick DK, Choudhri TF, Dailey AT, et al, American Association of Neurological Surgeons/Congress of Neurological Surgeons. Guidelines for the performance of fusion procedures for degenerative disease of the lumbar spine. Part 11: interbody techniques for lumbar fusion. J Neurosurg Spine 2005;2(6):692–9.

[36] Fritzell P, Hagg O, Wessberg P, et al, Swedish Lumbar Spine Study Group. 2001 Volvo Award Winner in Clinical Studies: Lumbar fusion versus nonsurgical treatment for chronic low back pain: a multicenter randomized controlled trial from the Swedish Lumbar Spine Study Group. Spine 2001;26(23):2521–32 [discussion: 2532–4].

[37] Brox JI, Sorensen R, Friis A, et al. Randomized clinical trial of lumbar instrumented fusion and cognitive intervention and exercises in patients with chronic low back pain and disc degeneration. Spine 2003;28(17):1913–21.

[38] Resnick DK, Choudhri TF, Dailey AT, et al, American Association of Neurological Surgeons/Congress of Neurological Surgeons. Guidelines for the performance of fusion procedures for degenerative disease of the lumbar spine. Part 7: intractable low-back pain without stenosis or spondylolisthesis. J Neurosurg Spine 2005;2(6):670–2.

[39] Connolly PJ, Grob D. Bracing of patients after fusion for degenerative problems of the lumbar spine—yes or no? Spine 1998;23(12):1426–8.

[40] Park P, Garton HJ, Gala VC, et al. Adjacent segment disease after lumbar or lumbosacral fusion: review of the literature. Spine 2004;29(17):1938–44.

[41] Blumenthal S, McAfee PC, Guyer RD, et al. A prospective, randomized, multicenter food and drug administration investigational device exemptions study of lumbar total disc replacement with the charite artificial disc versus lumbar fusion: part I: evaluation of clinical outcomes. Spine 2005;30(14):1565–75.

[42] de Kleuver M, Oner FC, Jacobs WC. Total disc replacement for chronic low back pain: background and a systematic review of the literature. Eur Spine J 2003;12(2):108–16.

[43] Lemaire JP, Carrier H, Sariali el-H, et al. Clinical and radiological outcomes with the charite artificial disc: a 10-year minimum follow-up. J Spinal Disord Tech 2005;18(4):353–9.

[44] Putzier M, Funk JF, Schneider SV, et al. Charite total disc replacement–clinical and radiographical results after an average follow-up of 17 years. Eur Spine J 2006;15(2):183–95.

[45] Van Buyten JP. Neurostimulation for chronic neuropathic back pain in failed back surgery syndrome. J Pain Symptom Manage 2006;31(4 Suppl):S25–9.

[46] Deer T, Chapple I, Classen A, et al. Intrathecal drug delivery for treatment of chronic low back pain: report from the National Outcomes Registry for Low Back Pain. Pain Med 2004;5(1):6–13.

[47] Gibson JN, Waddell G. Surgery for degenerative lumbar spondylosis: updated cochrane review. Spine 2005;30(20):2312–20.

[48] Freeman BJ, Fraser RD, Cain CM, et al. A randomized, double-blind, controlled trial: intradiscal electrothermal therapy versus placebo for the treatment of chronic discogenic low back pain. Spine 2005;30(21):2369–77 [discussion: 2378].

[49] van Kleef M, Barendse GA, Kessels A, et al. Randomized trial of radiofrequency lumbar facet denervation for chronic low back pain. Spine 1999;24(18):1937–42.

[50] Leclaire R, Fortin L, Lambert R, et al. Radiofrequency facet joint denervation in the treatment of low back pain: a placebo-controlled clinical trial to assess efficacy. Spine 2001;26(13):1411–6 [discussion: 1417].

ELSEVIER
SAUNDERS

Neurol Clin 25 (2007) 523–537

NEUROLOGIC
CLINICS

Physical Medicine and Complementary Approaches

Deborah A. Venesy, MD

*Department of Physical Medicine and Rehabilitation, Cleveland Clinic, 9500 Euclid Avenue,
C21, Cleveland, OH 44195, USA*

*Pain is real when you get other people to believe in it. If no one believes in it
but you, your pain is madness or hysteria.*

Naomi Wolf

Back pain is the second most common reason that patients come to a doctor, with lifetime prevalence for the general population between 60% and 80%. This back pain epidemic, as noted by Waddell and others, is the most common reason for filing for workers' compensation claims and is the number one disability for people under 45 years of age [1–4].

As health care costs continue to increase, although the variety of treatment options for back and neck pain remains extensive, the effectiveness of many therapeutic options never has been proved. A major challenge for researchers in the neuromuscular and spine field is to "provide evidence of which treatment, if any, is the most optimal for (subgroups of) patients with low back pain" [5]. This article reviews current complementary and noninterventional treatment options for back and neck pain. Acute pain is defined as 6 weeks or less and chronic pain as 12 weeks or more. In addition, the referenced evidence rating system is the one used by the Agency for Health Care Policy and Research (AHCPR) in its guidelines for acute low back problems in adults: clinical practice guideline no.14 (Box 1) [2]. The literature review is based mainly on systematic reviews, such as Cochrane reviews, when available, and other relevant studies. vanTulder and colleagues are quoted and referenced frequently, as they have contributed the preponderance of systematic reviews on this topic and established a standard of care. Divergent opinions abound in clinical practice and research and highlight the difficulty in managing this complex patient population. The research has generated what seem to be equivocal and conflicting

E-mail address: venesyd@ccf.org

0733-8619/07/$ - see front matter © 2007 Elsevier Inc. All rights reserved.
doi:10.1016/j.ncl.2007.02.004   *neurologic.theclinics.com*

Box 1. Panel ratings of available evidence supporting guideline statements

A = *Strong* research-based evidence (multiple relevant and high-quality scientific studies)

B = *Moderate* research-based evidence (one relevant, high-quality scientific study or multiple adequate scientific studies)

C = *Limited* research-based evidence (at least one adequate scientific study of patients who have low back pain [LBP])

D = Panel interpretation of information that did not meet inclusion criteria as research-based evidence

---

From Bigos S, Bowyer O, Braen G, et al. Acute low back problems in adults. Clinical practice guideline no. 14. Rockville (MD): Agency for Health Care Policy and Research, Public Health Service; December 1994. US Department of Health and Human Services, AHCPR Publication no. 95-0642. 1–160.

---

conclusions in some situations. Further clarification through large randomized trials may clarify some of this ambiguity.

Management of back pain is complicated by several factors. Many patients present with symptoms but without physical findings on examination or imaging studies. Other patients demonstrate structural abnormalities without clear clinical correlates. One study, for instance, demonstrated lumbar MRI scan structural changes (disc bulge, protrusion, and extrusion) in more than 50% of asymptomatic individuals [3]. There has been a proliferation of surgical and nonsurgical treatments without national or international standards of treatment. Factors, such as income, educational level, and job type, exert influences on the expression of symptoms and response to treatment.

In chronic LBP, where symptoms are present for more than 3 months, factors beyond imaging results and physical examination become important in the evaluation of the clinical picture and the selection of therapy. This is because illness behavior and subjective symptomatology contribute to the perpetuation of disability [6]. In addition to standard history and physical examination, other tools are used by specialists to assess spine impairment and disability fully. Pain diagrams or drawings are helpful in identifying radicular patterns, diffuse pain in soft tissue (such as fibromyalgia), or somatosensory patterns that can extend outside the lines of the body. Physiatrists also assess patients' functional impairments at home and work. Tools, such as the Oswestry Disability Index and the Roland-Morris Low Back Pain and Disability Questionnaire, facilitate assessment of functional impairments at home and work [7,8].

The physiatric approach to back pain assessment pays particular attention to psychosocial components of the history. In addition to looking for clinically significant physical findings, there is an assessment of personal beliefs that may have an impact on patients' manifestation of pain, their willingness to be compliant in treatment, or both. Several factors are associated with resistance to standard physical treatments of spine pain (Box 2) [9]. Box 3 lists specific illness behaviors identified by Waddell and coworkers [10].

The AHCPR has developed guidelines on acute low back problems in adults [2]. The acute LBP guidelines were federally mandated and developed in 1994 by a panel of 23 national experts and seven consultants and remain clinically instructive [1]. A summary of the panel's findings and recommendations is found in Table 1.

Complementary medicine treatment approaches

In a 1997 study, figures indicated $25 billion per year was spent on medical care for back pain and an additional $50 billion spent on disability and lost productivity [5,11]. Despite the prevalence of back pain, few treatments have proved effective in controlled trials [2,5,11]. Patients often consult with practioners of complementary and alterative medicine (CAM) in search of treatments, such as spinal manipulation, massage therapy, and acupuncture. A description of these treatments follows.

Spinal manipulation

Spinal manipulation is practiced by osteopathic physicians, chiropractors, and physical therapists. Spinal manipulation is described as the use of hands applied to patients incorporating instructions and maneuvers to achieve maximal painless movement [12]. Manipulation is promoted as a technique to restore joint movement by releasing entrapped synovial folds

---

Box 2. Factors that complicate management of back pain

1. Many patients who have back pain have no physical findings.
2. Many patients who have physical findings have no symptoms. For example, more than 50% of asymptomatic adults have structural changes noted on lumbar MRI.
3. There is an abundance of treatment options from which clinicians and patients can choose.
4. Approaches to back pain vary from country to country.
5. Income or education level.
6. Inappropriate illness behaviors (see Box 2).

Adapted from Waddell G, Newton M, Henderson I, et al. A fear-avoidance beliefs questionnaire (FABQ) and the role of fear-avoidance beliefs in chronic low back pain and disability. Pain 1993;52:157–68.

Box 3. Nonorganic physical signs (Waddell signs)

1. Tenderness
   Superficial
   Nonanatomic
2. Simulation
   Axial loading
   Rotation
3. Distraction (straight leg raising)
4. Regional
   Weakness
   Sensory
5. Over-reaction
   3 out of 5 positive

Adapted from Waddell G, McCulloch JA, Kummel E, et al. Nonorganic physical signs in low-back pain. Spine 1980;5(2):117–25.

---

or plica, relaxing hypertonic muscles, and disrupting articular or periarticular adhesions that develop as a result of trauma and inflammation, immobilization, and degenerative joint disease [13].

A *Cochrane Database of Systematic Reviews* report in 2006 assessed 33 randomized controlled trials (RCTs) and semirandomized controlled trials studying manipulation or mobilization treatment of cervical pain. The evidence did not favor manipulation or mobilization done alone or in combination with various other physical medicine agents; when compared with one another, neither was superior. There was insufficient evidence available to draw conclusions for neck disorders with radicular findings [12,14].

A Cochrane review in 2003 assessed manipulation for lumbar spine pain in 39 RCTs and found that spinal manipulation was superior only to sham therapy for patients who had acute LBP. They discovered that there is no evidence that spinal manipulation is better than other treatments of acute or chronic LBP [12,15,16]. Although this evidence suggests no scientific basis for the use of manipulation, debate continues because of claims of practitioners and patients as to the effectiveness of this type of therapy.

A recent study by Childs and colleagues assessed the predictive value of the effectiveness of lumbar manipulation based on a set of clinical criteria, which included (1) LBP fewer than 16 days (ie, acute LBP), (2) no pain or symptoms below the level of the knee, (3) low score (<19 points) on the Fear-Avoidance Beliefs Questionnaire, (4) at least one hypermobile segment in the lumbar spine, and (5) at least one hip joint with more than 35° of internal range of motion [9,17]. Patients were assigned randomly to have

Table 1
Review of the 1994 recommendations from the Agency for Health Care Policy and Research clinical guidelines regarding acute low back pain treatment in adults with associated levels of scientific evidence, levels A through D

	Recommendation for treatment or finding	Option for treatment or finding	Recommendation against treatment or finding
History and physical examination (34 studies)	• History (B) • History of cancer or infection (B) • History of trauma (C) • Cauda equina (C) • Straight leg raise (B) • Neurologic examination (B)	• Pain scale (D) • Pain drawing (D)	
Patient education (14 studies)	• Low back pain education (B) • Back schools in work setting (C)	• Back schools in non-work environment (C)	
Medications (23 studies)	• NSAIDs (B) • Acetaminophen (C)	• Muscle relaxants (C) • Opioids (C)	• Options for over 2 weeks (C) • Antidepressants (C)
Physical Treatment (42 studies)	Spinal manipulation during first month of acute LBP (B)	• Spinal manipulation for LBP over 1 month (C) • Manipulation for radicular pain (C) • Moist heat or cold (C) • Corset for back pain prevention at work (C)	• TENS (C) • Traction (B) • Biofeedback (C) • Corset for treatment of back pain (D) • Prolonged spinal manipulation (D)
X-ray of lumbar spine (18 studies)	Red flag present for fracture or symptoms of cancer or infection (C)		Routine use in acute LBP without red flags (B)

From Bigos S. Lower back pain: perils, pitfalls, and accomplishments of guidelines for treatment of back problems. Neurol Clin 1999;17(1):179–92; with permission.

either five sessions of spinal manipulation and exercise or exercise alone. Patients who met the criteria maintained their level of functional improvement after manipulation for at least 6 months [17,18]. Childs and colleagues' predictive model may improve future spinal manipulation study designs and classification systems [18].

Massage therapy

Massage is the second most common CAM therapy [19]. Cherkin and colleagues [11] performed a systematic review of RCTs published between 1995 and 2002 assessing manipulation, massage, and acupuncture for nonspecific back pain. They found three RCTs investigating therapeutic massage for back pain. All three studies noted that there was improvement in the subjects' level of function with therapeutic massage as a treatment of subacute and chronic back pain. One of the studies [20] randomly assigned 262 patients who had chronic LBP to therapeutic massage, traditional Chinese acupuncture, or self-care educational materials. These investigators noted reduced pain and improved function from massage (10-week study period; approximately eight massage visits) that continued for 1 year after the study [20]. Furthermore, Furlan and coworkers' [21] recent report in the *Cochrane Database of Systematic Reviews* suggests that acupressure or pressure point massage is more effective than classic or Swedish massage, but more research is required.

Acupuncture

The effectiveness of acupuncture remains unclear and controversial. Cherkin and colleagues [11] conclude that acupuncture is more effective than no treatment or sham treatment. In their 2003 review of 20 RCTs of acupuncture treatment of LBP, they found the study quality poor. Manheimer and colleagues' [22] 2005 meta-analysis of acupuncture and LBP concludes that acupuncture is an effective treatment of chronic LBP. The range for the number of acupuncture sessions and times per week for chronic LBP in their meta-analysis was 1 to 16 sessions and 1 to 2 times per week. They conclude that there was not enough data to recommend acupuncture for acute LBP. Acupuncture is less effective than manipulation, and there is no evidence that acupuncture is superior to other therapies. Comparisons among the various studies were hampered by lack of uniformity regarding patient selection, control selection, and selection of outcomes.

Other noninterventional treatment approaches

Exercise is one of the few effective treatments of back pain, although the scientific evidence in most studies suggests only modest improvements.

A brief description of several other noninterventional treatment options, including exercise therapy, follows.

Exercise therapy

In 2000, vanTulder and colleagues published a Cochrane review investigating the effectiveness of exercise for LBP [23]. They reviewed 39 RCTs of all types of exercise for patients experiencing acute and chronic LBP. They looked at how exercise had an impact on pain intensity, functional status, overall improvement, and return to work. vanTulder and colleagues concluded that there was no scientific evidence to support the effectiveness of exercise for acute LBP, yet exercise may be beneficial for chronic LBP [23].

Hayden and colleagues [23,24] updated the 2000 Cochrane review and published their critique of 61 RCTs (6390 subjects) evaluating exercise therapy. Many of the studies did not supply adequate clinical information. For example, 90% of the published studies described their population sufficiently, yet only 54% described their exercise intervention adequately. The majority, 43 of 61 studies, focused on exercise treatment of chronic LBP. Hayden and coworkers [23,24] conclude that exercise is slightly effective at lowering pain levels and improving overall function, especially those exercise programs that were designed individually. The exercise programs usually included strengthening or trunk/spine stabilization exercises.

Hayden and colleagues [23,24] also reviewed exercise therapy for subacute (6–12 weeks' duration) and acute LBP. They found moderate proof that a graded-activity exercise program improves work absentee outcomes for patients who have subacute LBP. Yet, there is no evidence that exercise is any more effective than any other treatment, including no treatment, of acute LBP.

If there is only moderate evidence that exercise is effective for chronic LBP, why are physical therapy and therapeutic exercise prescribed? Guidelines endorsed by the American Academy of Physical Medicine and Rehabilitation and the North American Spine Society recommend therapeutic exercise and education, and medication management, for patients who have subacute and chronic back pain. Goals of intervention for patients who have subacute back pain, between 6 weeks and 3 months, are to prevent progressive deconditioning and the materialization of psychosocial barriers, such as work absenteeism and impaired function at home [25]. Clinical experience shows that patients respond favorably to an individualized exercise program and feel that this type of program involves themselves in their own recovery.

Thus, goals of physical rehabilitation for patients who have persistent back pain include developing a plan for pain control, developing a home exercise program, establishing independence and self-care, and returning to regular or normal activities of daily living. Issues that conspire to delay or prevent success with a rehabilitation program include fear of reinjury and over-reliance on passive treatments, such as bed rest, local application of heat or cold, ultrasound, magnets, massage, corsets, and collars.

Historically, back pain disorders commonly were treated with aggressive and specific progressive resistance exercises (PRE) in the early twentieth century [26]. DeLorme and Watkins [26] introduced their theory of PRE in the 1940s. They were the first to quantify muscle strength objectively by controlling the intensity (repetition maximum), the number of sets and repetitions, and the frequency. DeLorme and Watkins [26] were careful that the spine extensor muscles were isolated during the PRE program. They prevented hip extension during the exercises. They discovered a gradual lessening of back pain as spinal strength improved [27].

Today, there are two popular exercise treatment approaches: the McKenzie Method and spinal stabilization. Unfortunately, there is no agreement as to which exercise protocol is more effective [28].

The McKenzie approach is one of the types of physical therapy for back and neck disorders used most frequently [29]. The McKenzie Method was developed by physical therapist, Robin McKenzie. He suggested a classification-based treatment approach for patients who have LBP: mechanical diagnoses and therapy, or the McKenzie Method. This classification is based on pain patterns noted during the evaluation. Centralization, moving pain from a leg or arm to the central back, is the most important and most studied pain pattern. McKenzie-trained therapists assess patients using a well-defined algorithm, which then leads to the spinal classification system. McKenzie identified three mechanical syndromes: postural, dysfunction (shortened segments related to scar or fibrosis), and derangement (disruption of a motion segment) [30]. McKenzie exercises not only are extension exercises but also dictate the direction of the exercise by "directional preference," or when the back/neck pain moves centrally and lessens when certain movements are performed [28]. The McKenzie Method uses self-generated movement and positioning strategies for the control of acute and chronic spine pain [31].

A typical McKenzie-based exercise program in one study consisted of performing six specific exercises, 5 times per day, with 5 to 10 repetitions of each exercise for an average of 15 days. The authors of that study found improved spine flexibility and less pain with their McKenzie therapeutic exercise protocol [32].

Another large trial of patients who had subacute and chronic back pain, 260 subjects, found that the McKenzie exercise approach, compared with dynamic strengthening exercises, was slightly more successful at improving patients' level of function at 2-months' follow-up, but the difference was not maintained at the longer follow-up evaluation [29].

Lumbar spinal stabilization exercises, including Pilates, also are popular [29]. The goal of dynamic spinal stabilization exercises is to re-educate and strengthen the deep postural spinal muscles, such as the multifidi and transverse abdominis, thereby decreasing pain and centralizing symptoms.

Theoretically, back injuries and back pain may be caused by the gradual degeneration of joints and other supporting spinal structures from repetitive microtrauma. Thus, if one strengthens and stabilizes, dynamically and statistically via stabilization exercises, the spinal muscles, one would note less back pain and improved spine function and strength [33].

Review of the literature found one small RCT of patients who had chronic back pain that demonstrated that stabilization exercises improved back pain and level of function [34].

Despite the popular prescription of exercise, there is limited research proving the efficacy of specific stabilization exercise and strengthening exercise. Theoretically, they make sense, and they are prescribed widely, but more outcome studies are needed.

Back schools

There are several systematic reviews regarding back schools. Linton and vanTulder [4] note that back and neck schools assume that patients are at higher risk for injury and complain more of pain because they do not know about proper posture and body mechanics. Thus, back schools are geared at lowering the risk for back injuries by increasing patients' or employees' fund of knowledge, such as how to lift properly [4]. Back and neck schools are attractive interventions, because they combine education with instruction, exercise, lifting techniques, and so forth, and they are inexpensive. Linton and vanTulder [4] identified nine RCTs and five non-RCTs regarding prevention and back school programs. There is strong evidence that back schools are not effective in preventing neck and back pain. Yet, in an occupational setting, there is moderate evidence that back schools reduce pain and improve return to work status and function [35].

Medications

Nonsteroidal anti-inflammatory drugs

Nonsteroidal anti-inflammatory drugs (NSAIDs) are an important pharmacologic class in the treatment of LBP. Relief of back pain from NSAIDs is not complete, but it is lasting and there is no drug tolerance effect demonstrated. The use of NSAIDs is limited by adverse side effects, such as gastrointestinal and cardiovascular complications. vanTulder and colleagues' 1997 systematic review of medications in the treatment of back pain found 19 RCTs, 10 of which were of high quality, related to the use of NSAIDs for LBP. vanTulder and colleagues [5] discovered the following strong (level 1) scientific evidence.

1. NSAIDs are more effective that placebo in patients who have acute LBP.
2. NSAIDs are not better or more effective than acetaminophen.
3. A variety of NSAIDs are equally as effective for the treatment of acute LBP.

vanTulder and colleagues' [5] Cochrane review also reviewed the literature regarding chronic LBP and NSAID use. They opined that there is moderate evidence (level 2), that NSAIDs are effective treatment of chronic LBP. Again, they concluded that different NSAIDs are equally effective for the treatment of chronic LBP.

Muscle relaxants

Approximately one third of patients complaining of LBP are prescribed muscle relaxants by a primary care provider. Prescription of muscle relaxants for nonspecific back pain is controversial, mainly because of their side effects. In addition to sedation, headaches, nausea, and vomiting, a potential for abuse and dependence is reported. There is strong scientific evidence that nonbenzodiazepine muscle relaxants are effective for acute LBP, but there is no proof that they are effective for chronic LBP [5,36]. vanTulder and colleagues [5,36,37] reviewed 30 trials going back to the 1960s: 8 trials used benzodiazepines, 23 antispasmodics, 3 benzodiazepines and antispasmodics, and 2 antispasticity medications. Twenty-three of the 30 RCTs were considered high-quality trials. Twenty-four studies were for acute LBP. The investigators concluded that there is strong support that nonbenzodiazepine muscle relaxants are effective for acute LBP. They found strong evidence that any muscle relaxant—benzodiazepine, nonbenzodiazepine, or antispasticity—was more effective than placebo for acute LBP. There is limited evidence for the effectiveness of muscle relaxants for chronic LBP. vanTulder and colleagues [37] recommended RCTs to study the effectiveness of muscle relaxants versus analgesic or NSAIDs.

Antidepressants

A new commissioned Cochrane review group will reinvestigate antidepressants treatment of LBP and compare them with placebo, analgesics, tricyclic antidepressants versus SSRIs, other medications, and physical therapy [38]. Currently, there are no systematic review conclusions on the effectiveness of antidepressants for LBP.

Lumbar supports

Linton and vanTulder [4] published a 2001 study reviewing back pain prevention, including lumbar supports. They found no scientific evidence that lumbar supports prevent back pain; however, the lumbar supports seemed to reduce the number of lost workdays when compared with no treatment. Moreover, they concluded that there is strong consistent evidence (level A) that lumbar supports are not effective in preventing back pain or back injury [4].

Transcutaneous electrical nerve stimulation

Transcutaneous electrical nerve stimulation (TENS) is a therapy that uses low-voltage electrical current for pain relief. TENS was developed in the

1970s as a technique to screen patients who have chronic pain to see who might respond to implanted stimulators [39]. TENS unit efficacy in the management of acute and chronic pain has been investigated and reviewed in more than 600 publications.

There are at least two good reviews of the literature published in the past 10 years, by Fishbain and colleagues and vanTulder and colleagues. Fishbain and colleagues [39] reviewed the literature on TENS unit efficacy in chronic pain. They found that nearly all of the TENS studies showed initial efficacy in 58% to 72% of patients who had intractable, chronic pain. The benefit of TENS seemed to decrease with time. They found 20 studies that reported the benefits of TENS in more than 7600 patients who had chronic pain. Only one of those 20 studies used a control group (sham TENS unit). Fishbain and colleagues [39] found six other studies that looked at other outcome measurements aside from decreased level of pain. Five of those studies demonstrated that long-term TENS unit use decreased the amount of medication patients took. One study showed improved socialization and another study showed improved sleep. Based on their literature review, Fishbain and colleagues and the Clinical Research Department at Empi, a TENS unit manufacturer, conducted a telephone outcome survey. They studied 506 randomly chosen TENS unit purchasers, most of whom had used the unit for more than 6 months. Empi contracted with an independent research firm to create a scientific survey and to conduct the study. The participants were questioned about how their functional status changed since using the TENS unit. The study participants reported statistically significant improvement in interference with work, home, and social activities and in activity level and pain management; decreased use of other therapies (ie, physical, occupational, and chiropractic); and decreased use of narcotics, muscle relaxants, NSAIDs, and steroids. Fishbain and colleagues' study showed that there is a group of patients who have chronic pain that benefits from long-term use (≥ 6 months) of TENS.

The meta-analysis of vanTulder and colleagues [5] did not support TENS unit efficacy. vanTulder and colleagues' 1997 review of RCTs found two studies, varying in quality, which looked at the effectiveness of TENS in acute LBP. They concluded that TENS is not effective for acute LBP. vanTulder and colleagues also studied the effectiveness of TENS in chronic LBP. They found three RCTs and stated that there is no evidence that TENS is effective for chronic LBP because of contradictory test results [5].

The cervical overview group for the Cochrane Library recently stated, "We cannot make any definitive statements on the effects of electrotherapy for people with acute or chronic mechanical neck disorders (MND). Based on the review of 11 trials and 525 people with MND, the current evidence on Galvanic current (direct or pulsed), iontophoresis, TENS, EMS, PTMF and permanent magnets is either lacking, limited, or conflicting" [40].

Interventional treatments

Spinal injections may be a useful tool in the evaluation and management of patients who have spinal disorders and increasingly are within the realm of physiatrists. Injections may be tried in several different structures, possible pain-generating structures, to decrease pain and improve overall level of function and patients' rehabilitation program. Injections should not be used alone, rather as an adjunct to rehabilitation exercise program. The benefits of epidural, facet, and sacroiliac joint injections in controlled prospective studies are variable and controversial.

Education

Time is a great healer. The majority of patients who have mechanical back pain improve(ie, they experience less pain and impairment within a few weeks). LBP does not equal pathology. Not every patient needs treatment, yet most patients benefit from education. Physiatrists' approach to the management of LBP is educating patients about the pain, the cause of their symptoms (if it can be determined), and the importance of staying as active as possible. Patients are afraid to hurt themselves because they have back pain and often stop exercising because they are not sure what to do and if their exercise contributes directly or indirectly to the pain itself. The physiatric approach involves stressing the importance of "motion as lotion." Physiatrists spend time counseling patients and families about appropriate exercise for back pain. Deconditioning increases their level of pain. Remaining active leads to more rapid recovery and less chronic back pain [41].

A primary focus should be to educate patients that approximately 90% of patients who have back pain improve within 4 to 6 weeks without treatment or intervention. They also should be informed that approximately two thirds experience another episode of back pain within the next year—this is the natural history. Improvement also is expected from each episode or flare-up of back pain. Bed rest is not recommended [2,5,41].

There is a variety of approaches to diagnosis and treatment of back pain. Physiatarists' medical vocabulary differs from chiropractors', therapists', and physicians', and this may confuse patients further.

This author provides written and verbal educational material to patients and also considers providing patient education brochures that emphasize decreasing fear and promoting self-management. The Internet also is a source of information for patients (eg, hospital Web sites, WebMD, and so forth).

Summary

There still is no gold standard for treatment or classification of back pain. Current evidence supports a few common interventions for the treatment of LBP: NSAIDs, muscle relaxants, active therapy, and exercise. Our job is to provide safe, reliable help to patients who have LBP. NSAIDs and muscle relaxants are efficacious for acute pain, and NSAIDs provide analgesia as the back pain becomes chronic. Therapeutic exercise is effective treatment of chronic LBP and for prevention of LBP [42]. Back schools and lumbar support do not prevent back injuries or pain. The evidence regarding TENS is equivocal, yet there is a group of patients who have chronic pain who do benefit from TENS. Therapeutic massage is more effective than acupuncture for subacute and chronic back pain. Spinal manipulation is effective for acute LBP, but it is no more effective than analgesics, physical therapy, exercise, or back school. Acupuncture seems effective for chronic pain but is less effective than manipulation.

Most systematic reviews suggest more research is needed. Researchers are developing clinical prediction rules for spinal manipulation and stabilization exercise programs. Hopefully, these clinical prediction rules will lead to the improvement in the designed quality outcome studies investigating all forms of treatment options. Deyo and Childs report "bewilderment" as to why large trials are scarce in musculoskeletal medicine. Delayed recovery from LBP is associated with enormous disability and health care costs. Patient education, activity, and exercise are pivotal to decreasing pain and disability associated with back pain, and additional research is needed to decrease the controversy associated with the many treatment options.

To know is one thing, and to think one knows is another. To know is science. To think one knows is ignorance.

Hippocrates

References

[1] Bigos S. Lower back pain: perils, pitfalls, and accomplishments of guidelines for treatment of back problems. Neurol Clin 1999;17(1):179–92.

[2] Bigos S, Bowyer O, Braen G, et al. Acute low back problems in adults. Clinical practice guideline no. 14. Rockville, MD: Agency for Health Care Policy and Research, Public Health Service; December 1994. US Department of Health and Human Services, AHCPR Publication no. 95-0642. 1–160.

[3] Jensen MC, Brant-Zawadzki MN, Obuchowski N, et al. Magnetic resonance imaging of the lumbar spine in people without back pain. N Engl J Med 1994;331(2):69–73.

[4] Linton SJ, vanTulder MW. Preventative interventions for back and neck pain problems: what is the evidence? Spine 2001;26(7):778–87.

[5] vanTulder MW, Koes BW, Bouter LM. Conservative treatment of acute and chronic non-specific low back pain: a systematic review of randomized controlled trials of the most common interventions. Spine 1997;22(18):2128–56.

[6] Waddell G, et al. Symptoms and signs: physical disease or illness behaviour? Br Med J 1984; 289:739–41.

[7] Yeomans S, et al. Outcome assessment. In: Craig Liebenson, editor. Rehabilitation of the spine: a practitioner's manual. 2nd edition. Baltimore (MD): Lippincott Williams & Wilkins; 2007. p. 146–68.

[8] Taylor SJ, Taylor AE, Foy MA, et al. Responsiveness of common outcome measures for patients with low back pain. Spine 24(17):1805–12.

[9] Waddell G, Sommerville D, Henderson I, et al. A fear-avoidance beliefs questionnaire (FABQ) and the role of fear-avoidance beliefs in chronic low back pain and disability. Pain 1993;52:157–68.

[10] Waddell G, et al. Nonorganic physical signs in low-back pain. Spine 5(2):117–25.

[11] Cherkin DC, Sherman KJ, Deyo RA, et al. A review of the evidence for the effectiveness, safety, and cost of acupuncture, massage therapy, and spinal manipulation for back pain. Ann Intern Med 2003;138(11):898–906.

[12] Ernst E, Canter PH. A systematic review of systematic reviews of spinal manipulation. J R Soc Med 2006;99(4):192–6.

[13] DeFranca G. Manipulation techniques for key joints. In: Craig Liebenson, editor. Rehabilitation of the spine: a practioner's manual. 2nd edition. Baltimore (MD): Lippincott Williams & Wilkins; 2007. p. 487–512.

[14] Gross AR, Hoving JL, Haines TA, et al. Cervical overview group. Manipulation and mobilization for mechanical neck disorders. Cochrane Database Syst Rev 2006;3.

[15] Assendelft WJJ, Morton SC, Yu EI, et al. Spinal manipulative therapy for low back pain: a meta-analysis of effectiveness relative to other therapies. Ann Intern Med 2003;138(11): 871–81.

[16] Assendleft WJJ, Morton SC, Yu EI, et al. Spinal manipulative therapy for low-back pain. Cochrane Database Syst Rev 2006;3 (ISSN 1464-780X).

[17] Childs JD, Fritz JM, Flynn TW, et al. A clinical prediction rule to identify patients with low back pain most likely to benefit from spinal manipulation: a validation study. Ann Intern Med 2004;141(12):920–8.

[18] Deyo RA. Treatments for back pain: can we get past trivial effects? Ann Intern Med 2004; 141(12):957–8.

[19] "2005 Industry Fact Sheet" from American Massage Therapy Association, fact sheet released January 2006. Available at: www.amtamassage.org. Accessed September 1, 2006.

[20] Cherkin DC, Eisenberg D, Sherman KJ, et al. Randomized trial comparing traditional Chinese medical acupuncture, therapeutic massage, and self-care education for chronic low back pain. Arch Intern Med 2001;161:1081–8.

[21] Furlan AD, Brosseau L, Imamura M, et al. Massage for low-back pain. Cochrane Database Syst Rev 2006;3.

[22] Manheimer E, White A, Berman B, et al. Meta-analysis: acupuncture for low back pain. Ann Intern Med 2005;142(8):651–63.

[23] Hayden JA, van Tulder MW, Malmivaara AV, et al. Meta-analysis: exercise therapy for nonspecific low back pain. Ann Intern Med 2005;142(9):765–75.

[24] Hayden JA, van Tulder MW, Malmivaara AV, et al. Meta-analysis: exercise therapy for nonspecific low back pain. Cochrane Database Syst Rev 2006;3.

[25] North American Spine Society (NASS). Phase III: clinical guidelines for multidisciplinary spine care specialists. Spinal stenosis version 1.0, vol. 202. LaGrange (IL): NASS. p. 91. Available at: www.guideline.gov. Accessed February 5, 2007.

[26] DeLorme T, Watkins A. Technics of progressive resistance exercise. Arch Phys Med 1948;29: 263–73.

[27] Carpenter DM, Nelson BW. Low back strengthening for the prevention and treatment of low back pain. Med Sci Sports Exerc 1999;31(1):18–24.

[28] Machado LAC, deSouza M, Ferreira PH, et al. The McKenzie method for low back pain. A systematic review of the literature with a meta-analysis approach. Spine 2006;31(9):E254–62.

[29] Moffet J, McLean S. The role of physiotherapy in the management of non-specific back pain and neck pain. Rheumatology 2006;45:371–8.

[30] Available at: http://www.mckenziemdt.org/. Accessed October 20, 2006.

[31] Jacob R, McKenzie R, Heffner S. McKenzie spinal rehabilitation methods. In: Craig Liebenson, editor. Rehabilitation of the spine: a practioner's manual. 2nd edition. Baltimore (MD): Lippincott Williams & Wilkins; 2007. p. 330–51.

[32] Skikic E, Suad T. The effects of McKenzie exercises for patients with low back pain, our experience. Bosn J Basic Med Sci 2003;3(4):70–5.

[33] Barr KP, Griggs M, Cadby T. Lumbar stabilization: core concepts and current literature, part 1. Am J Phys Med Rehabil 2005;84:473–80.

[34] Hides J, Jull G, Richardson C. Long-term effects of specific stabilizing exercises for first-episode low back pain. Spine 2001;26:243–8.

[35] Heymans MW, van Tulder MV, Esmail R, et al. Back schools for non-specific low-back pain. Cochrane Database Syst Rev 2006;3.

[36] vanTulder MV, Touray T, Furlan AD, et al. Muscle relaxants for non-specific low back pain. Cochrane Database Syst Rev 2003;2.

[37] vanTulder MW, Touray T, Furlan AD, et al. Muscle relaxants for non-specific low-back pain. Cochrane Database Syst Rev 2006;3.

[38] vanTulder MW, Hienkens EEM, Roland M, et al. Antidepressants for non-specific low-back pain. Cochrane Database Syst Rev 2006;3.

[39] Fishbain DA, Chabal C, Abbott A, et al. Transcutaneous electrical nerve stimulation (TENS) treatment outcome in long-term users. Clin J Pain 1996;12(3):201–14.

[40] Kroeling P, Gross A, Goldsmith CH. Cervical overview group. Electrotherapy for neck disorders. Cochrane Database Syst Rev 2006;3.

[41] Deyo RA, Rainville J, Kent DL. What can the history and physical examination tell us about low back pain? JAMA 1992;268(6):760–5.

[42] Linton SL, Bradley LA, Jensen I, et al. The secondary prevention of low back pain: a controlled study with follow-up. Pain 1989;36:197–207.

ELSEVIER
SAUNDERS

Neurol Clin 25 (2007) 539–566

NEUROLOGIC
CLINICS

Chronic Pain Management in Spine Disorders

Edward Covington, MD

*Section of Pain Medicine, Neurological Institute, Desk C-21, Cleveland Clinic,
9500 Euclid Avenue, Cleveland, OH 44195, USA*

In chronic spine-related pain, as in most other chronic noncancer pain conditions, a basic premise is that nonstructural factors are responsible for the predominance of pain and dysfunction and that structural corrections therefore are unlikely to be the most effective intervention. This premise also implies that at some point interminable searching for peripheral pathology that can explain the patient's status becomes futile and possibly even harmful. These ideas fly in the face of a health care system that is predicated on eliminating symptoms by identifying and correcting underlying tissue pathology, yet they are well supported by experimental findings and the results of treatment.

The source of pain

Causes of chronic spine-related pain are commonly believed to include such factors as strains and sprains, anulus tears, internal disc disruption, facet arthropathy, and bone pathology. Yet this condition, which causes more disability than any other pain problem in industrialized societies, is usually unexplained by examination or imaging. To further complicate matters, abnormal imaging is frequently found in asymptomatic subjects [1–3].

Some of the mystery is likely attributable to the inappropriate reliance on old concepts of nociceptive pain. In essence, they imply a more or less linear relationship between pain perception and peripheral stimulation: a nociceptor is activated, the signal is transmitted to the dorsal horn (DH), and from there by way of the thalamus to the cortex, where pain is appreciated. Pain is seen as an analog representation of some event (eg, a child stepping on one's

E-mail address: covinge@ccf.org

0733-8619/07/$ - see front matter © 2007 Elsevier Inc. All rights reserved.
doi:10.1016/j.ncl.2007.01.009

toe produces minimal pain, whereas an adult or an automobile would produce correspondingly greater pains). As a result, when a patient complains
of severe pain and no appropriate pathology is located the validity of the
complaints or the diagnosis is challenged.

Current evidence shows that pain is a creation of the nervous system and
not just a gauge of nociceptor activation. Nociceptive afferent signals are
subject to marked attenuation and amplification by descending facilitatory
and inhibitory tracts that have their action at the DH [4]. Further, the presence of prolonged nociceptive stimulation, inflammation, or nerve injury
can lead to sensitization of the neurons that relay pain, death of inhibitory
cells [5,6], loss of tonic inhibition, and structural neuroplastic changes. Activation of immune cells, including glia [7] that were previously thought of as
having only structural roles, produces exaggerated, widespread, and mirror-
image pains [8–10].

Cells in the rostroventral medulla that function to amplify incoming pain
signals at the level of the DH have been shown to fire in response to pain
vigilance, among other things. Animal models suggest that the simple facts
of anticipating a pain and expecting it to be important are sufficient to ac-
tivate these "on cells," in essence activating the amplifiers before the pain
stimulus has begun [11].

Increasing evidence points to genetic differences in pain appreciation and
responses to endogenous and exogenous opioids [12–14]. Furthermore,
there is compelling evidence that individuals reporting high/low pain in response to a standard stimulus demonstrate correspondingly high or low activation of somatosensory cortex, anterior cingulate gyrus (a likely index of
affective components of pain), and frontal cortex [15]. The conclusion is that
those who report unusual pain actually experience unusual pain in the absence of incentives for misrepresentation.

It has been found that patients who have idiopathic chronic low back
pain (CLBP) who are subjected to quantified thumb pressure report more
pain and show more functional MRI (fMRI) activation in brain areas likely
to reflect pain perception than controls, suggesting that at least some
portion of CLBP is related to central sensitization [16]. Evidence also implicates central sensitization as a significant factor in whiplash-associated pain
[17]. Spine pain can thus result from local tissue pathology or central
sensitization.

For many reasons it is therefore unrealistic to expect that reports of
chronic spine-related pain necessarily correlate with the presence or severity
of spine pathology.

Psychosocial issues

Factors unrelated to spine pathology play a major role in the onset of
spine pain, in the transition of acute into chronic spine-related disability,
and in recovery from organic spine conditions.

Environmental factors

In a 4-year prospective study of 3020 aircraft workers, job dissatisfaction and poor performance appraisals predicted reports of acute back pain at work [18]. Although the strongest predictor was a history of back problems, other factors were mostly psychosocial. Subjects who "hardly ever" enjoyed their job tasks were 2.5 times more likely to report a back injury than subjects who "almost always" enjoyed them.

Papageorgiou and colleagues [19] followed 1412 pain-free employees for 12 months. Primary care records were monitored to determine which patients sought care for low back pain (LBP), and questionnaires assessed which subjects had LBP without seeking care. The odds of reporting LBP were doubled in those dissatisfied with their work. Perceived inadequacy of income (odds ratio 3.6) and partly skilled/unskilled laborers (odds ratio 4.8) were strongly associated with consulting for a new episode of LBP.

Numerous subsequent investigations have confirmed this first report that a back injury at work is independently predicted by prior LBP, physical work stress, and psychologic intolerance of the job, whether because of factors in the workplace, the individual, or their interaction.

Investigators have sought predictors of chronicity in LBP in hopes that preventive efforts could be targeted. Typically, biomedical clinicians seek predictors in tissue pathology, behaviorists seek reinforcers that perpetuate pain behavior, and cognitive theorists posit that erroneous belief systems perpetuate disability and depression. Conclusions are impeded by the large number of cross-sectional studies in which changes induced by chronicity may be misinterpreted as causal.

In a review of prospective studies, Valat and colleagues [20] found that progression to chronic pain was more dependent on demographic, psychosocial, and occupational factors than on medical pathology. Chronicity was associated with multiple functional symptoms, evidence of nonorganic disease, pain in the legs, significant self-rated disability at onset, a protracted initial episode, multiple recurrences, and a history of low back pain or hospitalization. Occupational factors with major impact included blue-collar jobs, heavy labor, requirements beyond subjects' capabilities, job dissatisfaction, and poor working conditions. Those who were new at the job or not well rated by their superiors were more likely to develop chronic pain. Prior compensation for a spinal condition, receipt of work-related sickness payments, and litigation about compensation were associated with chronicity. Social and economic predictors included lack of schooling, language problems, low income, and unfavorable family status. Numerous studies found that elevation of Minnesota multiphasic personality inventory (MMPI) scale 3 early in the illness predicted chronicity, as did coping strategies. These and other studies show that chronicity is predicted by somatization, depression, catastrophizing, stress, and compensation. Job satisfaction and orthopedic impairment seem to independently predict outcome.

Dionne and colleagues [21] followed 569 HMO enrollees with acute (4-6 weeks) LBP for 2 years. Strongest predictors of chronic disability were somatization, depression, and the extent of disability at 1 month. Continuing disability was strongly predicted by catastrophizing, family stress, number/intensity of pain complaints, financial compensation, and frequency of medical contact in the preceding year. Medical factors (eg, sciatica, spondylolisthesis, osteoarthritis, degenerative disc disease) were largely nonpredictive, with the exception of prior back-related disability.

Even in patients who had such objective pathology as acute radicular pain and disc prolapse or protrusion, the only somatic factor found to predict outcome was the extent of disc displacement—the less the displacement, the worse the outcome [22]. Persistent pain was predicted by depression and four pain coping strategies. Application for retirement at 6 months was best predicted by depression and daily hassles at work.

The system. Ironically, much disability may be attributed to the systems designed to help. Workers' compensation systems may be especially toxic, with long delays in diagnosis and treatment, during which time workers must continually prove how sick they are to obtain care they believe they need. Physicians and attorneys for each side may take polarized and improbable positions [23]. The result is that patients receiving and applying for workers' compensation benefits seem to fare worse with virtually all interventions than those not so encumbered.

In 274 patients seen 1 to 5 years following posttraumatic LBP, Greenough and Fraser [24] found receipt of compensation to be associated with greater pain, disability, and nonphysiologic signs on examination and pain drawings. In a later study, Greenough and colleagues [25] found that compensation and nonphysiologic signs adversely affected outcome of anterior lumbar fusion at 2-year follow-up. When these patients were studied 10 to 12 years following surgery, the effects of compensation on outcome had dissipated, whereas those of nonphysiologic signs persisted [26]. Significantly, 41% of compensable patients were receiving social security benefits at this review, versus 17% of the noncompensable ones.

Rainville and colleagues [27] studied 85 CLBP patients who completed a spine rehabilitation program. At baseline, those receiving compensation reported more pain, depression, and disability than those without and at follow-up they had less improvement in depression and disability. After 12 months, pain scores improved only for those not receiving compensation.

Litigation may adversely affect recovery from trauma, perhaps especially when the pathology is ambiguous. This theory is indirectly supported by the rarity of whiplash in situations in which litigation is uncommon, compared with the United States where whiplash neck-sprain claims make up two thirds of all bodily injury claims [28]. It may be significant that the rate of compensated whiplash in Saskatchewan, which has a tort system, is 10 times that of Quebec, which has a no-fault system [29].

In a study of more than 2000 LBP patients who had one or no previous operations, Long [23] found that all those working at intake returned to work with the exception of those in litigation, of whom not one returned to work. Vocational failure occurred despite success on other outcome variables as good as in those not litigating.

Blake and Garrett [30] found that litigating patients improved as much as others in a pain rehabilitation program with the exception of the quality of life score, in which they showed no significant improvement.

Psychologic issues

Chronic pain syndrome (CPS) is a term (not a diagnosis) that has fallen into disfavor but is still often used. It characterizes a condition of severe intractable pain with marked functional impairment and other behavioral changes, yet no clear relationship to organic disorder. Typically these patients have inordinate use of medications and health care services, which are largely nonproductive. CPS is thus a nonspecific term for patients most typified by abnormal illness behaviors, primarily those of somatic preoccupation and regression into the sick role. The term is useful in that it properly directs therapy toward the reversal of regression and away from an exclusive focus on nociception. It does not, however, substitute for a careful diagnosis of the physiologic, psychologic, and environmental factors that produce the syndrome.

Long [23] studied more than 4000 patients who had LBP and sciatica and more than 2000 who had CPS and concluded that the primary determinant of vocational disability was the psychiatric status of the patient before the onset of the symptoms.

Carragee and colleagues [31] followed 100 patients who had mild CLBP and no prior spine-related disability for 5 years. Moderate or severe Modic change of the vertebral end plate was the only structural variable that weakly predicted adverse outcome. Provocative discography and baseline MR predicted no outcome variables, but were weakly associated with pain episodes. Psychosocial variables strongly predicted long- and short-term disability and health care visits for LBP. A model with normal DRAM (normal scores on Modified Zung Depression Test and Modified Somatic Pain Questionnaire), a score below the 25th percentile on the Fear Avoidance Beliefs Questionnaire (physical activity subscale), and non-smoker status identified 100% of long-term disability subjects, 88% of all disability subjects, and 75% of subjects having a remission.

It is reasonable to posit a stress-diathesis model in which the degree of disability from a given degree of organic pathology varies with the psychologic strengths of the individual, the stresses of the workplace, and incentives and disincentives for recovery. Clearly these variables overlap; the person with poor coping skills and limited education is unlikely to obtain the most desirable work situation.

Cognitive factors in chronic pain

Because we react less to events than to our understanding of them, cognition plays a major role in pain. Its aversive quality is modified by its interpretation. The cancer patient who is convinced "the surgeon got it all" is more content than the healthy person who fears occult pathology. The patient who fears that his back pain presages neurologic impairment likely experiences more pain and dysfunction than a patient with a more benign understanding. Pain tolerance is reduced by negative thoughts, such as those emphasizing the aversiveness of the situation, the person's inability to tolerate it, or the physical harm that could occur.

Cognitive influences include not only beliefs about pain but also beliefs about the self. A person's sense of power and competence strongly modifies coping. The "learned helplessness" model of depression suggests that those who feel unable to control events in their life eventually stop trying. In patients who have chronic pain, those who perceive themselves as helpless are likely to be depressed and passive, which increases disability and pain. Conversely, beliefs in self-efficacy are associated with higher function in painful conditions [32,33], and increases in such beliefs predict recovery [34].

Locus of control refers to the perception that events are determined by one's own behavior (internal control) or by such outside forces as other people or fate (external control). Those whose locus of control is internal recognize their role in determining their future. They feel and function better than those who have external locus of control. Chronic pain patients with a "chance external" locus of control reported more depression and anxiety, felt helpless to deal with their pain, and relied on maladaptive coping strategies [35]. The sense of having no control may explain much of the relationship between pain and depression.

Acceptance has recently been recognized as playing a major role in rehabilitation from chronic pain. Although chronic pain patients often persevere in trying to control a fundamentally uncontrollable experience [36], acceptance is a disengagement from the struggle and an engagement in positive everyday activities. In 230 pain center–type patients, acceptance correlated with less pain, depression, anxiety, and downtime and with less physical, social, and work disability [37].

Pain as behavior

Major advances in pain management resulted from the behavioral conceptualization of pain [38], which attributed many behaviors associated with chronic pain to environmental reinforcers. Pain behaviors—complaining, moaning, holding body parts, and other activities that communicate pain to others—usually begin as involuntary reflexes or respondents, but increase in response to reinforcement and become less contingent on sensations than on rewards. Through this process of operant conditioning behaviors may increase over time unrelated to nociception.

Reinforcers, commonly referred to as secondary gains, include such perquisites of the sick role as caretaking, drugs, and financial compensation. Perhaps more importantly, they include escape from noxious influences, such as a hazardous job, odious work environments, or critical or demanding supervisors. Conditioning of this sort usually occurs without the knowledge of the subject and does not constitute faking. The impact of reinforcement on the sick role is demonstrated by behaviorally oriented pain units, where severely disabled patients rapidly regain function in response to changed reinforcement contingencies.

Motivation to preserve or recover function may depend on the balance between the gains of the sick role and those of wellness. Those who derive substantial gratification and remuneration at work are less easily disabled than those with little to lose. Conversely, in a declining economy with insecure employment, the dependability of even modest disability income (and health insurance) may be preferable to the uncertainty of competitive employment, especially for those who are marginally qualified and who have back pain. It is likely that disability is less a function of health than of incentives and disincentives for vocational recovery.

Although it has long been known that reinforcement of pain behavior led to an increase in that behavior, recent studies suggest that such reinforcement increases actual pain perception. In patients who have LBP who are known to have a solicitous spouse, the presence of the spouse led to an increased report of pain from noxious electrical stimulation of the back and more than doubled cingulate activation [39]. Hölzl and colleagues [40] found that negative reinforcement altered pain sensitization processes in healthy subjects.

Fear and deconditioning

The profound impairment that results from prolonged inactivity is often attributable to fear of injury. As patients lose strength and range of motion they increase their susceptibility to strains and sprains. Kori and colleagues [41] suggested that pain behavior often has more to do with phobic processes than neurologic ones. Fear of injury is compounded by a person's beliefs that he or she is ill and in some fashion fragile. Unwarranted fear of personal injury is one of the more easily treatable causes of regression and dysfunction.

Psychiatric illness in chronic pain

The most frequent nonsomatoform psychiatric illnesses in pain center patients are anxiety disorders, depression, and substance abuse. In 200 patients who had CLBP entering a functional restoration program, Polatin and colleagues [42] found that 77% of patients met lifetime diagnostic criteria and 59% demonstrated current symptoms for at least one psychiatric diagnosis (excluding somatoform disorders). The most common were those listed.

Fifty-one percent met criteria for personality disorder. Substance abuse and anxiety disorders seemed to precede CLBP, whereas major depression could either precede or follow it. Studies vary as to the prevalence of psychiatric disorder; however, they tend to agree about those that are most common.

Depression, anxiety, and anger

Estimates of the prevalence of depression in chronic pain patients range from 10% to 83%. This extreme variance reflects variable settings, populations, and diagnostic criteria. In a Canadian general population survey of 118,533 people, CLBP was present in 9%. Major depression was present in 5.9% of those who did not have pain and in 19.8% of those who had CLBP. The rate of major depression increased in a linear fashion with pain severity [43]. It is likely that the arrow of causality can point in either direction; there is evidence that pain predicts depression and depression predicts pain, and to similar degrees [44].

In a probability sample of 5692 United States adults, 35% of those who had CLBP had comorbid mental disorders. Major depression was present in 12.6%, dysthymia in 5.6%, any anxiety disorder in 26.5%, and any substance use disorder in 4.8%. There was no increased prevalence of (nonalcohol) drug abuse [45].

Major affective disorder can present with pain, in which case treatment of the mood disorder often provides relief. More commonly, however, depression appears as a consequence of pain, although not necessarily a direct result of it. Rudy and colleagues [46] showed that the link between pain and depression could be mediated by perceived life interference (loss of gratifying activities) and loss of self-control.

There seems to be a vicious cycle in which pain behavior, loneliness, inactivity, helplessness, depression, withdrawal, loss of reinforcers and distractions, inactivity, and pain are mutually reinforcing. Improving one element in this series often benefits the others. These issues, of course, are not resolved by pharmacotherapy, but do respond to successful rehabilitation.

Anxiety can amplify pain and provide disincentives for recovery (ie, illness may permit escape from feared or stressful situations). Chronic tension can lead to muscle contractions and other physiologic responses that worsen pain. Nociceptors that are normally unaffected by norepinephrine become sensitive to it following injury, so that neuropathic pains are often exacerbated by anxiety, fear, anger, or excitement.

Although less studied, anger also plays an important role in chronic pain. It may relate to issues of blame attribution, an important modifying factor in recovery from injury. DeGood and Kiernan [47] found that patients who blamed others for their pain reported greater mood distress and behavioral disturbance, poorer response to past treatments, and lower expectations of future benefits than those who attributed their pain to their own actions or to chance.

Addictive disorders

Chemical dependence, including alcoholism, is an important contributor to pain-related dysfunction [48–50]. Drug craving provides an incentive for pain behavior, whereas withdrawal produces hyperalgesia. Addiction impairs coping and fosters regression. Although evidence suggests that the prevalence of addiction (excluding nicotine [51]) is not significantly higher in those who have chronic pain than in normal subjects, those who have addictive disorder are overrepresented in physicians' offices and hospitals, and perhaps especially in pain clinics. Kouyanou and colleagues [52], using strict diagnostic criteria in a population of 125 South London pain clinic patients, found that 12% met *Diagnostic and Statistical Manual of Mental Disorders, Third Edition* criteria for active abuse/dependence and an additional 10% met criteria for a substance use disorder in remission. Hoffman and colleagues [53] administered a structured diagnostic interview to 414 chronic pain patients at the Åre Hospital in Sweden and found that 23.4% met *Diagnostic and Statistical Manual of Mental Disorders, Revised Third Edition* criteria for active misuse or dependency, and an additional 9.4% met criteria for remission. Experience suggests that comorbid addiction renders most treatments for chronic pain ineffective unless the addiction is controlled first. It leads to obvious difficulties and hazards associated with opioid prescribing.

Somatoform disorders

Psychogenic pain (not a current diagnostic term) is a concept whose existence is disputed, yet pains of various sorts are clearly prominent features in somatization disorder. The terminology has changed multiple times and the current term for what was called psychogenic pain is "pain disorder associated with psychologic factors." The criteria require that pain cause significant distress or impairment in functioning; that psychologic factors be judged to have an important role in the onset, severity, exacerbation, or maintenance of the pain; and that the symptom or deficit not be intentionally produced or feigned [54]. The method for determining that psychologic factors are causative is unspecified.

Psychogenic pain is akin to conversion disorders, such as blindness and paralysis, and is similarly typified by nonphysiologic findings on examination and behavioral inconsistencies. Patients may demonstrate behaviors that are incompatible with the degree of impairment they describe, and a plethora of complaints and marked functional impairment may coexist with well-preserved muscle definition. It may be that the term is used for several unrelated conditions, given that some diagnosed with psychogenic pain seem euthymic and animated and sleep well, whereas others seem to suffer severely, cannot sleep, and even attempt suicide.

One clue to the presence of somatization is apparent reluctance to discuss nonsomatic issues. If asked about family, work, or politics, the response inevitably and rapidly diverges to talk about doctors, symptoms, and treatments. This behavior is not typically seen even in severe physical illness. Another clue is the sense of immediacy in the recounting of the traumatic event; a minor remote event is described as though it occurred yesterday.

There is evidence of a continuum between symptoms of posttraumatic stress disorder, dissociation, somatization, and affect dysregulation. These interrelated symptoms commonly follow major trauma and there seems to be a hierarchy of traumas, such that natural disasters lead to fewer symptoms than do adult interpersonal traumas, with childhood trauma causing the most severe symptoms [55]. Rome and Rome [56] hypothesized that a process akin to kindling follows psychic trauma, leading to symptom amplification, spontaneous symptoms, anatomic spreading, and cross-sensitization. These are processes that also characterize pain following neurologic trauma. They noted a melding of sensory and affective symptoms and a "polymodal allodynia" that rendered these people sensitized to physical and emotional stressors.

Other psychiatric conditions that may present with pain include hypochondriasis, dementia, psychosis, and factitious disorder. Experience suggests that new onset of conversion or somatization in the elderly is rare, and when present it may herald dementia. Malingering is by definition not a psychiatric illness. Although believed to be uncommon in chronic pain (based on no data), it does occur.

Treatment

One great conundrum in chronic spine pain is that a myriad of treatments help temporarily; however, the condition persists for decades, begging the question of the value of transient relief in intransigent conditions. This is a question of judgment, economics, and personal preference. We must challenge the value of, for example, a month of good relief for a condition that lasts many years. And we must ask whether the answer varies depending on whether we are the payer, the clinician, or the parent of the person suffering. In no case is the answer unconflicted.

A second conundrum in these conditions is that immediate effects may be in a direction opposite to those of long-term outcomes. Most patients who have back pain feel definite symptom relief with an opioid, a benzodiazepine, and a bed, yet the effects of these over time may well be adverse.

A third issue in assessing treatments is the question of what should be measured. The obvious answer, that pain reduction is the primary outcome variable, may be wrong. For example, a treatment that enabled a person isolated in bed with a pain level of 7 on a scale of 10 to begin playing golf with the same pain level would clearly be beneficial, perhaps more so than one that only improved the level of pain in bed. Not only pain, but also function must be assessed. In fact, given that most chronic pain is not associated with neurologic or anatomic deficits, it can be argued that essentially all of the functional impairments seen result from pain itself, and that it is only in functional change that one can assess analgesia. Certainly documentation of improved function is more persuasive than a report that a drug "took the edge off."

Because a multiplicity of influences combine to create spine pain–related disability, an intervention that addresses only one of them is likely to be low yield except in the case in which one cause is very predominant. This situation may be a reason for the often disappointing long-term outcomes of spine surgery whose goal is pain reduction. This outcome is often puzzling to clinicians in situations in which, for example, there is excellent evidence of facet arthropathy, but its denervation leads only to transient benefit. The procedure, of course, does not remediate central sensitization that may have occurred, nor does it correct the deconditioning and psychosocial components of the pain syndrome.

The outcome of many treatments for chronic spine pain may be unsatisfactory when used individually. It also follows that the most successful treatment may be a "shotgun approach." Such strategies have the ability to address multiple components of the pain syndrome; however, they suffer from difficulties in scientific validation—when multiple treatments are combined, it is difficult to demonstrate the efficacy of any one of them.

Pharmacotherapy

Opioids

Decades of controversy regarding the appropriate role of opioids in chronic noncancer pain have led to important research and insights but have left important questions unanswered, mostly because the duration of studies is typically short in comparison with the duration of the problem being addressed. The issues, as with all treatments, concern risks and benefits. Traditionally the risk for chronic opioid therapy (chiefly addiction) was believed to be high and the benefit low because of the inevitable development of analgesic tolerance. Both beliefs have been challenged.

Risks. Respiratory depression, which must always be considered in aggressive acute opioid therapy, is one of the opioid effects to which tolerance develops most rapidly. Patients are regularly seen taking thousands of milligrams of morphine equivalents daily with no respiratory impairment whatsoever and no sedation, for that matter. Organ toxicity is another non-issue with opioids. Patients using methadone for upward of 40 years for addiction management have shown no adverse renal, hepatic, or neurologic effects. There are hormone changes, most notably decreased testosterone, leading to loss of libido and often requiring replacement [57].

Cognitive changes are unclear. Cancer patients show slowed performance, but not necessarily with more errors, after an increase in opioid dosing; however, this tends to normalize after a few weeks as tolerance develops. A confounding factor is that cognitive performance is markedly impaired by unrelieved pain, so that at times morphine can seem to improve cognition in patients who have LBP [58]. Most studies detect little or no cognitive decrement from stable doses of opioids and there is no increase in vehicle accidents [59]. Yet clinical experience with patients who have failed aggressive opioid treatment and therefore require weaning is that many describe a sense of "coming out of a fog" as opioids are eliminated and that their families perceive them as having recovered their previous personalities. A reasonable conclusion would be that most patients on moderate dose opioids can perform complex tasks effectively and safely; however, there are some adverse effects that remain poorly defined.

Addiction was once believed to be an almost inevitable consequence of long-term opioid exposure. It is now often thought of as something like an allergy (ie, an idiosyncratic reaction to a substance that occurs in a minority of people on exposure). The change in understanding results from two factors. The first is a recognition that physical dependence, most manifestations of which seem to arise in the locus ceruleus, is distinct from addiction, which seems related more to changes in the nucleus accumbens reward centers. In fact, addiction occurs without physical dependence (eg, hallucinogens) and the converse is equally true (eg, phenytoin). Sudden, severe relapses in addicts or alcoholics who have been abstinent for years often occur on re-exposure to minimal amounts of their drug of choice, which further demonstrates that addictive behaviors may be unrelated to physical dependence.

The second reason for reduced concern about iatrogenic addiction from therapeutic opioid use is that data from short-term studies demonstrate that this is actually rare, probably occurring in less than 0.3% of patients exposed. Addiction is a disease that is influenced by biology, environment, and psychology. It seems clear that the risk for addiction in those using substances recreationally is far higher than in those using them therapeutically. It is not clear whether it is also influenced by chronology (ie, whether the risk from taking high-dose opioids for a month differs from the risk from doing so for 5 years).

Porter and Jick [60], as part of the Boston Collaborative Drug Surveillance Program, examined files of 39,946 hospitalized monitored medical patients. Among 11,882 who received one or more narcotic doses there were four cases of apparently new addiction, considered major in only one.

Perry and Heidrich [61] sent questionnaires to burn facilities in an investigation of analgesia for débridement. The authors noted that of 181 respondents, representing the knowledge of at least 10,000 hospitalized burn patients, no cases of iatrogenic addiction were reported, and state that, "the 22 patients reported to abuse drugs after discharge all had a prior history of drug abuse."

Both of these studies suffer from serious deficiencies in the way addiction was defined and assessed, and neither followed patients after hospitalization to determine whether evidence of addiction surfaced following discharge. In addition, they have been widely cited as evidence for the safety of chronic opioid therapy, which they do not address. They so suggest that acute opioid therapy has only a remote chance of inducing obvious addiction.

In a retrospective study of 48 patients hospitalized for addiction to Oxy-Contin, Potter and colleagues [62] found that 31% began OxyContin by use of a legitimate prescription; however, 77.1% reported prior nonopioid substance use problems (including alcohol) and 48% had prior problems with other opioids. Similarly, among a sample of 200 patients who had CLBP, substance abuse was found to have preceded pain in 94% of patients who had substance abuse [42].

Benefits. The major lingering concern regarding the usefulness of chronic opioid analgesia is that it is unclear to what extent there is sustained analgesia, or expressed negatively, to what extent do analgesic tolerance and opioid-induced hyperalgesia mitigate the pain reduction otherwise anticipated from these agents.

Brown and colleagues [63] reviewed the literature on opioid maintenance for CLBP in 1996, at which time they found no controlled studies. Case series reports on a total of 566 patients were positive overall. Most studies of opioid therapy are short term [64], however, and those that extend beyond 18 months typically show dropout rates of 50% or higher [65–68] and pain reductions of less than 30% of baseline [65], even when used intrathecally [69]. It is apparent that even when opioids are necessary, they are rarely sufficient for the treatment of chronic pain patients in general, and this is even more the case in those who have comorbid addiction. Fitness, psychologic counseling, and use of adjuvant analgesics are essential for most patients.

There have been particular fears concerning the use of chronic opioids in those who have addictive disorders; however, there are reports of success with this method (see Refs. [70,71]). Dunbar and Katz [72] studied 20 patients who had chronic nonmalignant pain and a history of substance abuse in an effort to identify predictors of successful opioid maintenance. Patients were treated for more than a year, and those who abused the treatment did so early. Nonabusers were more likely to be active in Alcoholics Anonymous, to have stable support systems, and to be free of recent polysubstance abuse.

Enthusiasm for use of chronic opioids is tempered by studies that show pain reduction following opioid elimination [73,74]. In behaviorally oriented chronic pain rehabilitation programs, patients who are severely dysfunctional and in severe pain despite substantial quantities of opioids often are more comfortable and functional after opioid weaning.

When Moulin and colleagues [75] treated myofascial, musculoskeletal, and rheumatic pain with morphine ($\leq$20 mg/d) versus placebo (benztropine), there was substantial pain reduction after dose titration. At end of the evaluation phase, however, there was only small pain reduction and no improvement in function. At least in some, chronic use of opioids does lead to loss of efficacy.

In a tertiary care multidisciplinary pain program, Harden and colleagues [76] compared a random sample of 100 patients taking daily opioids with an equal number taking no opioids. The groups were similar regarding pain type, duration, location, and surgical history, but those on opioids were more often taking anxiolytics and muscle relaxants, reported more current pain, and more frequently reported current or past clinical depression or anxiety. No significant differences were noted in pain, psychologic status, or functioning. It was concluded that daily opioids lack efficacy in chronic pain with regard to analgesia, decreased adjunctive medication use, or functional recovery.

Eriksen and colleagues [77] identified 1906 chronic nonmalignant pain patients from a survey of 12,684 random adult Danes. In this group, opioid use (versus nonopioid use) was associated with moderate to very severe pain, poor self-rated health, vocational disability, health care use, and lower quality of life on all items in the SF-36(r) health survey.

Anti-inflammatory agents

The nonsteroidal anti-inflammatory drugs (NSAIDs) are most often used for acute pains, especially musculoskeletal pains and headaches; however, they also play a role in several chronic noncancer pains, including those related to the spine (see review by Airaksinen and colleagues [78]). In addition, human disc substance has been shown to contain proinflammatory substances (eg, phospholipase A2, cytokines) that may produce perineural inflammation, explaining why some neuropathic pains respond to NSAIDs [79,80]. They also have an opioid-sparing effect in severe pain. The doses used for analgesia are commonly substantially less than those required to reduce inflammation in inflammatory disorders, and this may result from their central action, given that NSAIDs given intrathecally are 200 to 500 times as potent as those given systemically [81], and processes of central sensitization depend in part on synthesis and diffusion of prostanoids through the spinal cord [82].

The tendency to select NSAIDs over opioids because of safety concerns must be tempered by the fact that gastrointestinal complications of NSAID therapy are the most prevalent category of adverse drug reactions in the United States; they are responsible for 16,500 deaths [83] and 103,000 hospitalizations annually [84]. Serious adverse events occur predominantly in high-dose and prolonged use but can occur in briefer and lower-dose use, especially in the elderly [85].

Antiepileptic drugs

Antiepileptic drugs are widely used for treatment of neuropathic pain and migraine [86–88]. Some reduce aberrant firing by blocking fast-acting voltage-gated Na channels (eg, carbamazepine), others increase inhibition through GABAergic mechanisms (eg, valproic acid, tiagabine), others interfere with excitatory amino acids (topiramate), and still others affect the $\alpha 2\delta$ subunit of the calcium channels on DH neurons (gabapentin, pregabalin).

These agents have not been shown to be useful for CLBP, although they may have efficacy in spine-related neuropathic pains, such as radiculitis, arachnoiditis, and postlaminectomy syndrome. Much of the evidence of efficacy has been in rodents with spinal root ligations.

Low-dose (1200 mg/d) gabapentin was not found to relieve LBP in a randomized controlled trial (RCT) [89]. Pregabalin was also found to be ineffective in two independent RCTs of 661 patients who had CLBP [90]. A RCT found that topiramate ≤300 mg/d reduced pain, functional impairment, and weight in patients who had CLBP. Leg pain was not an exclusion factor, but neurologic deficits were [91]. Khoromi and colleagues [92] treated lumbar radicular pain with topiramate up to 400 mg/d (mean 200) and found statistically significant but minor (19%) pain reduction and high (31%) dropouts. An open study of lamotrigine suggested that higher doses (400 mg/d) may be effective for sciatica [93].

Antidepressants

Antidepressants have been used for more than 30 years for various pain syndromes, primarily those related to neuropathic pain, headaches, and central sensitization [94–101]. There have also been many studies of their use in back pain; however, these have often been difficult to interpret because they either failed to exclude depression (so that improvement could be attributable to mood alteration) or they failed to exclude sciatica (so that improvement could be attributable to effects on neuropathic pain).

There have been several reviews of this question. Fishbain [101] reviewed 10 trials with serotonin-norepinephrine reuptake inhibitors, of which 7 found analgesia. Five studies with norepinephrine (NE) reuptake inhibitors were reviewed, and 4 found analgesia. Two trials of SSRIs were negative. Salerno and colleagues [102] performed a meta-analysis, from which they concluded that evidence supported an analgesic effect in LBP but that improvement in activities of daily living was not substantiated. Staiger and colleagues [103] found that among NE reuptake inhibitors (tricyclics and tetracyclics) 4 of 5 studies demonstrated significant improvement in at least one outcome measure, whereas none of 3 studies of non–NE reuptake inhibitors found significant benefit.

A well-controlled study of maprotiline did exclude patients who had depression and controlled for the presence of radicular pain. It found that maprotiline ≤150 mg/d was analgesic for axial pain, whereas paroxetine ≤30 mg/d was not [104].

Topical agents

Over-the-counter agents, such as salicylates and menthol, are widely used for temporary soothing effects. There are few data on other medications used for back pain. A 6-week open-label study found topical lidocaine patches to be effective for acute and chronic LBP [105]. A single randomized trial (N = 320) found capsicum plaster to provide relief that was statistically and clinically significant in patients who had LBP [106].

Muscle relaxants

Most drugs marketed for muscle relaxation in fact have no effect on muscles, but are central sedatives or analgesics. In 14 RCTs there was good evidence of efficacy for acute LBP, with apparently equal efficacy among the various agents [107]. There is little evidence of efficacy in chronic use, although most seem to be benign.

Baclofen, a GABA-B agonist, does reduce muscle spasm, inhibits nociceptive input at the DH, activates the descending noradrenergic inhibitory system, and inhibits ascending noradrenergic and dopamine pathways. In mice, it is analgesic in the tail flick latency model and acid-induced writhing, but not in ischemic myelopathy [108]. Oral baclofen has failed to relieve most pain in humans [109]. It has been most useful for patients in whom pain results from spasticity, in which case oral and spinal administration are efficacious. Greatest effects are with intrathecal administration, which has reduced musculoskeletal pain [110] among others [111,112]. Inadvertent abrupt withdrawal of intrathecal baclofen has led to fatalities.

Tizanidine relieves pain attributable to muscle spasticity and is analgesic intrathecally in animal neuropathic pain. Several reports indicate benefit in acute LBP, with an effect on acute spasm superior to that of Valium, but there are no studies in CLBP [113,114].

Interventional pain management

Interventional pain management had its origins in regional anesthesia but developed beyond its roots to include such treatments as intradiscal electrothermal therapy, epidural lysis of adhesions, and neuroaugmentation. Its role in nonspecific LBP has recently been reviewed [78]. Strategies in chronic spine-related pain include diagnostic nerve blocks, therapeutic blocks and neuroablation, neuroaugmentation, and intraspinal drug delivery.

Diagnostic blocks may be used to identify a myofascial pain component, to confirm sympathetically mediated pain, to distinguish visceral from somatic pain, and to locate a pain generator (eg, to distinguish discogenic pain from that of facet arthropathy).

Therapeutic blocks may be temporary or permanent, the latter involving glycerol, alcohol, freezing, or radiofrequency ablation. Permanent is a relative term, because reinnervation occurs after a variable period of time. Acute radiculitis may respond to selective root injections with steroids. Steroid injections also relieve focal inflammatory conditions, such as tendonitis and bursitis. (See reviews of epidural steroid injections for LBP [115] and sciatica [116]).

Neuroaugmentation refers to techniques based on stimulation of neural tissues, for purposes of this discussion, to relieve pain, although there are other indications, such as movement disorders and psychiatric illness. Spinal cord stimulation involves placement of an electrode, energized by a (usually) implanted programmable generator, against the posterior spinal cord. Most important indications are neuropathic pains. The role of motor cortex stimulation for chronic pain remains to be defined and is under investigation.

Surgical spine pain management is addressed elsewhere and includes not only stabilization procedures but also such techniques as anterolateral cordotomy, dorsal root entry zone lesions, and rhizotomy, among others. They are generally reserved for patients who have failed less aggressive treatments. Detailed discussion is beyond the scope of this article.

Reconditioning therapies

Acute and chronic LBP are worsened by bed rest and inactivity and improved by activity, fitness, and general conditioning. Much of the syndrome of CLBP is attributable to processes of deconditioning and deactivation with attendant losses in range of motion, impairments in posture, abdominal weakness, and so forth. Not only does deactivation ultimately increase pain but it also precludes pursuing many healthy interests, leaving patients with few distracters from the pain. Although it may seem obvious that no acceptable treatment of disabling CLBP should ignore physical rehabilitation, a remarkable number of patients have undergone various sorts of passive therapies, from oral medications to implantable technology, with minimal attention to this.

Brox and colleagues [117] randomly assigned patients who were greater than 1 year post herniation to either fusion with pedicle screw fixation or to back education plus three exercise sessions per day for 3 weeks. The two treatments were equally effective in improving function.

There is controversy concerning the best sort of exercise program for spine pain of varying mechanisms, which is addressed elsewhere. Numerous studies confirm the benefit of exercises that address aerobic conditioning, strength, and flexibility for patients who have LBP [118]. What may be overlooked is that reconditioning also has psychologic benefits in reducing anxiety and depression while improving learned helplessness and sense of personal fragility [119–122]. Patients understandably misinterpret chronic pain as an indicator of bodily danger, to which they respond with self-protection strategies, chiefly inactivity. Graduated exposure to exercises helps overcome the fear and thereby restores function [123].

Psychologic interventions

Education

Mystery and uncertainty about the cause of pain worsens its severity. The suffering of back patients is intensified when doctors are unable to identify its cause. In LaCroix's [124] study, illness understanding predicted return to work. Waddell and colleagues [125] found that more of the variance of disability attributable to back pain was accounted for by fear avoidance beliefs than by pain itself. These beliefs seem related not to disease severity but to uncertainty of diagnosis [126]. This fact of clinical worsening by diagnostic ambiguity is a special challenge in those who have CLBP, because a precise anatomic source of the pain is not identifiable in probably 80%. The role of unrealistic fears of self-injury in increasing dysfunction has been described.

An essential role for every clinician treating patients who have back pain is to educate them about their pathology if known, about the current inability of medicine to explain most LBP, about the benign nature of LBP, and about the difference between hurt and harm, so that they are not inappropriately deterred from reconditioning programs that may at first increase pain.

Education must also involve families, who often promote regression in the mistaken belief that it is necessary to protect the patient from harmful, excessive activity. They may also accept the patient's sense of helplessness as valid and therefore provide unnecessary caretaking. Families should be helped to understand that rest can be toxic and that activity is beneficial.

Operant conditioning

The first multidisciplinary pain rehabilitation programs were based on Fordyce's operant conditioning model, in which social reinforcers of pain behavior were systematically withdrawn and wellness behaviors, such as exercising and conversing about nonmedical issues, were consistently rewarded with attention and compliments [38]. Although this may not be easily provided in an outpatient office-based practice, families can be educated about the advantages of attending more to the person and less to the symptoms. They should be encouraged to resume their roles of spouse, lover, playmate, companion, or child, and to relinquish the role of caretaker. Social behavioral reinforcers can be effective despite being subtle (eg, a spouse can be taught to consistently maintain eye contact if the patient is discussing emotions, activities, sports, and so forth, and to look elsewhere during reiterations of symptoms). Family must be reminded that small immediate reinforcers are often more powerful than large delayed ones. At the same time, the person's life situation can be reviewed to seek disincentives to recovery and to seek ways of replacing them with rewards, if possible.

Cognitive behavioral therapies

In cognitive behavioral therapy (CBT) patients are trained to identify, challenge, and alter automatic maladaptive thinking patterns. In a 1988 study Turner and Clancy [127] compared operant behavioral treatment with CBT in a randomly assigned sample of 81 mildly impaired CLBP patients. Both treatments were superior to controls in physical and social disability. At 1-year follow-up there was no difference between the two treatments.

Four RCTs of CBT reviewed by Compas and colleagues [128] all showed improved activity and psychologic function. Three found reductions in pain and one found reductions in medication use. Based on meta-analysis of 25 RCTs, Morley and colleagues [129] concluded that CBT is effective (compared with waiting list control) in chronic pain (excluding headache) in the domains of pain experience, depression, other mood or affect, cognitive coping and appraisal, behavioral activity level, and social role functioning. There were fewer studies of behavioral (operant) treatment, but sufficient to conclude that efficacy was shown for pain, mood other than depression, social role function, and expressed pain behavior. There were also few studies of relaxation and biofeedback training, but efficacy was shown for pain, depression, coping and social role functioning. Catastrophizing was reduced by cognitive therapy, relaxation training, and operant conditioning.

A remarkable study by McQuay and colleagues [130] in 1997 reviewed more than 15,000 randomized studies with pain as an outcome, along with others that were not randomized. Despite impediments to investigation, evidence from 35 trials supported CBT for pain, mood, catastrophizing, other coping self-statements, pain behavior, and functional impairment. The high-quality trials demonstrated large and sustainable changes in targeted outcomes.

More recently, Thieme and colleagues [131] compared operant behavioral therapy (OBT) with CBT in 125 patients who had fibromyalgia. Both groups reported reduced pain. The CBT group had improvements in cognitive and affective variables, and the OBT group had improved physical function and behavior. Controls actually showed deterioration. Benefits were maintained at 12-month follow-up. In a controlled trial of CBT with temporomandibular dysfunction patients, intent-to-treat analysis showed substantial improvements in pain, activity interference, jaw function, depression, pain beliefs, catastrophizing, and coping that were maintained at 12-month follow-up [132].

Biofeedback and relaxation training

In biofeedback training, such parameters as digital temperature, surface electromyogram (EMG), and palmar electrodermal response are monitored and visual or audio feedback is provided to the patient. With training, the person learns to modify these functions voluntarily. This technique has been used to abort migraine headache and to improve sphincter control following neurologic injury. Paraspinal EMG feedback is commonly used with CLBP patients. The process of learning to reduce muscle tension, sweating, and vasoconstriction leads to generalized relaxation. There is overlap in the clinical effects of such therapies as biofeedback training, relaxation training, self-hypnosis, and meditation, and all may induce states of muscular relaxation and reduced autonomic activity. In practice, techniques are often combined.

The National Institutes of Health Technology Assessment Panel on Integration of Behavioral and Relaxation Approaches [133] found strong evidence for the use of relaxation techniques in reducing chronic pain in several medical conditions. There was moderate evidence for the effectiveness of cognitive-behavioral techniques and biofeedback in chronic pain.

Flor and Birbaumer [134] randomly assigned a relatively functional group of patients (73% CLBP) to biofeedback training, CBT, or conservative medical treatment (heterogeneous interventions, including massage, nerve blocks, analgesics, and exercises). At 24-month follow-up the biofeedback group had significant reductions in pain, interference with life activities, affective distress, health care use, and catastrophizing. They showed less muscular reactivity under stress. Differences were substantial: 40% of the biofeedback training groups had two or more SD reductions in pain severity, life interference, and affective distress, compared with 17% of the cognitive-behavioral group and 8% of the medical group. Van Tulder's [107] review was less positive. They found only five low-quality RCTs of EMG biofeedback training for CLBP, four of which were negative.

Our clinical experience in a multidisciplinary pain rehabilitation program is that mixed chronic pain patients generally rate biofeedback training and physical therapy as the most helpful program components.

Multidisciplinary pain rehabilitation programs

Many patients who have chronic nonmalignant pain fail to achieve reasonable comfort and function despite appropriate treatment with single or even several therapies. Multidisciplinary pain rehabilitation programs (MPRPs) typically combine many of the previously described treatments into programs that range from a few hours a week to inpatient in intensity. Early programs were based largely on Fordyce's behavioral approach, including operant conditioning and exercises [38]. Although methods have evolved, there remains in most programs a focus on replacing sick role–type behaviors with normal activities, which staff attempt to reinforce.

Targets for MPRP treatment include not only pain but also function (work, play, socialization, sex), affect (depression, anger, anxiety), inappropriate health care use, and comorbid psychiatric illness. Although programs differ, common elements typically include the following:

Education
Reconditioning physical therapy
Biofeedback and relaxation training
Medications
Psychotherapies: individual, group, family
Treatment of psychiatric comorbidity, including addiction
Drug weaning

Some programs provide interventional therapies, whereas others prefer that these be completed, if indicated, before MPRP treatment. Some offer treatments, such as massage or myofascial release, yoga, and martial arts exercises, and some do not provide addiction treatment.

It seems a truism in medicine that the more treatments that have failed, the less is the likelihood that the next one will succeed. Despite this, and although MPRPs typically treat only patients who have failed multiple single interventions, their success rate is high. In a review of outcome studies, Turk found that such programs produce 14% to 60% pain reduction, up to 73% decrease in opioid use, dramatic increases in activity levels, 43% more working after treatment than before (twice the untreated rate), a 90% reduction in physician visits (one study), 50% to 65% fewer surgeries than untreated patients, 65% fewer hospitalizations than untreated, and 35% fewer receiving disability income [135]. Deardorff and colleagues [136] review found pain reductions of 14% to 42% and improvements in physical reconditioning. Forty-nine percent had reduced narcotics use and 65% were drug free at one year. Health care use was reduced, and 47% to 90% were seeking no additional care at 1 year. Work or vocational rehabilitation was successful in 55% mean. Treatment results were usually maintained at 2.5 to 3 years. In a meta-analysis of 65 studies of chronic pain rehabilitation programs, Flor and colleagues [137] found improvements in pain, mood, and interference with life activities, including work. Health care use declined. Benefits were stable over time. The authors found most studies to be of marginal quality.

Turk compared costs of returning a patient to work with various treatments, including drugs, conservative care, surgery, spinal cord stimulators, implantable drug delivery systems, and pain rehabilitation programs. He found that chronic pain rehabilitation programs led to comparable pain reduction, but superior outcomes in medication use, health care use, functional activities, return to work, closure of disability claims, iatrogenic consequences, and adverse events [138]. Using 1995 dollars, he found 27 fewer surgeries per 100 patients leading to $4050 saved per patient (at $15,000/operation). Annual medical costs had averaged more than $13,000/year pretreatment, which dropped to $5,600 in the year after treatment, leading to $7,700/year/patient saved following treatment. This savings was in addition to $400,000 saved per person removed from permanent disability.

Addressing LBP more specifically, Guzmán and colleagues [139] found 10 trials with 12 randomized comparisons of chronic pain rehabilitation programs versus controls. There was strong evidence of improved function versus inpatient/outpatient nonmultidisciplinary treatments. There was moderate evidence of reduced pain versus outpatient nonmultidisciplinary rehabilitation or usual care. There was contradictory evidence of vocational outcomes: some reported improvements in work readiness, whereas others showed no significant reduction in sickness leaves. Less intensive outpatient psychophysical treatments did not improve pain, function, or vocational outcomes.

It is reasonable to conclude that when "everything has failed," many patients can be restored to good function and quality of life with MPRP treatment. Unfortunately, many such programs have ceased to exist because of lack of reimbursement or low return on investment, which leads health care facilities to close them down. Current provision of pain care services often seems based more on incomes than on outcomes.

Summary

Chronic nonmalignant pain is less a symptom of a disease than a disease in itself. Accordingly, successful treatments rely less on identifying underlying pathology than on treating neural causes of pain amplification, psychologic causes of disability, and the sequelae of deconditioning and psychiatric illness. The outcome, when such treatment is provided, is remarkably favorable.

References

[1] Wiesel SW, Tsourmas N, Feffer HL, et al. A study of computer assisted tomography. 1. The incidence of positive CT scans in an asymptomatic group of patients. Spine 1984;9(6): 549–55.

[2] Boden SD, Davis DO, Dina TS, et al. Abnormal magnetic resonance scans of the lumbar spine in asymptomatic subjects. J Bone Joint Surg Am 1990;72(3):403–8.

[3] Jensen M, Brant-Zawadzld M, Obuchowski N, et al. MRI of lumbar spine in people without back pain. N Engl J Med 1994;331:69–73.

[4] Fields HL, Heinricher MM. Anatomy and physiology of a nociceptive modulatory system. Philos Trans R Soc Lond B Biol Sci 1985;308:361–74.

[5] Arvidsson J, Ygge J, Grant G. Cell loss in lumbar dorsal root ganglia and transganglionic degeneration after sciatic nerve resection in the rat. Brain Res 1986;373:15–21.

[6] Sugimoto T, Bennett GJ, Kajander KC. Transsynaptic degeneration in the superficial dorsal horn after sciatic nerve injury: effects of a chronic constriction injury, transection, and strychnine. Pain 1990;42:205–13.

[7] Watkins LR, Maier SF. Beyond neurons: evidence that immune and glial cells contribute to pathological pain states. Physiol Rev 2002;82:981–1011.

[8] Woolf CJ. Central mechanisms of acute pain. In: Bond MR, Charlton JE, Woolf CJ, editors. Pain research and clinical management, vol. 4, Proc Vth World Congress on pain. Amsterdam: Elsevier; 1991. p. 25–34.

[9] Torebjörk HE, Lundberg L, LaMotte R. Neural mechanisms for capsaicin-induced hyperalgesia (abstract). Pain 1990;41(Supplement 1):S114.

[10] Coderre TJ, Katz J, Vaccarino AL, et al. Contribution of central neuroplasticity to pathological pain: review of clinical and experimental evidence. Pain 1993;52:259–85.

[11] Duncan GH, Bushnell MC, Bates R, et al. Task-related responses of monkey medullary dorsal horn neurons. J Neurophysiol 1987;57(1):289–310.

[12] Zubieta JK, Heitzeg MM, Smith YR, et al. COMT val 158 met genotype affects μ-opioid neurotransmitter responses to a pain stressor. Science 2003;299(5610):1240–3.

[13] Uhl GR, Sora I, Wang Z. The μ opiate receptor as a candidate gene for pain: polymorphisms, variations in expression, nociception, and opiate responses. Proc Natl Acad Sci U S A 1999;96(14):7752–5.

[14] Devor M, Raber P. Heritability of symptoms in an experimental model of neuropathic pain. Pain 1990;49:51–67.

[15] Coghill RC, McHaffie JG, Yen YF. Neural correlates of interindividual differences in the subjective experience of pain. Proc Natl Acad Sci U S A 2003;100(14):8538–42.

[16] Giesecke T, Gracely RH, Grant MAB, et al. Evidence of augmented central pain processing in idiopathic chronic low back pain. Arthritis Rheum 2004;50(2):613–23.

[17] Curatolo M, Arendt-Nielsen L, Petersen-Felix S. Evidence, mechanisms, and clinical implications of central hypersensitivity in chronic pain after whiplash injury. Clin J Pain 2004; 20(6):469–76.

[18] Bigos SJ, Battie MC, Spengler DM, et al. A prospective study of work perceptions and psychosocial factors affecting the report of back unjury. Spine 1991;16(1):1–6.

[19] Papageorgiou AC, Macfarlane GJ, Thomas E, et al. Psychosocial factors in the workplace—do they predict new episodes of low back pain? Evidence from the South Manchester Back Pain Study. Spine 1997;22(10):1137–42.

[20] Valat JP, Goupille P, Vedere V. Low back pain: risk factors for chronicity. Rev Rhum Engl Ed 1997;64(3):189–94.

[21] Dionne CE, Koepsell TD, Von Korff M, et al. Predicting long-term functional limitations among back pain patients in primary care settings. J Clin Epidemiol 1997;50(1):31–43.

[22] Hasenbring M, Marienfeld G, Kuhlendahl D, et al. Risk factors of chronicity in lumbar disc patients. A prospective investigation of biologic, psychologic, and social predictors of therapy outcome. Spine 1994;19(24):2759–65.

[23] Long DM. Effectiveness of therapies currently employed for persistent low back and leg pain. PRN Forum 1995;4(2):122–5.

[24] Greenough CG, Fraser RD. The effects of compensation on recovery from low-back injury. Spine 1989;14(9):947–55.

[25] Greenough CG, Taylor LJ, Fraser RD. Anterior lumbar fusion. A comparison of noncompensation patients with compensation patients. Clin Orthop 1994;300:30–7.

[26] Penta M, Fraser RD. Anterior lumbar interbody fusion. A minimum 10-year follow-up. Spine 1997;22(20):2429–34.

[27] Rainville J, Sobel JB, Hartigan C, et al. The effect of compensation involvement on the reporting of pain and disability by patients referred for rehabilitation of chronic low back pain. Spine 1997;22(17):2016–24.

[28] Schrader H, Obelieniene D, Bovim G, et al. Natural evolution of late whiplash syndrome outside the medicolegal context. Lancet 1996;347:1207–11.

[29] Spitzer WO, Skovron ML, Salmi LR, et al. Scientific monograph of the Quebec Task Force on Whiplash-Associated Disorders: redefining "Whiplash" and its management. Spine 1995;20(8S):3S–73S.

[30] Blake C, Garrett M. Impact of litigation on quality of life outcomes in patients with chronic low back pain. Ir J Med Sci 1997;166(3):124–6.

[31] Carragee EJ, Alamin TF, Miller JL, et al. Discographic, MRI and psychosocial determinants of low back pain disability and remission: a prospective study in subjects with benign persistent back pain. The Spine Journal 2005;5:24–35.

[32] Buckelew SP, Huyser B, Hewett JE, et al. Self-efficacy predicting outcome among fibromyalgia subjects. Arthritis Care Res 1996;9(2):97–104.

[33] Rejeski WJ, Craven T, Ettinger WH Jr, et al. Self-efficacy and pain in disability with osteoarthritis of the knee. J Gerontol B Psychol Sci Soc Sci 1996;51(1):24–9.

[34] Turner JA, Holtzman S, Mancl L. Mediators, moderators, and predictors of therapeutic change in cognitive-behavioral therapy for chronic pain. Pain 2007;127(3):276–86. Epub 2006 Oct 27.

[35] Crisson JE, Keefe FJ. The relationship of locus of control to pain coping strategies and psychological distress in chronic pain patients. Pain 1988;35:147–54.

[36] Aldrich S, Eccleston C, Crombez G. Worry about chronic pain: vigilance to threat and misdirected problem solving. Behav Res Ther 2000;38:457–70.

[37] McCracken LM, Eccleston C. Coping or acceptance: what to do about chronic pain? Pain 2003;105:197–204.

[38] Fordyce WE. Behavioral methods for chronic pain and illness. St. Louis (MO): CV Mosby Co; 1976.

[39] Flor H, Lutzenberger W, Knost B, et al. Spouse presence alters brain response to pain. Orlando (FL): Society for Neuroscience; 2002.

[40] Hölzl R, Kleinböhl D, Huse E. Implicit operant learning of pain sensitization. Pain 2005; 115(1–2):12–20.

[41] Kori SH, Miller RP, Todd DD. Kinesophobia: a new view of chronic pain behavior. Pain Management 1990;3(1):35–43.

[42] Polatin PB, Kinney RK, Gatchel RJ, et al. Psychiatric illness and chronic low-back pain. The mind and the spine—which goes first? Spine 1993;18(1):66–71.

[43] Currie SR, Wang JL. Chronic back pain and major depression in the general Canadian population. Pain 2004;107(1–2):54–60.

[44] Gureje O, Simon GE, Von Kor M. A cross-national study of the course of persistent pain in primary care. Pain 2001;92:195–200.

[45] Von Korff M, Crane P, Lane M, et al. Chronic spinal pain and physical–mental comorbidity in the United States: results from the national comorbidity survey replication. Pain 2005; 113:331–9.

[46] Rudy TE, Kerns RD, Turk DC. Chronic pain and depression: toward a cognitive-behavioral mediation model. Pain 1988;35(2):129–40.

[47] DeGood DE, Kiernan B. Perception of fault in patients with chronic pain. Pain 1996;64(1): 153–9.

[48] Savage SR. Preface: pain medicine and addiction medicine—controversies and collaboration. J Pain Symptom Manag 1993;8:254–6.

[49] Adams LL, Gatchel RJ, Robinson RC, et al. Development of a self-report screening instrument for assessing potential opioid medication misuse in chronic pain patients. J Pain Symptom Manag 2004;27:440–59.

[50] Covington EC, Kotz MK. Psychological approaches to the treatment of pain in addiction. In: Graham AW, Schultz TK, Mayo-Smith M, Ries RK, editors. Principles of Addiction Medicine. 3rd Edition. Washington, DC: American Society of Addiction Medicine; 2003. p. 1421–37.

[51] Kaila-Kangas L, Leino-Arjas P, Riihimaki H, et al. Smoking and overweight as predictors of hospitalization for back disorders. Spine 2003;28:1860–8.

[52] Kouyanou K, Pither CE, Wessely S. Medication misuse, abuse and dependence in chronic pain patients. J Psychosom Res 1997;43:497–504.

[53] Hoffmann NG, Olofsson O, Salen B, et al. Prevalence of abuse and dependency in chronic pain patients. Int J Addict 1995;30:919–27.

[54] American Psychiatric Association. DSM-IV. Diagnostic and statistical manual of mental disorders. 4th edition. Washington, DC: American Psychiatric Association; 1994.

[55] van der Kolk BA, Pelcovitz D, Roth S, et al. Dissociation, somatization, and affect dysregulation: the complexity of adaptation to trauma. Am J Psychiatry 1996;153(7 Suppl): 83–93.

[56] Rome HP, Rome JD. Limbically augmented pain syndrome (laps): kindling, corticolimbic sensitization, and the convergence of affective and sensory symptoms in chronic pain disorders. Pain Med 2000;1(1):7–23.

[57] Daniell HW, Lentz R, Mazer NA. Open-label pilot study of testosterone patch therapy in men with opioid-induced androgen deficiency. J Pain 2006;7(3):200–10.

[58] Jamison R, Schein J, Vallow S, et al. Neuropsychological effects of long-term opioid use in chronic pain patients. J Pain 2003;4(2 Suppl):1–104 [abstract 604].

[59] Tassain V, Attal N, Fletcher D, et al. Long term effects of oral sustained release morphine on neuropsychological performance in patients with chronic non-cancer pain. Pain 2003; 104(1–2):389–400.

[60] Porter J, Jick H. Addiction rare in patients treated with narcotics. N Engl J Med 1980;302: 123.

[61] Perry S, Heidrich G. Management of pain during debridement: a survey of US burn units. Pain 1982;13:267–80.

[62] Potter JS, Hennessy G, Borrow JA, et al. Substance use histories in patients seeking treatment for controlled-release oxycodone dependence. Drug Alcohol Depend 2004;76:213–5.

[63] Brown RL, Fleming MF, Patterson JJ. Chronic opioid analgesic therapy for chronic low back pain. J Am Board Fam Pract 1996;9(3):191–204.

[64] Ballantyne JC, Mao J. Medical progress: opioid therapy for chronic pain. N Engl J Med 2003;349:1943–53.

[65] Roth SH, Fleischmann RM, Burch FX, et al. Around-the-clock, controlled-release oxycodone therapy for ostearthritis-related pain: placebo-controlled trial and long-term evaluation. Arch Intern Med 2000;160:853–60.

[66] Robbins L. Long-acting opioids for severe chronic daily headache. Headache Q 1999;10: 135–9.

[67] Saper JR, Lake AE 3rd, Hamel RL, et al. Daily scheduled opioids for intractable head pain: long-term observations of a treatment program. Neurology 2004;62:1687–94.

[68] Kalso E, Edwards JE, Moore RA, et al. Opioids in chronic non-cancer pain: systematic review of efficacy and safety. Pain 2004;112:372–80.

[69] Brown J, Klapow J, Doleys D, et al. Disease-specific and generic health outcomes: a model for the evaluation of long-term intrathecal opioid therapy in noncancer low back pain patients. Clin J Pain 1999;15:122–31.

[70] Covington EC. Pain and addictive disorder: Challenge and opportunity. In: Benzon HT, Rathmell J, Wu C, Turk DC, Argoff CE, editors. Raj's Practical Management of Pain, 4th Edition. New York: Elsevier-Mosby.

[71] Kennedy JA, Crowley TJ. Chronic pain and substance abuse: a pilot study of opioid maintenance. J Subst Abuse Treat 1990;7:233–8.

[72] Dunbar SA, Katz NP. Chronic opioid therapy for nonmalignant pain in patients with a history of substance abuse: report of 20 cases. J Pain Symptom Manage 1996;11(3):163–71.

[73] Schofferman J. Long-term use of opioid analgesics for the treatment of chronic pain of nonmalignant origin. J Pain Symptom Manage 1993;8(5):279–88.

[74] Rome JD, Townsend CO, Bruce BK, et al. Chronic noncancer pain rehabilitation with opioid withdrawal: comparison of treatment outcomes based on opioid use status at admission. Mayo Clin Proc 2004;79(6):759–68.

[75] Moulin DE, Iezzi A, Amireh R, et al. Randomised trial of oral morphine for chronic noncancer pain. Lancet 1996;347:143–7.

[76] Harden RN, Bruehl S, Siegler J, et al. Pain, psychological status, and functional recovery in chronic pain patients on daily opioids: a case comparison. J Back Musculoskeletal Rehab 1997;9:101–8.

[77] Eriksen J, Sjøgren P, Bruera E, et al. Critical issues on opioids in chronic non-cancer pain: an epidemiological study. Pain 2006;125(1–2):172–9.

[78] Airaksinen O, Brox JI, Cedraschi C, et al. Chapter 4: European guidelines for the management of chronic nonspecific low back pain. Eur Spine J 2006;15(Suppl 2):S192–300.

[79] Franson RC, Saal JS, Saal JA. Human disc phospholipase A2 is inflammatory. Spine 1992;(6 Suppl):S129–32.

[80] Genevay S, Gabay C. Is disk-related sciatica a TNFα-dependent inflammatory disease? Joint Bone Spine 2005;72(1):4–6.

[81] Malmberg AB, Yaksh TL. Hyperalgesia mediated by spinal glutamate or substance P receptor blocked by spinal cyclooxygenase inhibition. Science 1992;257:1276–8.

[82] Coderre TJ, Gonzales R, Goldyne ME, et al. Noxious stimulus-induced increase in spinal prostaglandin E2 is noradrenergic terminal-dependent. Neurosci Lett 1990;115:253–8.

[83] Singh G, Triadafilopoulos G. Epidemiology of NSAID induced gastrointestinal complications. J Rheumatol Suppl. 1999;56:18–24.

[84] Wolfe MM, Lichtenstein DR, Singh G. Gastrointestinal toxicity of nonsteroidal antiinflammatory drugs. N Engl J Med 1999;340(24):1888–99.

[85] Dubois RW, Melmed GY, Henning JM, et al. Risk of upper gastrointestinal injury and events in patients treated with cyclooxygenase (COX)-1/COX-2 nonsteroidal antiinflammatory drugs (NSAIDs), COX-2 selective NSAIDs, and gastroprotective cotherapy: an appraisal of the literature. J Clin Rheumatol 2004;10(4):178–89.

[86] McQuay H, Carroll D, Jadad AR, et al. Anticonvulsant drugs for management of pain: a systematic review. BMJ 1995;311:1047–52.

[87] Gilron I, Watson CP, Cahill CM, et al. Neuropathic pain: a practical guide for the clinician. CMAJ 2006;175(3):265–75.

[88] Colombo B, Annovazzi PO, Comi G. Medications for neuropathic pain: current trends. Neurol Sci 2006;27(Suppl 2):S183–9.

[89] McCleane GJ. Does gabapentin have an analgesic effect on background, movement and referred pain? A randomized, double-blind, placebo controlled study. The Pain Clinic 2001; 13:103–7.

[90] Remmers AE, Sharma U, LaMoreaux L, et al. Pregabalin treatment of patients with chronic low back pain [American Pain Society 2000 Poster 660]. Available at: http://ampainsoc. org/db2/abstract/view?poster_id=730#660. Accessed March 12, 2007.

[91] Muehlbacher M, Nickel MK, Kettler C, et al. Topiramate in treatment of patients with chronic low back pain: a randomized, double-blind, placebo-controlled study. Clin J Pain 2006;22(6):526–31.

[92] Khoromi S, Patsalides A, Parada S, et al. Topiramate in chronic lumbar radicular pain. J Pain 2005;6(12):829–36.

[93] Eisenberg E, Damunni G, Hoffer E, et al. Lamotrigine for intractable sciatica: correlation between dose, plasma concentration and analgesia. Eur J Pain 2003;7(6):485–91.

[94] Sindrup SH, Otto M, Finnerup NB, et al. Antidepressants in the treatment of neuropathic pain. Basic Clin Pharmacol Toxicol 2005;96:399–409.

[95] Cayley WE Jr. Antidepressants for the treatment of neuropathic pain. Am Fam Physician 2006;73(11):1933–4.

[96] Lynch ME. Antidepressants as analgesics: a review of randomized controlled trials. J Psychiatry Neurosci 2001;26(1):30–6.

[97] Perrot S, Maheu E, Javier RM, et al. Guidelines for the use of antidepressants in painful rheumatic conditions. Eur J Pain 2006;10:185–92.

[98] Rowbotham MC, Goli V, Kunz NR, et al. Venlafaxine extended release in the treatment of painful diabetic neuropathy: a double-blind, placebo-controlled study. Pain 2004;110(3): 697–706.

[99] Goldstein DJ, Lu Y, Detke MJ, et al. Duloxetine vs. placebo in patients with painful diabetic neuropathy. Pain 2005;116(1–2):109–18.

[100] Sullivan MD, Robinson JP. Antidepressant and anticonvulsant medication for chronic pain. Phys Med Rehabil Clin N Am 2006;17(2):381–400.

[101] Fishbain D. Evidence-based data on pain relief with antidepressants. Ann Med 2000;32(5): 305–16.

[102] Salerno SM, Browning R, Jackson JL. The effect of antidepressant treatment on chronic back pain: a meta-analysis. Arch Intern Med 2002;162(1):19–24.

[103] Staiger TO, Gaster B, Sullivan MD, et al. Systematic review of antidepressants in the treatment of chronic low back pain. Spine 2003;28(22):2540–5.

[104] Atkinson JH, Slater MA, Wahlgren DR, et al. Effects of noradrenergic and serotonergic antidepressants on chronic low back pain intensity. Pain 1999;83(2):137–45.

[105] Gimbel J, Linn R, Hale M, et al. Lidocaine patch treatment in patients with low back pain: results of an open-label, nonrandomized pilot study. Am J Ther 2005;12(4):311–9.

[106] Frerick H, Keitel W, Kuhn U, et al. Topical treatment of chronic low back pain with a capsicum plaster. Pain 2003;106(1–2):59–64.

[107] Van Tulder MW, Koes BW, Bouter LM. Conservative treatment of acute and chronic nonspecific low back pain. A systematic review of randomized controlled trials of the most common interventions. Spine 1997;22(18):2128–56.

[108] Aley KO, Kulkarni SK. Baclofen analgesia in mice: a GABA-B mediated response. Methods Find Exp Clin Pharmacol 1991;13(10):681–6.

[109] Terrence CF, Fromm GH, Tenicela R. Baclofen as an analgesic in chronic peripheral nerve disease. Eur Neurol 1985;24(6):380–5.

[110] Loubser PG, Akman NM. Effects of intrathecal baclofen on chronic spinal cord injury pain. J Pain Symptom Manage 1996;12:241–7.

[111] Herman RM, D'Luzansky SC, Ippolito R. Intrathecal baclofen suppresses central pain in patients with spinal lesions. A pilot study. Clin J Pain 1992;8(4):338–45.

[112] Taira T, Kawamura H, Tanikawa T, et al. A new approach to control central deafferentation pain: spinal intrathecal baclofen. Stereotact Funct Neurosurg 1995;65(1–4): 101–5.

[113] Berry H, Hutchinson DR. Tizanidine and ibuprofen in acute low-back pain: results of a double-blind multicenter study in general practice. J Int Med Res 1988;16(2):83–91.

[114] Fryda-Kaurimsky Z, Muller-Fassbender H. Tizanidine (DS 103-282) in the treatment of acute paravertebral muscle spasm: a controlled trial comparing tizanidine and diazepam. J Int Med Res 1981;9(6):501–5.

[115] Samanta A, Samanta J. Is epidural injection of steroids effective for low back pain? BMJ 2004;328:1509–10.

[116] Koes BW, Scholten RJ, Mens JM, et al. Efficacy of epidural steroid injections for low back pain and sciatica: a systematic review of randomized clinical trials. Pain 1995;63: 279–88.

[117] Brox JI, Reikeras O, Nygaard O, et al. Lumbar instrumented fusion compared with cognitive intervention and exercises in patients with chronic back pain after previous surgery for disc herniation: a prospective randomized controlled study. Pain 2006;122(1–2):145–55. Epub 2006 Mar 20.

[118] Liddle SD, Baxter GD, Gracey JH. Exercise and chronic low back pain: what works? Pain 2004;107:176–90.

[119] Trivedi MH, Greer TL, Grannemann BD, et al. Exercise as an augmentation strategy for treatment of major depression. J Psychiatr Pract 2006;12(4):205–13.

[120] Dunn AL, Trivedi MH, Kampert JB, et al. Exercise treatment for depression: efficacy and dose response. Am J Prev Med 2005;28(1):1–8.

[121] Ströhle A, Feller C, Onken M, et al. The acute antipanic activity of aerobic exercise. Am J Psychiatry 2005;162:2376–8.

[122] Salmon P. Effects of physical exercise on anxiety, depression, and sensitivity to stress: a unifying theory. Clin Psychol Rev 2001;21(1):33–61.

[123] De Jong JR, Vlaeyen JWS, Onghena P, et al. Fear of movement/(re)injury in chronic low back pain education or exposure in vivo as mediator to fear reduction? Clin J Pain 2005; 21:9–17.

[124] Lacroix JM, Powell J, Lloyd GJ, et al. Low-back pain. Factors of value in predicting outcome. Spine 1990;15(6):495–9.

[125] Waddell G, Newton M, Henderson I, et al. A fear-avoidance beliefs questionnaire (FABQ) and the role of fear-avoidance beliefs in chronic low back pain and disability. Pain 1993;52: 157–68.

[126] Klenerman L, Slade PD, Stanley IM, et al. The prediction of chronicity inpatients with an acute attack of low back pain in a general practice setting. Spine 1995;20(4):478–84.

[127] Turner JA, Clancy S. Comparison of operant behavioral and cognitive-behavioral group treatment for chronic low back pain. J Consult Clin Psychol 1988;56(2):261–6.

[128] Compas BE, Haaga DA, Keefe FJ, et al. Sampling of empirically supported psychological treatments from health psychology: smoking, chronic pain, cancer, and bulimia nervosa. J Consult Clin Psychol 1998;66(1):89–112.

[129] Morley S, Eccleston C, Williams A. Systematic review and meta-analysis of randomized controlled trials of cognitive behavior therapy and behavior therapy for chronic pain in adults, excluding headache. Pain 1999;80:1–13.

[130] McQuay HJ, Moore RA, Eccleston C, et al. Systematic review of outpatient services for chronic pain control. Health Technol Assess 1997;1(6):i–iv,1–135.

[131] Thieme K, Flor H, Turk DC. Psychological pain treatment in fibromyalgia syndrome: efficacy of operant behavioural and cognitive behavioural treatments. Arthritis Research &

Therapy 2006, 8:R121. Available at: http://arthritis-research.com/content/8/4/R121. Accessed March 12, 2007.

[132] Turner JA, Mancl L, Aaron LA. Short- and long-term efficacy of brief cognitive-behavioral therapy for patients with chronic temporomandibular disorder pain: a randomized, controlled trial. Pain 2006;121(3):181–94.

[133] NIH Technology Assessment Panel on integration of behavioral and relaxation approaches into the treatment of chronic pain and insomnia: integration of behavioral and relaxation approaches into the treatment of chronic pain and insomnia. JAMA 1996;276(4):313–8.

[134] Flor H, Birbaumer N. Comparison of the efficacy of electromyographic biofeedback, cognitive-behavioral therapy, and conservative medical interventions in the treatment of chronic musculoskeletal pain. J Consult Clin Psychol 1993;61(4):653–8.

[135] Turk DC. Efficacy of multidisciplinary pain centers in the treatment of chronic pain. In: Cohen MJM, Campbell JM, editors. Pain treatment centers at a crossroads: a practical and conceptual reappraisal. Progress in pain research and management, vol. 7. Seattle (WA): IASP Press; 1996. p. 257–73.

[136] Deardorff WW, Rubin HS, Scott DW. Comprehensive multidisciplinary treatment of chronic pain: a follow-up study of treated and non-treated groups. Pain 1991;45(1):35–43.

[137] Flor H, Fydrich T, Turk DC. Efficacy of multidisciplinary pain treatment centers: a meta-analytic review. Pain 1992;49:221–30.

[138] Turk DC. Clinical effectiveness and cost-effectiveness of treatments for patients with chronic pain. Clin J Pain 2002;18(6):355–65.

[139] Guzmán J, Esmail R, Karjalainen K, et al. Multidisciplinary rehabilitation for chronic low back pain: systematic review. Br Med J 2001;322(7301):1511–6.

ELSEVIER
SAUNDERS

Neurol Clin 25 (2007) 567–575

NEUROLOGIC
CLINICS

Index

Note: Page numbers of article titles are in **boldface** type.

0733-8619/07/$ - see front matter © 2007 Elsevier Inc. All rights reserved.
doi:10.1016/S0733-8619(07)00042-4

Moving?

Make sure your subscription moves with you!

To notify us of your new address, find your **Clinics Account Number** (located on your mailing label above your name), and contact customer service at:

E-mail: elspcs@elsevier.com

800-654-2452 (subscribers in the U.S. & Canada)
407-345-4000 (subscribers outside of the U.S. & Canada)

Fax number: 407-363-9661

Elsevier Periodicals Customer Service
6277 Sea Harbor Drive
Orlando, FL 32887-4800

*To ensure uninterrupted delivery of your subscription, please notify us at least 4 weeks in advance of move.